# STATISTICS IN EPIDEMIOLOGY

## Methods, Techniques, and Applications

**Hardeo Sahai**
Department of Biostatistics and Epidemiology
University of Puerto Rico
San Juan, Puerto Rico

**Anwer Khurshid**
Department of Mathematical Statistics
and Operational Research
University of Exeter
Exeter, United Kingdom

CRC Press
Boca Raton New York London Tokyo

**Library of Congress Cataloging-in-Publication Data**

Sahai, Hardeo.
Statistics and epidemiology: methods, techniques, and applications/ by Hardeo Sahai and Anwer Khurshid.
p. cm.
Includes bibliographical references and index.
ISBN 0-8493-9444-9 (permanent paper)
1. Epidemiology—Statistical methods. I. Khurshid, Anwer.
RA652.2.M3S24 1995
614'.072—dc20 95-349
CIP



Direct all inquiries to CRC Press LLC, 2000 N.W. Corporate Blvd., Boca Raton, Florida 33431.


International Standard Book Number 0-8493-9444-9
Library of Congress Card Number 95-349
Printed in the United States of America 2 3 4 5 6 7 8 9 0
Printed on acid-free paper

General impressions are never to be trusted. Unfortunately when they are of long standing they become fixed rules of life, and assume a prescriptive right not to be questioned. Consequently those who are not accustomed to original inquiry entertain a hatred and a horror of statistics. They cannot endure the idea of submitting their sacred impressions to cold-blooded verification. But it is the triumph of scientific men to rise superior to such superstitions to desire tests by which the value of beliefs may be ascertained, and to feel sufficiently masters of them to discard contemptuously whatever may be found untrue.

*Sir Francis Galton*

No aphorism is more frequently repeated in connection with field trials, than that we must ask Nature few questions or, ideally, one question, at a time. The writer is convinced that this view is wholly mistaken. Nature, he suggests, will best respond to a logical and carefully thought out questionnaire; indeed, if we ask her a single question, she will often refuse to answer until some other topic has been discussed.

*Sir Ronald A. Fisher*

...comparisons which are really comparisons between two social classes with different standards of nutrition and education are palmed off as comparisons between the results of a certain medical treatment and its neglect. Thus, it is easy to prove that the wearing of tall hats and the carrying of umbrellas enlarges the chest, prolongs life and confers comparative immunity from disease; for the statistics show that the classes which use these articles are bigger, healthier, and live longer than the class which never dreams of possessing such things. It does not take much perspicacity to see that what really makes this difference is not the tall hat and the umbrella, but the wealth and nourishment of which they are evidence, and that a gold watch or membership of a club in Pall Mall might be proved in the same way to have the like sovereign virtues. A university degree, a daily bath, the owning of thirty pairs of trousers, a knowledge of Wagner's music, a pew in the church, anything, in short, that implies more means and better nurture than the mass of laborers enjoy, can be statistically palmed off as a magic-spell conferring all sort of privileges.

*George Bernard Shaw: The Doctor's Dilemmas*

"What is fate?" Nasruddin was asked by a scholar.

"An endless succession of intertwined events, each influencing the other."

"That is hardly a satisfactory answer. I believe in cause and effect."

"Very well," said the Mulla, "look at that." He pointed to a procession passing in the street.

"That man is being taken to be hanged. Is that because someone gave him a silver piece and enabled him to buy the knife with which he committed the murder; or because someone saw him to do it; or because nobody stopped him?"

*Anonymous*

Through my acquaintance with the late Karl Pearson I was early impressed with the necessity of mathematics in biology and indeed in all branches of science. Pearson, always smiling and charming, would not admit that anyone who was not a mathematician could claim any scientific authority whatsoever. I subscribed faithfully to his journal Biometrika without understanding any of its equations or more than, say, five per cent of its sentences. But I found that the biometricians, though their technical skill and subtlety seemed wonderful to me, were as credulous, as prejudiced, as thoughtless as to the facts they were measuring and the assumptions from which they started, as Isaac Newton himself. Even their counting was not to be depended on; for they added up facts and opinions indiscriminately, and cooked their calculation by 'weighing' them with fancy frequencies which represented nothing but their personal guesses and tastes.

*George Bernard Shaw: Everybody's Political What's What?*

I will also tell you of an experiment that has been made in this Kingdom of Kerman.

The people of Kerman, then, are good, very humble, peaceful, and as helpful to one another as possible. For this reason, one day that the King of Kerman was surrounded by his wise men, he said to them: "Gentlemen, I am greatly astonished at not knowing the reason of the following fact: namely that, whereas in the Kingdom of Persia, so near to our land, people are so wicked and treacherous that they constantly kill one another, with us, who, yet are almost one with them, there hardly ever occur outbursts of wrath or disorder." The wise men answered him that the cause lay in the soil. Then the King sent some of his men into Persia, and particularly to the Kingdom of Isfaan above mentioned, whose inhabitants surpassed all the others in the wickedness. Here, on the advice of his wise men, he had seven ships loaded with earth, and brought to his kingdom. When the earth arrived, he had it sprinkled, after the manner of pitch, on the floor of certain much frequented rooms; and had it covered with carpets, in order that its softness should not soil those present. Then they sat down to a banquet, and straightway, at the very first course, they began offending one another with words and deeds, and wounding one another mortally. Then the king declared that truly the cause of the fact lay in the soil.

*The Travels of Marco Polo*

"The cause of lighting," Alice said very decidedly, for she felt quite sure about this, "is the thunder — no, no!" she hastily corrected herself, "I meant it the other way."

"It's too late to correct it," said the Red Queen. "When you've once said a thing, that fixes it, and you must take the consequences."

*Lewis Carroll*

"Whenever we use mathematics in order to study some observational phenomena we must essentially begin by building a mathematical model (deterministic or probabilistic) for these phenomena. Of necessity, the model must simplify matters and certain details must be ignored. The success of the model depends on whether or not the details ignored are really unimportant in the development of the phenomena studied. The solution of the mathematical problem may be correct and yet be in considerable disagreement with the observed data simply because the underlying assumptions made are not warranted. It is usually quite difficult to state with certainty, whether or not a given mathematical model is adequate before some observational data are obtained. In order to check the validity of a model, we must deduce a number of consequences of our model and then compare these predicted results with observations".

*J. Neyman: University of California Publications in Statistics, Vol. 1, 1954*

The role of modern statistical theory and practice vis-a-vis the other sciences has been sometimes likened to the role of pure mathematics and sometimes to that of inductive logic, within the general framework of the philosophy of science. The first comparison or analogy would be, in one sense, an enormous overstatement and, in another sense, an understatement. The second one is closer to the mark in the sense that modern statistical theory and practice have added important elements to classical inductive logic, or rather, brought out more clearly and developed very considerably certain elements that were already there in a very latent form in classical inductive logic.

*S. N. Roy: An unfinished manuscript; quoted in R. D. Bock: Multivariate Statistical Methods in Behavioral Research, 1975*

The unhappy statistician has to try to disentangle the effect from the ravelled skein with which he is presented. No easy matter this, very often, and a matter demanding not merely a knowledge or method, but all the best qualities that an investigator can possess — strong common sense, caution, reasoning power and imagination, and when he has come to his conclusion the statistician must not forget this caution: he should not be dogmatic. "You can prove anything by statistics" is a common gibe. Its contrary is more nearly true — you can never prove anything by statistics. The statistician is dealing with the most complex cases of multiple causation. He may show the facts are in accordance with this hypothesis or that. But it is quite another thing to show all other possible hypotheses are excluded, and that the facts do not admit of any other interpretation than the particular one he may have in mind.

*George Undy Yule*

Thc normal law of error stands out in the experience of mankind as one of the broadest generalizations of natural philosophy. It serves as the guiding instrument in researches in the physical and social sciences and in medicine, agriculture and engineering. It is an indispensable tool for the analysis and the interpretation of the basic data obtained by observation and experiment.

*W. J. Youden*

# Foreword

Epidemiologic research, having to do with frequencies of occurrence, is by its very nature *statistical* science. It is, therefore, most natural and very important that persons with full statistical competence take an active role in its development, teaching, and textbook writing, notably in data analysis. Accordingly, epidemiology has been greatly enriched by textbooks authored by statistical heavyweights, most notably, Breslow and Day.

This text by Sahai and Khurshid falls in the Breslow and Day class of ambition and learnedness, though not of originality. It aims to address the entire range of data-analytic topics in epidemiology; it is up-to-date and rich in references to original literature. For a rather advanced epidemiologic data analyst, therefore, this text is a most valuable resource in the desk reference sense.

I congratulate Sahai and Khurshid for a major accomplishment in delineation of the present stage of development in epidemiologic data analysis.

**Olli S. Miettinen**
Montreal, Canada

# Preface

The purpose of this volume is to present a thorough treatment of statistical methods and techniques that are commonly employed in epidemiologic data analysis involving prospective, retrospective, and cross-sectional studies of disease occurrence. The core of a course in epidemiologic statistics usually focuses on these topics, although due to limitation of time, it is not possible to cover any topic in great detail. Prospective studies for cohorts that take into account person-time of observations, which is likely to vary between cohort members when cases occur, are also considered. The analyses of epidemiologic effect measures involving risk difference, risk ratio and odds ratio, including measures based on incidence rates per number of person-years of observations, are presented. In presenting these methods we have taken note of the common conceptual foundation and the methods of analysis, underlying prospective, retrospective, and cross-sectional approaches to epidemiologic studies, so that statistical methods and techniques appropriate to one design can be carried over to the other with very little or no change. Further, although we have emphasized the necessity of taking into account the particular design in the choice of appropriate methods of data analysis, there is very little discussion of various designs and their planning and execution. This volume deals mainly with the analysis of epidemiologic data and with related quantitative issues. The interested reader is referred to other sources where appropriate discussion on these topics can be found.

The risk difference, incidence rate difference, risk ratio, incidence rate ratio, and odds ratio have been used extensively in epidemiologic investigations as measures of strength of association between a condition and a risk factor. There are other measures of associations that can also be employed, but these are the most useful and widely used in epidemiologic and clinical investigations. A considerable amount of statistical methodology has been devoted to developing both exact and approximate techniques for the estimation of these effect measures. The purpose of this work is to present in a unified manner some important results for constructing point and interval estimates for these epidemiologic effect measures. We focus our presentation on mainly large sample interval estimation techniques, since most such procedures produce reasonably valid results. The consideration of large sample intervals is also primarily a matter of necessity since no viable and practical methods exist for determining exact intervals for certain epidemiologic effect measures. However, whenever feasible, we also discuss the construction of exact types of confidence intervals emphasizing their usefulness for small and moderate size data sets.

The use of confidence interval formulas is illustrated with appropriate numerical examples taken from the literature. Although the major emphasis in this volume is on methods of constructing confidence intervals, the relevant results on point estimation are also discussed and illustrated in full detail. Tests of hypotheses involving epidemiologic effect measures are generally not covered. In this regard, we have been guided by the epidemiologic wisdom of Professor Kenneth J. Rothman, who remarked that the notion of statistical significance could be expunged from the lexicon of epidemiology without any loss.[1] However, whenever deemed appropriate, pertinent results on tests of hypotheses are also included. Furthermore, it is assumed that the reader is familiar with standard statistical techniques on estimation and hypothesis testing covered in a one or two semester introductory biostatistics course at the level of Woolson[2] or Rosner.[3] We have endeavored to present these methods in as clear and concise manner as possible so that epidemiologists and other researchers, without extensive statistical background, can appreciate their usage and can apply them to their own work.

**Hardeo Sahai**
San Juan, Puerto Rico
**Anwer Khurshid**
Exeter, United Kingdom

---

[1] Kenneth J. Rothman, *Modern Epidemiology*. Boston: Little, Brown, 1986.

[2] Robert F. Woolson, *Statistical Methods for the Analysis of Biomedical Data*. New York: John Wiley & Sons, 1987.

[3] Bernard Rosner, *Fundamentals of Biostatistics,* 4th ed. Boston: PWS-KENT, 1994.

# Acknowledgments

A work of this nature is never done in isolation and we want to express our sincere appreciation to all individuals who directly or indirectly helped us at various stages of the development of this work. We wish to give our special thanks to Professor Olli S. Miettinen of McGill University for his many pioneering and fundamental research contributions in quantitative epidemiology, for his numerous constructive comments and criticisms and for kindly consenting to write a Foreword for this volume. We also would like to express our appreciation to Professor Peter Armitage of the University of Oxford, Professor Alvan R. Feinstein of Yale University School of Medicine, Professor Charles H. Hennekens and Dr. Julie Buring of the Harvard Medical School and Brigham and Women's Hospital, Dr. Michael Hills of the London School of Hygiene and Tropical Medicine, Professor Nathan Mantel of the American University, and Professor James J. Schlesselman of the University of Pittsburgh for reading preliminary drafts of the manuscripts and making some helpful comments and suggestions.

The first author wishes to thank to the many students of the EPID 6530 — Epidemiologic Methods course, offered at the University of Puerto Rico Graduate School of Public Health, who have waded through earlier drafts of the preprinted versions while the text was being written. He also gratefully acknowledges a sabbatical (1993–1994) granted by the Administrative Board of the University of Puerto Rico Medical Sciences Campus which finally made possible the completion of a perennially evolving manuscript into a book. He would like to thank Dr. Robert P. Hirsch, Division of Biostatistics and Epidemiology at the George Washington University Health Sciences Center, for some helpful discussions and suggestions during the course of the first author's sabbatical visit to that university in the autumn of 1993. He also expresses his gratitude to Professor Antonio Martin Andrés, Division of Biostatistics at the University of Granada Medical and Dental Faculties, for many helpful discussions and remarks when the first author held a visiting professorial appointment there in the fall of 1993, and for all his kindness and hospitality extended during the author's stay in Spain.

Portions of the manuscript were written and revised during the course of the first author's sabbatical visit to the Veracruzana University, Mexico, during the Spring of 1994 and he is especially thankful to Dr. Mario M. Ojeda and other university authorities for organizing and hosting the visit and making his sojourn pleasant and enjoyable. A group of students and professors from the Department of Mathematics and Statistics of the National University of Colombia participated in a seminar devoted to mathematical and statistical aspects of the topics covered in the text and their comments have been extremely valuable. We have also greatly benefitted by the comments and criticisms received from a group of participants in a short course on multivariate analysis of epidemiologic data offered by the first author at the Symposium on Multivariate Data Analysis held in Santafé de Bogota, Colombia in June 1994, where portions of the manuscript were used as resource material. We would particularly like to thank Dr. Jorge Martínez and Professor Constanza Quintero for organizing and hosting these activities, their constant interest and enthusiasm in promoting them, and for all their help and cooperation in bringing these events to fruitful completion. The first eight chapters of the manuscript were also used as primary reference material in a short course on categorical data analysis offered by the first author at the National University of Trujillo, Peru during the course of his visiting professorial appointment in the summer of 1994. We are especially grateful to Professor Segundo M. Chuquilin Teran and other university authorities for an invitation to visit that institution and to Professor Carlos A. Minchón Medina who as an active participant in the course checked all the numerical computations of most of the worked examples appearing in the text.

Of course, we did not address all the comments, suggestions, and criticisms brought to our attention, and any remaining shortcomings are our own fault and responsibility.

We would also like to thank the editorial and production staff at the CRC Press, especially Bob Stern, Nora Konopka, Carolyn Lea, and Julie Haydu, for their help and cooperation, which is so essential in bringing the project to completion and in the final production of the book.

Much of our own introduction to topics covered in this volume came from some existing works, e.g., Breslow and Day (1980, 1987), Kahn and Sempos (1989), Kelsey, Thompson and Evans (1986), Kleinbaum, Kupper and Morgenstern (1982), Miettinen (1985), Rothman (1986), Schesselman (1982) and Selvin (1991), which have been extensively used by the first author during the course of his teaching, research and consulting activities, and we are deeply indebted to these authors for their contributions. Both referenced and unreferenced assertions to statements and formulas in this book are usually documented in one or more of these sources in somewhat greater detail, and the readers wanting further discussions and details are advised to consult them. We have made every attempt to acknowledge any materials, formulas, examples, and data sources utilized to the original sources and any subsequent works referring to those sources for the sake of wide accessibility. However, there is no guarantee for any accuracy or completeness, and any omission or oversight to due credit or priority is deeply regretted and would be rectified in any further revision of this work.

The authors and CRC Press wish to acknowledge the associations, societies, journals, and publishers which kindly granted us permission to reprint their previously published copyrighted materials. Sources are noted where they appear in text.

Finally, some words of appreciation and gratitude are in order for our family members, who have been helpful when we needed it, have been tolerant to our idiosyncrasies, and perhaps, one day, would agree with us that all this effort was worth it. Hardeo Sahai wishes to thank his children, Amogh, Mrisa, and Pankaj, for providing a peaceful environment and for their patience and understanding throughout the time that the work was in progress. Anwer Khurshid wants to thank his parents for their love and affection and encouragement to pursue higher education which led to a career in statistics. A vote of thanks is also due to his daughter, Sumayya, and son, Sohaib, who cheerfully accepted Dad's excessive devotion to his third child, "the book". Finally, and most importantly, he is indebted to his wife, Shehla, who cheerfully attended to all the domestic chores while he was preoccupied with this task. At times she was the only one who believed that the project would ever be completed.

# About the Authors

**Hardeo Sahai, Ph.D**, is Professor of Biostatistics at the Medical Sciences Campus of the University of Puerto Rico and Honorary Professor of Statistics at the National University of Trujillo (Perú). He obtained a M.S. in Mathematical Statistics from the University of Chicago and a Ph.D. in Statistics from the University of Kentucky. He was a Senior Operations Research Analyst at the Defense Logistics Agency, a Senior Mathematical Statistician at the U.S. Bureau of the Census, Chief Statistician at the U.S. Army Recruiting Command, Senior Research Statistician at the Travenol Laboratories, Inc., and a member of the Technical Staff of the Burroughs Corporation before joining the Medical Sciences Campus of the University of Puerto Rico. He has held visiting professorships at the Federal University of Ceará (Brazil), National University of Colombia, National University of Trujillo (Perú), Veracruzana University (México), University of Cádiz (Spain) and the University of Granada (Spain). He is a former recipient of the Fulbright Scholar Award, the Department of Army Certificate of Achievement Award, and the University of Kentucky Outstanding Alumnus Award and has lectured extensively in several other universities in Latin America and Spain. He is the author or co-author of over 100 scientific papers published in a variety of mathematical, statistical, educational, public health and epidemiology journals. Dr. Sahai's other books include, *A Dictionary of Statistical, Scientific and Technical Terms* (with José Berríos, Wadsworth, 1982) and *Tablas y Formulas Estadísticas para las Ciencias Biológicas, Sociales y Físicas* (with Wilfredo Martínez, Grupo Editorial Iberoamerica, 1996). He is a fellow of the American Association for the Advancement of Science, the Royal Statistical Society (U.K.), Institute of Statisticians (Chartered Statistician) and the Institute of Mathematics and Its Applications (Chartered Mathematician); an elected member of the International Statistical Institute; and a member of the American Statistical Association, Institute of Mathematical Statistics, Bernoulli Society, International Biometric Society, and Epidemiologic Research Society. Dr. Sahai has been cited in *American Men and Women of Science, Who's Who in Science and Engineering, Who's Who in American Education, Who's Who in the South and Southwest, Who's Who in America,* and *Who's Who in the World.*

**Anwer Khurshid, Ph.D.**, is Assistant Professor of Statistics at the University of Karachi (Pakistan). He is currently affiliated with the University of Exeter (U.K.). He earned his B.A. and M.A. in Statistics from the University of Karachi and his Ph.D. in Statistics from the University of Exeter (U.K.). He is the author or co-author of several papers published in mathematical, statistical, and methodological journals, with articles appearing in *International Forum on Information and Documentation, Journal of Clinical Computing, Computers in Nursing, Statistics: A Journal of Theoretical and Applied Statistics, Biometrical Journal, Collegiate Microcomputer, Pi-Mu-Epsilon: National Honorary Mathematics Society Journal, Quality and Quantity: International Journal of Methodology, Statistica Applicata: Italian Journal of Applied Statistics, The New Zealand Statistician, Journal of Biopharmaceutical Statistics, Statistics in Medicine, Journal of Official Statistics*, and *Computers in Biology and Medicine.* He is a Fellow of the Royal Statistical Society (U.K.) and a member of the American Statistical Association, the International Biometric Society, and the International Association of Official Statistics of the International Statistical Institute.

# Contents

AUTISM
COALITION

www.autismcoalition.org

# 1 Introduction

Considered in this text is the problem of investigating the association between a dichotomous risk factor and a measurable outcome or endpoint of interest such as development of a particular disease or death due to the disease. Special consideration is given to the question of measuring the association between a dichotomous risk factor and a dichotomous disease state or endpoint.

Methods are presented for point and interval estimates for risk difference, incidence rate difference, risk ratio, incidence rate ratio, and odds ratio, the most useful and widely used measures of association in epidemiologic and clinical investigations. The techniques of obtaining confidence intervals based on point estimates of epidemiologic effect measures are described. These estimates can come from a cross-sectional study, in which, for example, the frequency of a certain disease is compared in two well-defined groups of subjects; from a retrospective study, in which a group of patients with a certain condition of interest (the case) is compared to another group of individuals without the condition (the control); or from a prospective study, in which samples of exposed and unexposed individuals, according to certain potentially etiologic antecedents of disease (the risk factor), are followed in order to observe the results of positive or negative conditions of a certain disease state.

Prospective studies may involve cohorts that take into account the person-time of observations. This time is likely to vary between different cohort members, when cases or points of outcome occur at different points in time. In such a cohort, the person-time of observations will generally vary as a function of both the time of admission into the study and the duration of the follow-up for the subjects remaining alive or free of the disease of interest. For these studies, the frequency of a condition or disease is computed based on the number of new cases or incidence during the time interval of follow-up and is expressed as per number of person-years of observation. This measure or quantity is often referred to as *disease rate, incidence rate, incidence density,* or *hazard rate.* For simplicity the term *incidence rate* is employed herein.

A numerical example is included for each method to illustrate computational procedures. All the calculations have been carried out in full arithmetical detail, although in some cases certain straightforward steps have been omitted. Most of the required calculations are fairly simple and can be readily performed using a handheld scientific calculator. Based on our experience with epidemiologists and other health science researchers and practitioners, it appears that even when they do have access to adequate computer hardware and software, they prefer to conduct their preliminary analysis of the data by employing handheld calculators, especially for small and moderate data sets. In addition, pertinent information is provided on the availability of suitable software, particularly for maximum likelihood and other procedures based on exact inferences which tend to be computationally complex, and the results obtained by using the software are compared to those obtained manually.

Most of the methods discussed are to be used for large sample approximations and are not reliable for analyses involving small samples. However, whenever appropriate, we discuss exact types of confidence intervals and illustrate their computations, which generally entail complex numerical algorithms that necessitate the use of a computer program. Although we attempt to provide some appreciation of the statistical principles and theory related to a particular procedure, the major emphasis of the text is methodological, with minimal mathematical and technical detail. In addition, some additional background material and results, including certain mathematical derivations of some of the main formulas used in the text, have been included in appendices. While some of the methods described in the text can be considered relatively advanced (e.g., maximum likelihood estimation, "exact" type intervals, and other related procedures), appropriate care has been taken to present them in such a manner that they can be understood easily and applied by readers with a nonmathematical background with the assistance of a suitable computing device.

# 2 Types of Epidemiologic Study Designs

Consider a dichotomous risk factor and a dichotomous disease state. In order to investigate whether an association exists between them, it is important to determine the type of sampling design employed in the study. Three basic sampling designs are employed in epidemiologic studies; prospective, retrospective, and cross-sectional designs.

## 2.1 PROSPECTIVE VS. RETROSPECTIVE STUDY DESIGNS

Prospective and retrospective studies can be viewed as different methods of sampling from a given study population, the collection of individuals to whom we would like to apply the results of the study. In prospective studies, also called cohort studies, we focus on risk factor groups and take samples of exposed and unexposed subjects; in retrospective studies, also called case-control studies, we focus on outcome groups and take samples of cases and noncases (controls). For example, consider Table 2.1, which gives the distribution of the number of subjects in a reference population according to the risk of exposure and the status of a disease. In a prospective study we would take samples from the exposed group (A + C) and the unexposed group (B + D). In a retrospective study we would take samples from the group with cases (A + B) and the group without cases (C + D). The sampling schemes of prospective and retrospective studies are illustrated in Figures 2.1 and 2.2.

## 2.2 CROSS-SECTIONAL VS. LONGITUDINAL STUDY DESIGNS

The main difference between the sampling design of prospective and retrospective studies is the choice of a particular distinguishing characteristic on the basis of which subjects are selected in the study. For prospective studies, this characteristic is likely an etiologic antecedent of disease (the risk factor), and for retrospective studies it is the disease state. Sometimes a study is undertaken in which people are chosen without regard to either risk factor or disease. A study that selects a sample from the study population and then classifies the

**TABLE 2.1**
**A 2 × 2 Display of a Reference Population in an Epidemiologic Study**

| | Exposed | Unexposed | Total |
|---|---|---|---|
| Cases | A | B | A + B |
| Noncases | C | D | C + D |
| Total | A + C | B + D | A + B + C + D |

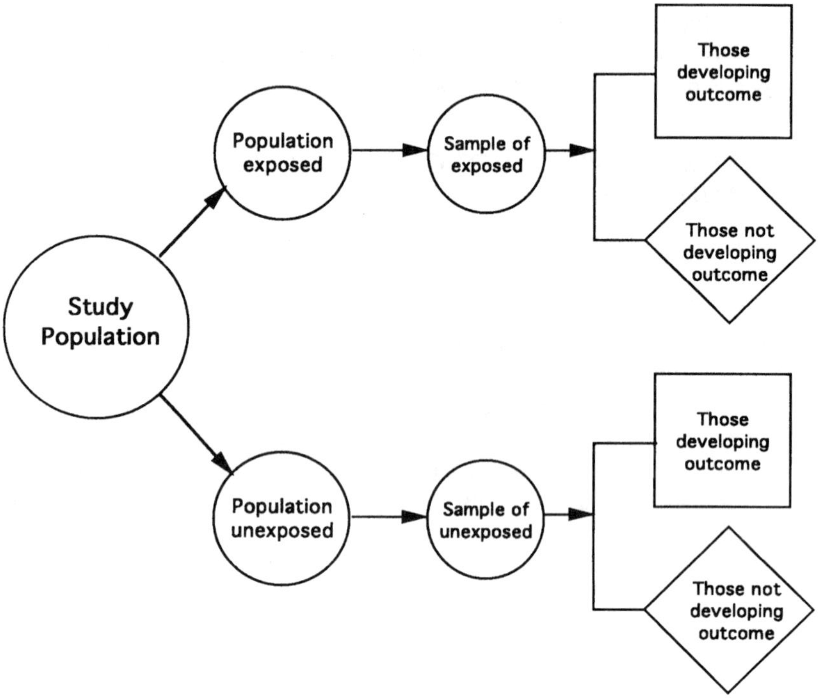


**FIGURE 2.1.** A prospective study design.

subjects according to risk factor and disease state is referred to as a cross-sectional study. In terms of the notations of Table 2.1, in a cross-sectional study a sample would be taken from the entire population A + B + C + D. The sampling design for this type of study is illustrated in Figure 2.3.

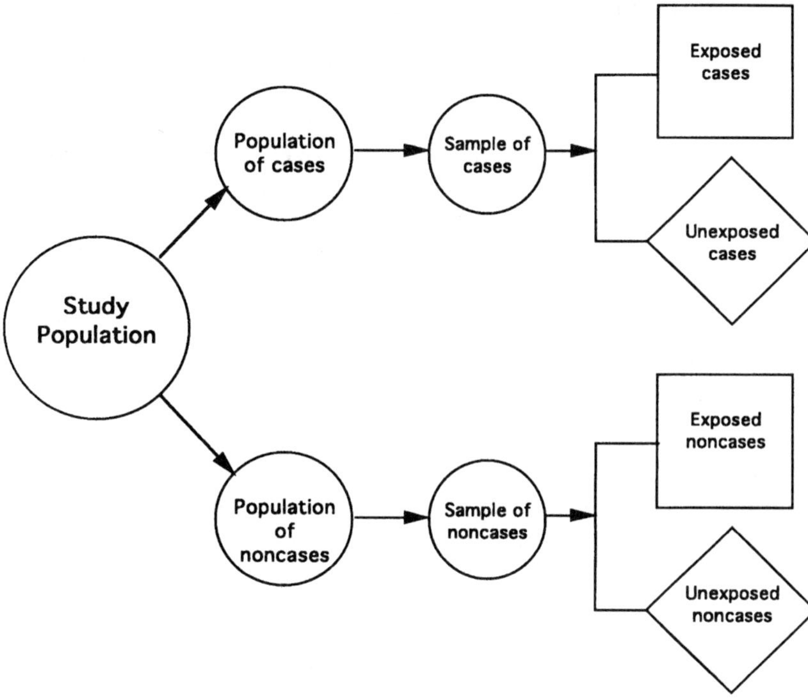


**FIGURE 2.2.** A retrospective study design.

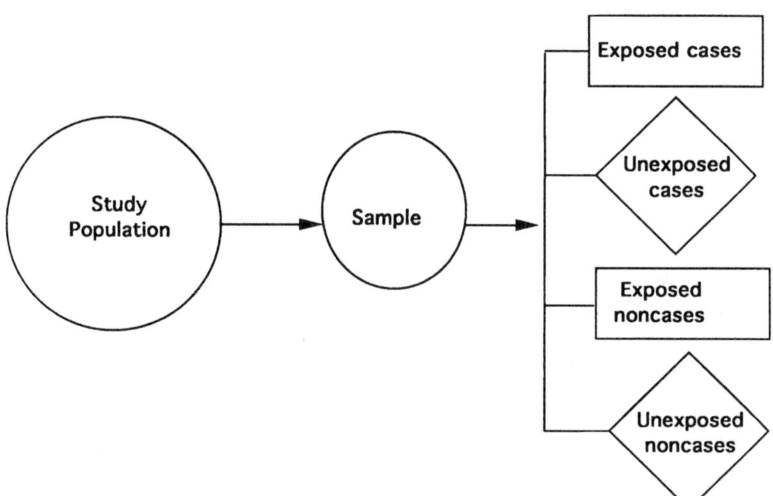


**FIGURE 2.3.** A cross-sectional study design.

## 2.3 A NOTE ON TERMINOLOGY

In epidemiologic literature some confusion seems to exist with regard to the use of the words *prospective* and *retrospective.* This confusion occurs usually because the terms may be used to describe either the selection of samples according to previous exposure (risk factor), to an effect, or to the chronology of the data collection work. For example, a study may involve a selection of two groups of individuals, exposed and unexposed to a certain risk in the past, through the use of medical records. The groups are followed, and the occurrence of any condition in the two groups is determined by a subsequent examination of the records. This study is essentially prospective in nature, although the individuals were drawn chronologically in retrospect.

Throughout this volume, we use the terms *prospective* and *retrospective* to designate whether the sampling design being with respect to *cause* or *effect.* The terms *cohort* and *follow-up* are also used as alternatives to *prospective.* This is because the essential feature of the method entails subsets of the population, known as cohorts, to describe well-defined groups of population, exposed or unexposed to a risk factor. These groups are followed to estimate reliable incidence or mortality rates in the population under study. Similarly, the term *case-control** is used to describe a retrospective study because the study starts with the identification of individuals with a disease (cases) of interest and a suitable reference or comparison group (control). Some disagreement exists among epidemiologists regarding the use of the term *retrospective* rather than *case-control study* because cases and controls may also be accumulated *prospectively;* i.e., each new case enters the study as it is diagnosed. Nevertheless, such a study may still be called *retrospective* because it looks backward in time from the outcome to its causes. For a further discussion of terminology in this area, see Feinstein (1973).

Finally, prospective and retrospective studies involve stratified sampling procedures.** This is always the case for retrospective studies; however, some prospective studies exist in which the groups of exposed and unexposed individuals are formed subsequent to the selection of the sample simply by splitting the sample into groups of exposed and unexposed subjects, respectively. It can be shown that the parameters and the statistical properties of such unstratified prospective studies are identical to those from cross-sectional studies.

* Miettinen (1976) suggested the use of the term *case-referent study* in place of *case-control study.* The point made by Miettinen is that the controls in a case-control study serve an entirely different purpose from the controls in a laboratory experiment or in a comparison group in a prospective study.

** The use of the term *stratified* is not generally in accord with with the principles of stratified sampling theory, but simply denotes a division or grouping of populations into subpopulations or strata of interest.

## 2.4 THE MEASUREMENT OF EFFECT

We consider mainly measures of risk effect based on count data (proportion type) and person-time observations (incidence density or incidence rates). In the epidemiologic literature measures of risk based on count (real) numerators and sampling-based count (quasi) denominators have been termed quasi (incidence) rates. It has been shown that the ratio of quasi rates is incidence rate ratio. For such measures, the statistical analysis follows that of the odds ratio in practice but not in principle. For further discussion and details in this area, refer to Miettinen (1976, 1985).

## 2.5 DESIGN-BASED VS. MODEL-BASED INFERENCE

Design-based and model-based inferences are two alternative conceptual frameworks used to address the question of the generalizability of the conclusions from investigations that include randomized experimental studies, observational studies involving subjects from a naturally defined group of individuals or judgmental and convenient samples, and sample surveys of randomly selected individuals. Studies that require the assumption of random selection of units from a well-defined target population are said to generate design-based inferences. In design-based inference formal conclusions are restricted to a finite population of subjects from which a sample (sampled population) has been drawn. Model-based inference requires making an assumption external to the study design in order to extend inferences to some target population of potential subjects beyond the study population. Thus, the main difference between design-based and model-based inference is the population to which the results can be generalized. Design-based inferences are more appropriate for sample surveys in which the target population is the same from which subjects have been randomly selected. For observational studies, including prospective and retrospective studies, model-based inferences are more appropriate because the target population is broader and more pervasive than the study population. In addition, the group of subjects included in the study are not usually randomly selected. For a detailed discussion of various aspects of inferences for observational studies, see Fairley and Mosteller (1977), Anderson et al. (1980), Breslow and Day (1980, 1987) and Rothman (1986).

A complete and thorough introduction to various aspects of prospective, retrospective, and cross-sectional studies, including their relative merits and demerits, can be found in books by Breslow and Day (1980, 1987), Kleinbaum et al. (1982), Schesselman (1982), and Kelsey et al. (1986). Brief accounts of these studies are given in the articles by McKinlay (1985) and Greenberg (1986, 1988). For an excellent and comprehensive review of observational studies in general, see McKinlay (1975).

# References

**Anderson, S., Auquer, A., Hauck, W., Oakes, D., Vandaele, W., and Weisberg, H. I.** (1980). *Statistical Methods for Comparative Studies.* John Wiley & Sons, New York.

**Breslow, N. E. and Day, N. E.** (1980). *Statistical Methods in Cancer Research, Vol. 1, The Analysis of Case-Control Studies.* International Agency for Research on Cancer, Lyons, France.

**Breslow, N. E. and Day, N. E.** (1987). *Statistical Methods in Cancer Research, Vol. 2, The Design and Analysis of Cohort Studies.* International Agency for Research on Cancer, Lyons, France.

**Fairley, B. and Mosteller, F.** (1977). *Statistics and Public Policy.* Addison-Wesley, Reading, MA.

**Feinstein, A. R.** (1973). "Clinical Biostatistics, XX: The Epidemiologic Trohoc, The Ablative Relative Risk Ratio and 'Retrospective' Research", *Clin. Pharmacol. Ther.,* 14, 291–307.

**Greenberg, R. S.** (1986). "Prospective Studies", In: *Encyclopedia of Statistical Sciences.* Vol. 7, pp. 315–319 (Eds. S. Kotz and N. L. Johnson). John Wiley & Sons, New York.

**Greenberg, R. S.** (1988). "Retrospective Studies (Including Case-Control)", In: *Encyclopedia of Statistical Sciences,* Vol. 8, pp. 120–124 (Eds. S. Kotz and N. L. Johnson). John Wiley & Sons, New York.

**Kelsey, J. L., Thompson, W. D., and Evans, A. S.** (1986). *Methods in Observational Epidemiology.* Oxford University Press, New York.

**Kleinbaum, D. G., Kupper, L. L., and Morgenstern, H.** (1982). *Epidemiologic Research: Principles and Quantitative Methods.* Lifetime Learning Publications, Belmont, CA.

**McKinlay, S. M.** (1975). "The Design and Analysis of the Observational Study: A Review", *J. Am. Stat. Assoc.* 70, 503–520 (comments, pp. 521–523; correction; *ibid,* 71, p. 255).

**McKinlay, S. M.** (1985). "Observational Studies", In: *Encyclopedia of Statistical Sciences,* Vol. 6, pp. 397–401 (Eds. S. Kotz and N. L. Johnson). John Wiley & Sons, New York.

**Miettinen, O. S.** (1976). "Estimability and Estimation in Case-Referent Studies", *Am. J. Epidemiol.* 103, 226–235.

**Miettinen, O. S.** (1985). *Theoretical Epidemiology: Principles of Occurrence Research in Medicine.* John Wiley & Sons, New York.

**Rothman, K. J.** (1986). *Modern Epidemiology.* Little, Brown, Boston.

**Schesselman, J. J.** (1982). *Case-Control Studies.* Oxford University Press, New York.

# 3 Prospective (Cohort) Studies

In prospective or cohort studies individuals with different levels of exposure are identified and subsequently followed up in time to determine their disease or health status. Prospective studies may entail count or cumulative incidence type data representing a cohort, which has been followed over a specified period of time, or person-time observations arising from a cohort in which the follow-up period is likely to vary between different cohort members. This chapter considers epidemiologic effect measures involving count data.

For example, each subject in a large population is classified as exposed or unexposed according to certain risk factors and as positive (case) or negative (noncase) according to some disease state. Suppose also that samples of exposed and unexposed cases are followed with the results shown in Table 3.1. Let $p_1$ and $p_2$ be the probabilities denoting risks for developing cases in the population for exposed and unexposed groups, respectively. The most commonly used sample estimates for $p_1$ and $p_2$ are obtained as

$$\hat{p}_1 = a/n_1 \quad \text{and} \quad \hat{p}_2 = b/n_2 .$$

## 3.1 MEASURES OF RISK

When any two numerical quantities are compared, a decision must be made regarding how they should be compared. Two approaches commonly used are calculate the difference between the two quantities or calculate the ratio of one quantity to the other. When comparing risks, a difference between risks is called *risk difference* and any ratio comparison of two risks is called a *risk ratio* or *relative risk.* If a risk is expressed in terms of odds* rather than probability, the ratio comparison of two risks is called an *odds ratio.*

### 3.1.1 RISK DIFFERENCE

The risk difference (RD) for exposed vs. unexposed groups is defined as

* The ratio of probability or proportion of a group experiencing an event to the probability of its complement (1-probability) is referred to as odds. For a further discussion of the relationship between probability and odds of an event see Appendix C.

**TABLE 3.1**
**A 2 × 2 Display of Sample Data in a Prospective Study**

| | Exposed | Unexposed | Total |
|---|---|---|---|
| Cases | $a$ | $b$ | $m_1$ |
| Noncases | $c$ | $d$ | $m_2$ |
| Total | $n_1$ | $n_2$ | $n$ |

$$\text{RD} = p_1 - p_2. \tag{3.1}$$

#### 3.1.1.1 Point Estimation

A sample estimate of the RD, which is also the maximum likelihood estimate, is obtained as

$$\hat{\text{RD}} = \hat{p}_1 - \hat{p}_2. \tag{3.2}$$

#### 3.1.1.2 Confidence Intervals

It is easily shown, using the result of the variance of the difference of two sample proportions, that the standard error* (SE) of $\hat{\text{RD}}$ is

$$\text{SE}\left(\hat{\text{RD}}\right) = \sqrt{\frac{p_1(1-p_1)}{n_1} + \frac{p_2(1-p_2)}{n_2}}, \tag{3.3}$$

with a good sample estimate

$$\hat{\text{SE}}\left(\hat{\text{RD}}\right) = \sqrt{\frac{\hat{p}_1(1-\hat{p}_1)}{n_1} + \frac{\hat{p}_2(1-\hat{p}_2)}{n_2}}. \tag{3.4}$$

The estimator (Equation 3.4) is the *maximum likelihood estimator* of $\text{SE}(\hat{\text{RD}})$. An unbiased estimator of $\text{Var}\left(\hat{\text{RD}}\right)$ is obtained by replacing $n_1$ and $n_2$ by $n_1 - 1$ and $n_2 - 1$, respectively.

* Standard error of an estimate (statistic) is defined as the standard deviation (SD) of the sampling distribution of the statistic. Some writers use the term *standard error* to designate an estimate of the SD of the sampling distribution which we call estimated standard error. By assuming that the estimate is normally distributed about the parameter value, a desired confidence interval can be obtained by adding and subtracting from the estimate an appropriate multiple of its standard error.

We now consider some methods of determining confidence intervals for the RD.

*Standard Error-Based Method*

For large *n*, the statistic $(\hat{\text{RD}} - \text{RD})/\hat{\text{SE}}(\hat{\text{RD}})$ can be treated as a standard normal variate. Thus, a 100(1 – α)% confidence interval (CI) for the RD is obtained as

$$\hat{\text{RD}} \pm Z_{\alpha/2}\,\hat{\text{SE}}\left(\hat{\text{RD}}\right)$$

$$= \hat{\text{RD}} \pm Z_{\alpha/2}\sqrt{\frac{\hat{p}_1\left(1-\hat{p}_1\right)}{n_1} + \frac{\hat{p}_2\left(1-\hat{p}_2\right)}{n_2}}, \tag{3.5}$$

where $Z_{\alpha/2}$ is the upper 100(α/2)th percentile of the standard normal distribution.

*Test-Based Method*

According to this method, the estimate of the standard error of the sampling distribution of $\hat{\text{RD}}$, obtained at the null value, is taken as an estimate of the standard error elsewhere along the scale. The rationale for this procedure is as follows. Consider the test of hypothesis:

$$H_0:\ \text{RD} = \text{RD}_0 \quad \text{vs.} \quad H_1:\ \text{RD} \neq \text{RD}_0.$$

Let $\hat{\text{RD}}$ be a sample estimator for the RD. Then, a large sample test statistic for testing the above hypothesis is

$$Z = \left(\hat{\text{RD}} - \text{RD}_0\right) / \hat{\text{SE}}_0\left(\hat{\text{RD}}\right).$$

The above statistic can also be written as

$$Z^2 = \left(\hat{\text{RD}} - \text{RD}_0\right)^2 / \left\{\hat{\text{SE}}_0\left(\hat{\text{RD}}\right)\right\}^2$$

or

$$\chi_1^2 = \left(\hat{\text{RD}} - \text{RD}_0\right)^2 / \left\{\hat{\text{Var}}_0\left(\hat{\text{RD}}\right)\right\},$$

where $\chi_1^2$ is a chi-square statistic with one degree of freedom.

An estimate of $\text{Var}_0(\hat{\text{RD}})$ or $\text{SE}_0(\hat{\text{RD}})$ can then be obtained as

$$\hat{\text{Var}}_0\left(\hat{\text{RD}}\right) = \left(\hat{\text{RD}} - \text{RD}_0\right)^2 / \chi_1^2$$

or

$$\hat{SE}_0(\hat{RD}) = \sqrt{(\hat{RD} - RD_0)^2 / \chi_1^2}.$$

The $\chi_1^2$ in the above expression is generally taken as the value of the Mantel-Haenszel chi-square statistic* under the null hypothesis $H_0 : RD = RD_0$. (Appendix A contains the definition of Mantel-Haenszel chi-square.)

One usually sets $RD_0 = 0$. Thus, a $100(1 - \alpha)\%$ CI for the RD is obtained as

$$\hat{RD} \pm Z_{\alpha/2} \sqrt{(\hat{RD})^2 / \chi_{MH}^2}, \tag{3.6}$$

where $\chi_{MH}^2$ is the Mantel-Haenszel chi-square statistic given by (also see Appendix A)

$$\chi_{MH}^2 = \frac{(n-1)(ad - bc)^2}{n_1 n_2 m_1 m_2}. \tag{3.7}$$

Although we have formulated Equation 3.6 in terms of a chi-square statistic, the real issue is the square of a standard normal statistic defined by $\chi = (a - E(a))/\sqrt{\mathrm{Var}(a)}$. The expression (3.6) can be rewritten in terms of $\chi$ more simply as

$$\hat{RD}(1 \pm Z_{\alpha/2}/\chi).$$

### *An Exact Method*

An exact CI for the RD can be calculated from the double binomial model. Construction of an exact CI is quite difficult, however, because the exact distribution of the difference in sample proportions is quite complicated. The calculation would involve iterative determination of the exact tail probability via elimination of a nuisance parameter. For a discussion of some methods and computational algorithms for determining small sample CIs for the difference of two proportions, see Thomas and Gart (1977), Santner and Snell (1980), Soms (1989a, b), Coe and Tamhane (1993), and Santner and Yamagani (1993). A FORTRAN program for implementing the Coe and Tamhane algorithm is given in Coe (1989). Another FORTRAN program, which implements the Santner and Yamagani algorithm, is available from the authors of said algorithm. The StatXact (1995) software implements the Santer and Snell (1980) algorithm for determining an exact CI for the RD rather conveniently.

* Miettinen (1976) recommended the use of any statistic that represents an equally efficient test of the null hypothesis based on the same data.

**TABLE 3.2**
**Data from the Evans County Heart Disease Study**

| | High CAT | Low CAT | Total |
|---|---|---|---|
| CHD | 27 | 44 | 71 |
| No CHD | 95 | 443 | 538 |
| Total | 122 | 487 | 609 |

From Kleinbaum, D. G., Kupper, L. L., and Morgenstern, H. (1982). *Epidemiologic Research: Principles and Quantitive Methods*, pp. 8–9. Lifetime Learning Publications, Belmont, CA. With permission.

*Other Methods*

In the statistical literature several other approximate methods are available for constructing approximate CIs for the risk difference. For example, Mee (1984), Nurminen (1986), and Beal (1987) used the scoring theory to construct CIs for the difference in two proportions, and Gart and Nam (1990) proposed using skewness corrections for the scoring-based procedures. However, the scoring-based procedures tend to be rather complex and in general require the use of an iterative algorithm. Anbar (1983) proposed a procedure that uses the quadratic formula to obtain the CI for the difference in two binomial parameters, while Mee (1984) pointed out that the procedure depends on the arbitrary choice of one of the two parameters used in the construction of the CI. More recently, Peskun (1993) put forth a new method based on normal theory which uses a Lagrange multiplier in the constrained minimization of the difference between two proportions.

*Example 3.1*

Consider the follow-up study data from the Evans County (Georgia) Heart Disease Study described by Cassels (1971) and further discussed in Kleinbaum et al. (1982). The data pertain to a cohort of 609 healthy white males between the ages of 40 and 76 who were residents of Evans County in 1960. The cohort was followed for 7 years, after which new cases of coronary heart disease (CHD) were identified. The level of circulating catecholamine (CAT) is the exposure variable of interest, the values of which were artificially generated for the purpose of illustration. The purpose of the study was to assess the putative association between CAT (as measured in 1960) and the subsequent 7-year incidence of CHD. The data are summarized in Table 3.2.

First, calculate an estimate of the RD and its standard error. From the data of Table 3.2, we obtain

$$\hat{p}_1 = 27/122 = 0.221$$

and

$$\hat{p}_2 = 44/487 = 0.090.$$

Thus, an estimate of the RD and its standard error are

$$\hat{\text{RD}} = \hat{p}_1 - \hat{p}_2 = 0.131$$

and

$$\hat{\text{SE}}(\hat{p}_1 - \hat{p}_2) = \sqrt{\frac{0.221(1-0.221)}{122} + \frac{0.090(1-0.090)}{487}}$$
$$= 0.040.$$

We now obtain 95% CIs for the RD using the standard error-based and the test-based procedures.

**Standard error-based method** — A 95% CI for the RD using this method is

$$0.131 \pm 1.96 \times 0.040 = (0.053, 0.209).$$

**Test-based method** — To obtain a CI for the RD using the test-based method, note that

$$\chi^2_{\text{MH}} = \frac{(609-1)(27 \times 443 - 44 \times 95)^2}{122 \times 487 \times 71 \times 538} = 16.220.$$

Therefore, a 95% CI for the RD using this method is given by

$$0.131 \pm 1.96\sqrt{(0.131)^2/16.220} = (0.067, 0.195).$$

### 3.1.2 Risk Ratio

A measure of association employed frequently in many epidemiologic investigations is the risk ratio, or relative risk. The risk ratio (RR) for exposed vs. unexposed groups is defined as

$$\text{RR} = p_1/p_2. \tag{3.8}$$

In other words, it is the likelihood of disease in those exposed to the risk factor relative to those who are not exposed to the risk factor. It represents how many more times the disease is likely to occur in the exposed group as compared to the unexposed group.

#### 3.1.2.1 Point Estimation

A sample estimate of the RR, which is also the maximum likelihood estimate, is obtained as

$$\hat{RR} = \hat{p}_1 / \hat{p}_2. \tag{3.9}$$

#### 3.1.2.2 Confidence Intervals

Although it is possible to directly derive a CI for the RR by first arriving at an approximate expression for $\hat{SE}(\hat{RR})$, it is generally not recommended. The reason is the imbalance of possible ranges for the interval. If RR > 1, it can go anywhere from 1 to ∞, but if RR < 1, the range is restricted to the interval from 0 to 1. For this reason, many mathematical approaches for constructing a CI for the RR employ the natural logarithm of the risk ratio. (Note that $-\infty < \log_e(RR) < \infty$.)

A 100(1 – α)% CI for $\log_e$(RR) can be obtained as

$$\log_e\left(\hat{RR}\right) \pm Z_{\alpha/2}\, \hat{SE}\left\{\log_e\left(\hat{RR}\right)\right\}. \tag{3.10}$$

From which a 100(1 – α)% CI for the RR can be obtained by taking antilogarithms of the corresponding endpoints of the CI for $\log_e$(RR).

*Taylor Series Method*

The method is essentially standard error based and employs an expression of the variance of the estimate derived from Taylor series approximation.

It can be shown that for large sample sizes ($n_1 \to \infty$, $n_2 \to \infty$) (see Appendix B)

$$SE\left\{\log_e\left(\hat{RR}\right)\right\} \approx \sqrt{\frac{(1-p_1)}{n_1 p_1} + \frac{(1-p_2)}{n_2 p_2}}, \tag{3.11}$$

with a good sample estimate

$$\hat{SE}\left\{\log_e\left(\hat{RR}\right)\right\} \approx \sqrt{\frac{(1-\hat{p}_1)}{n_1 \hat{p}_1} + \frac{(1-\hat{p}_2)}{n_2 \hat{p}_2}}. \tag{3.12}$$

Therefore, a 100(1 – α)% CI for $\log_e$(RR) is given by

$$\log_e\left(\hat{RR}\right) \pm Z_{\alpha/2} \sqrt{\frac{(1-\hat{p}_1)}{n_1 \hat{p}_1} + \frac{(1-\hat{p}_2)}{n_2 \hat{p}_2}}, \tag{3.13}$$

from which a 100(1 – α)% CI for the RR can be obtained by taking antilogarithms of the corresponding endpoints.

The above CI method was recommended by Katz et al. (1978) on the basis of results of extensive simulation studies and is sometimes referred to as the Katz method.

*Test-Based Method*

The rationale for this procedure is as follows. Consider the test of hypothesis:

$$H_0 : \text{RR} = \text{RR}_0 \quad \text{vs.} \quad H_1 : \text{RR} \neq \text{RR}_0$$

Let $\hat{\text{RR}}$ be a sample estimator for the RR. Then, a large sample test statistic for testing the above hypothesis is*

$$Z = \left(\hat{\text{RD}} - \text{RD}_0\right) / \hat{\text{SE}}_0\left(\hat{\text{RD}}\right).$$

The above statistic can also be written as

$$Z^2 = \left(\hat{\text{RR}} - \text{RR}_0\right)^2 / \left\{\hat{\text{SE}}_0\left(\hat{\text{RR}}\right)\right\}^2$$

or

$$\chi_1^2 = \left(\hat{\text{RR}} - \text{RR}_0\right)^2 / \hat{\text{Var}}_0\left(\hat{\text{RR}}\right),$$

where $\chi_1^2$ is a chi-square statistic with one degree of freedom.

An estimate of $\text{Var}_0(\hat{\text{RR}})$ or $\text{SE}_0(\hat{\text{RR}})$ can be obtained as

$$\hat{\text{Var}}_0\left(\hat{\text{RR}}\right) = \left(\hat{\text{RR}} - \text{RR}_0\right)^2 / \chi_1^2$$

or

$$\hat{\text{SE}}_0\left(\hat{\text{RR}}\right) = \sqrt{\left(\hat{\text{RR}} - \text{RR}_0\right)^2 / \chi_1^2}.$$

* As stated earlier, because of the asymmetric distribution of the RR, the test statistic is generally based on the logarithmic transformation:

$$Z = \left\{\log_e\left(\hat{\text{RR}}\right) - \log_e\left(\text{RR}_0\right)\right\} / \hat{\text{SE}}_0\left\{\log_e\left(\hat{\text{RR}}\right)\right\}.$$

As before, the $\chi_1^2$ in the above expression is generally taken as the value of the Mantel-Haenszel chi-square statistic* under the null hypothesis $H_0 : \mathrm{RR} = \mathrm{RR}_0$.

One usually sets $\mathrm{RR}_0 = 1$, or $\log_e(\mathrm{RR}_0) = 0$ if the CI is obtained using the logarithm of the test statistic. Thus, a $100(1 - \alpha)\%$ CI for $\log_e(\mathrm{RR})$ is obtained:

$$\log_e\left(\hat{\mathrm{RR}}\right) \pm Z_{\alpha/2}\sqrt{\left\{\log_e\left(\hat{\mathrm{RR}}\right)\right\}^2 / \chi^2_{\mathrm{MH}}}, \tag{3.14}$$

where $\chi^2_{\mathrm{MH}}$ is the Mantel-Haenszel chi-square statistic defined in Equation 3.7.

Again, note that the expression (3.14) is more readily formulated in terms of the standard normal statistic $\chi$ as

$$\log_e\left(\hat{\mathrm{RR}}\right)\left(1 \pm Z_{\alpha/2}/\chi\right).$$

From which a $100(1 - \alpha)\%$ CI for the RR can be written as

$$\left(\hat{\mathrm{RR}}\right)^{\left(1 \pm Z_{\alpha/2}/\chi\right)}.$$

*A Poisson Model Method*

An approximate CI for the RR also can be obtained by assuming that the individual risks of developing a case between the exposed and unexposed groups are sufficiently low so that the observed outcomes $a$ and $b$ in Table 3.1 can be considered as emanating from the Poisson populations with parameters $\lambda_1$ and $\lambda_2$, respectively. Noting that the Poisson distribution with parameter $\lambda$ can be considered as the limiting form of the binomial distribution — as $n \to \infty$, $p \to 0$ such that $np \to \lambda$ — the RR is determined by

$$\mathrm{RR} = \frac{p_1}{p_2} = \left(\frac{n_2}{n_1}\right)\frac{\lambda_1}{\lambda_2}.$$

Thus, a CI for the RR can be obtained by first determining a confidence interval for $\lambda_1/\lambda_2$. An "exact" CI for $\lambda_1/\lambda_2$ can be obtained readily by using the results based on a binomial probability interval (e.g., see Sahai and Khurshid, 1993). The resulting $100(1 - \alpha)\%$ lower and upper confidence limits for the RR, for example, $\mathrm{RR}_\mathrm{L}$ and $\mathrm{RR}_\mathrm{U}$, are then determined by

$$\mathrm{RR}_\mathrm{L} = \left(\frac{n_2}{n_1}\right)\left(\frac{a}{b+1}\right)\frac{1}{F_{\alpha/2,2(b+1),2a}} \tag{3.15}$$

* Miettinen (1976) recommended the use of any statistic that represents an equally efficient test of the null hypothesis based on the same data.

and

$$\mathrm{RR_U} = \left(\frac{n_2}{n_1}\right)\left(\frac{a+1}{b}\right)F_{\alpha/2,2(a+1),2b},$$

where $F_{\alpha/2,\nu_1,\nu_2}$ represents the upper $100(\alpha/2)$th percentile of the $F$ distribution with $\nu_1$ and $\nu_2$ degrees of freedom.

This method, based on Poisson distribution, was first suggested by Bross (1954). Simulation studies for this method have shown that the method produces reasonable results, although the limits tend to be somewhat conservative.

*An Exact Method*

An exact CI for the RR entails the total number of cases and the use of two independent binomial models. The determination of exact confidence limits would thus involve iterative evaluation of the exact tail probability via elimination of a nuisance parameter. For a description of an "exact" method based on a hypergeometric model, refer to Appendix D. Santer and Snell (1980) and Coe and Tamhane (1993) proposed new methods and computational algorithms for constructing a small sample CI for the risk ratio. A FORTRAN program for implementing the Coe and Tamhane algorithm is given in Coe (1989). The StatXact (1995) software implements the Santer and Snell (1980) algorithm rather conveniently.

It would be seen later that under certain conditions, the odds ratio as a measure of risk provides a reasonable approximation of the relative risk. The exact confidence limits for the odds ratio can be determined using a statistical model involving a noncentral hypergeometric distribution. The computations are somewhat complicated, but not nearly as complicated as the computation of exact confidence limits for the RR involving a statistical model of two independent binomial variates. Inasmuch as the odds ratio is only an approximation of the RR, the calculation of exact limits for the odds ratio does not yield exact confidence limits for the RR. However, for rare diseases for which risks are quite small, the exact confidence limits for the odds ratio can be used as reasonable surrogate values for confidence limits of the RR.

*Other Methods*

Several other approximate methods are available for determining CIs for the RR. Some of these methods are described in Appendix D. For a review of some additional methods and their numerical comparison, see Gart and Nam (1988).

*Example 3.2*

Consider again the Evans County Heart Disease Study, described in Example 3.1. An estimate of the RR and its standard error are

$$\hat{\mathrm{RR}} = \hat{p}_1/\hat{p}_2 = 2.456$$

and

$$\hat{\text{SE}}\left\{\log_e\left(\hat{\text{RR}}\right)\right\} = \sqrt{\frac{(1-0.221)}{122(0.221)} + \frac{(1-0.090)}{487(0.090)}} = 0.223.$$

We now illustrate the computation of the CIs for the RR using the Taylor series, test-based, and Poisson model methods.

**Taylor series method** — A 95% CI for $\log_e$(RR) using the Taylor series method is

$$\log_e(2.456) \pm 1.96 \times 0.223 = (0.461, 1.336),$$

from which a 95% CI for the RR is given as (1.586, 3.804). Note that the interval does not include 1.

**Test-based method** — To obtain a CI for the RR using the test-based method, note that (from Example 3.1), $\chi^2_{\text{MH}} = 16.220$. Therefore, a 95% CI for $\log_e$(RR) using this method is

$$\log_e(2.456) \pm 1.96\sqrt{\left\{\log_e(2.456)\right\}^2/16.220} = (0.461, 1.336).$$

From which a 95% CI for the RR is given as (1.586, 3.804). Note that these limits are the same as those obtained using the Taylor series method. However, in general, the two methods may yield different results.

**Poisson model method** — To obtain a 95% CI for the RR using the Poisson model assumptions, note that using the data in Table 3.1, we have

$$a = 27,\ n_1 = 122,$$

$$b = 44,\ n_2 = 487,$$

$$F_{\alpha/2,2(b+1),2a} = F_{0.025,90,54} = 1.6421,$$

and

$$F_{\alpha/2,2(a+1),2b} = F_{0.025,56,88} = 1.5922.$$

Thus, using Equation 3.15, the lower and upper confidence limits for the RR, for example, $\text{RR}_\text{L}$ and $\text{RR}_\text{U}$, are given by

$$\text{RR}_\text{L} = \left(\frac{487}{122}\right)\left(\frac{27}{44+1}\right)\frac{1}{1.6421} = 1.459$$

and

$$\mathrm{RR}_{\mathrm{U}} = \left(\frac{487}{122}\right)\left(\frac{27+1}{44}\right)1.5922 = 4.045.$$

Note that these limits provide a rather poor approximation in comparison to the Taylor series and the test-based results because the requirements of the Poisson model are not observed.

### 3.1.3 Odds Ratio

Another measure of association that is used frequently is the odds ratio (OR). The OR for exposed vs. unexposed groups is defined as

$$\mathrm{OR} = \frac{p_1/(1-p_1)}{p_2/(1-p_2)}. \tag{3.16}$$

The OR is clearly a ratio of the odds of the disease in those exposed to the risk factor to the odds of the disease among those who are not exposed to the risk factor. It is frequently of interest to note that for rare diseases, the numerical values of RR and OR will be very nearly equal. In such a case, the odds ratio is often referred to as *approximate risk ratio* or relative risk.

Mathematically it is fairly easy to see that for rare diseases, when the probability is very small that the exposed group will develop the outcome, the OR closely approximates the RR. Thus, when $p_1$ and $p_2$ are fairly small; in other words, $p_1 \approx p_2 \approx 0$ and $1 - p_1 \approx 1 - p_2 \approx 1$, we have

$$\mathrm{OR} \approx p_1/p_2.$$

For example, if the incidence of a particular disease in a group exposed to some condition is 30/100,000 as compared to an incidence of 10/100,000 in a group unexposed to the condition, the RR, for exposed vs. unexposed groups, is

$$\mathrm{RR} = \frac{30/100{,}000}{10/100{,}000} = 3.$$

The OR for exposed vs. unexposed groups is

$$\mathrm{OR} = \frac{30/99{,}970}{10/99{,}990} = 3.0006,$$

which is nearly the same as the RR.

#### 3.1.3.1 Point Estimation

A sample estimate of the OR is obtained as

$$\hat{\text{OR}} = \frac{\hat{p}_1/(1-\hat{p}_1)}{\hat{p}_2/(1-\hat{p}_2)} = \frac{(a/n_1)\div(c/n_1)}{(b/n_2)\div(d/n_2)} = \frac{ad}{bc}. \tag{3.17}$$

$\hat{\text{OR}}$ is calculated as the ratio of the products *ad* and *bc* of entries from cells that are diagonally opposite. Thus, the OR is also referred to as the cross-product ratio or cross ratio. Note also that the estimator (3.17) can always be used as an estimator of the OR, whether the disease is rare or common. When the disease is rare, the OR is sufficiently close to the RR so that Equation 3.17 can be used as an estimate of RR as well as the OR.

#### 3.1.3.2 Confidence Intervals

In principle, as indicated earlier in the case of RR, it is possible to derive an approximate CI for the OR by first deriving an approximate expression for $\hat{\text{SE}}(\hat{\text{OR}})$; it is, however, not recommended, and a logarithmic transformation is generally employed. Thus, a 100(1 – α)% CI for $\log_e$(OR) can be obtained as

$$\log_e\left(\hat{\text{OR}}\right) \pm Z_{\alpha/2}\,\hat{\text{SE}}\left\{\log_e\left(\hat{\text{OR}}\right)\right\}. \tag{3.18}$$

From which a 100(1 – α)% CI for the OR can be obtained by taking antilogarithms of the corresponding endpoints of the CI for $\log_e$(OR).

*Taylor Series Method*

Given a sample estimate of the OR as

$$\hat{\text{OR}} = \frac{ad}{bc}, \tag{3.19}$$

it can be shown, using asymptotic theory for the maximum likelihood estimator, that for large sample sizes (Haldane, 1955; Gart, 1962; Breslow and Day, 1987)

$$\begin{aligned} \text{SE}\left(\hat{\text{OR}}\right) &\approx \text{OR}\left(\frac{1}{n_1p_1} + \frac{1}{n_1(1-p_1)} + \frac{1}{n_2p_2} + \frac{1}{n_2(1-p_2)}\right)^{1/2} \\ &= \text{OR}\left(\frac{1}{n_1p_1(1-p_1)} + \frac{1}{n_2p_2(1-p_2)}\right)^{1/2}, \end{aligned} \tag{3.20}$$

and

$$\begin{aligned}\mathrm{SE}\left\{\log_e\left(\hat{\mathrm{OR}}\right)\right\} &\approx \left(\frac{1}{n_1 p_1} + \frac{1}{n_1(1-p_1)} + \frac{1}{n_2 p_2} + \frac{1}{n_2(1-p_2)}\right)^{1/2} \\ &= \left(\frac{1}{n_1 p_1(1-p_1)} + \frac{1}{n_2 p_2(1-p_2)}\right)^{1/2}.\end{aligned} \tag{3.21}$$

Upon substituting the sample estimates $\hat{p}_1 = a/n_1$ and $\hat{p}_2 = b/n_2$ into the above equations, the standard errors (3.20) and (3.21) are reasonably well estimated by (Gart and Zweifel, 1967; Breslow and Day, 1987)

$$\hat{\mathrm{SE}}\left(\hat{\mathrm{OR}}\right) \approx \hat{\mathrm{OR}}\left(\frac{1}{a} + \frac{1}{b} + \frac{1}{c} + \frac{1}{d}\right)^{1/2} \tag{3.22}$$

and

$$\hat{\mathrm{SE}}\left\{\log_e\left(\hat{\mathrm{OR}}\right)\right\} \approx \left(\frac{1}{a} + \frac{1}{b} + \frac{1}{c} + \frac{1}{d}\right)^{1/2}. \tag{3.23}$$

From these results, a 100(1 – α)% CI for $\log_e(\mathrm{OR})$ is obtained as

$$\log_e \frac{ad}{bc} \pm Z_{\alpha/2}\left(\frac{1}{a} + \frac{1}{b} + \frac{1}{c} + \frac{1}{d}\right)^{1/2}. \tag{3.24}$$

Given the CI for $\log_e(\mathrm{OR})$, the CI for the OR can be obtained as the antilogarithms of the corresponding endpoints. Note that the estimated standard errors of the sample odds ratio and log odds ratio given by Equations 3.22 and 3.23 show that the precision of the estimates depends not only on the sample sizes $n_1$ and $n_2$, but also on the individual cell counts. Although $\mathrm{SE}(\hat{\mathrm{OR}})$ and $\hat{\mathrm{SE}}(\hat{\mathrm{OR}})$ are generally of no particular interest for making formal inferences, they do provide a descriptive measure of the precision with which the underlying parameter has been estimated.

From Equation 3.19, $\hat{\mathrm{OR}}$ is equal to 0 or ∞ if any of the cell entries equal to zero. Naturally, these are undesirable estimates of the odds ratio. A modification that avoids this problem is due to Haldane (1955) and Anscombe (1956), who suggested adding 0.5 to each cell entry in the calculation of the OR. If the subjects in each row are randomly selected, $\hat{\mathrm{OR}}$ and $\hat{\mathrm{SE}}\{\log_e(\hat{\mathrm{OR}})\}$ have smaller asymptotic bias and mean square error if 0.5 is added to each cell entry in the calculation of $\hat{\mathrm{OR}}$ and $\hat{\mathrm{SE}}\{\log_e(\hat{\mathrm{OR}})\}$ (Gart and Zweifel, 1967).

Cox and Snell (1989), Mantel (1980), and Miettinen (personal communication, 1994) prefer to ignore the 1/2 correction factor. If one encounters a situation in which $\hat{\mathrm{OR}}$ is infinite as a consequence of division by zero, one may compute a lower confidence limit for the OR using Equation 4.14, obtained from the exact conditional distribution. The use of the 1/2 correction factor in this calculation is not recommended.

The method described above is also sometimes called the *logit method* and was first devised by Woolf (1955). It is widely recommended as a satisfactory approximation except when any one of the cell entries *a, b, c, d* is very small, and then a more accurate but complex procedure (described in Chapter 4) should be used. The results of the CI usually do not need to agree with the customary chi-square test of OR without the continuity correction.

*Test-Based Method*

As discussed earlier, a 100(1 – α)% CI for $\log_e$(OR) can be obtained as

$$\log_e\left(\hat{\mathrm{OR}}\right) \pm Z_{\alpha/2}\sqrt{\left\{\log_e\left(\hat{\mathrm{OR}}\right)\right\}^2 / \chi^2_{\mathrm{MH}}}, \tag{3.25}$$

where $\chi^2_{\mathrm{MH}}$ designates the Mantel-Haenzel chi-square statistic with one degree of freedom. Again, note that the expression (3.25) is more readily formulated in terms of the standard normal statistic $\chi$ as

$$\log_e\left(\hat{\mathrm{OR}}\right)\left(1 \pm Z_{\alpha/2}/\chi\right),$$

from which a 100(1 – α)% CI for the OR can be written more simply as

$$\left(\hat{\mathrm{OR}}\right)^{\left(1 \pm Z_{\alpha/2}/\chi\right)}.$$

*An Exact Method*

The method of determining an exact CI for the OR is the same for both the prospective and retrospective data and is described for the retrospective study in Section 4.1.1.2.

*Example 3.3*

Refer to the Evans County Heart Disease Study, described in Example 3.1. An estimate of the OR and its standard error are

$$\hat{\mathrm{OR}} = \frac{27 \times 443}{95 \times 44} = 2.862,$$

$$\hat{\mathrm{SE}}\left\{\log_e\left(\hat{\mathrm{OR}}\right)\right\} = \left(\frac{1}{27} + \frac{1}{95} + \frac{1}{44} + \frac{1}{443}\right)^{1/2} = 0.269,$$

and

$$\hat{SE}\left(\hat{OR}\right) = 2.862 \times 0.269 = 0.770.$$

We now illustrate the computation of the CIs for the OR using the Taylor series and the test-based methods.

**Taylor series method** — Using the value of $\hat{SE}\{\log(\hat{OR})\}$, a 95% CI for $\log_e$(OR) is obtained as

$$\log_e(2.862) \pm 1.96 \times 0.269 = (0.524, 1.579),$$

which yields a 95% CI for the OR as (1.688, 4.851).

**Test-based method** — Using the logarithmic transformation, a 95% CI for $\log_e$(OR) is obtained as

$$\log_e(2.862) \pm 1.96\sqrt{\left(\log_e(2.862)\right)^2 / 16.220} = (0.540, 1.563),$$

which yields a 95% CI for the OR as (1.716, 4.773).

Note that the test-based limits obtained via logarithmic transformation compare favorably with those obtained by the Taylor series method.

### 3.1.4 A Comparison of the Taylor Series and Test-Based Methods

This section presents a brief summary of the results involving a comparison of properties of the Taylor series and test-based methods of constructing CIs for RD, RR, and OR. Both methods employ a large sample normal approximation and make use of the asymptotic variance of the estimate. The duality at issue between the two methods is the conditions under which variance is estimated. A variance estimate is by definition a "local" estimate, in which the parameter condition coincides with the point estimate. In test-based intervals the null condition is involved in variance estimation instead of the more general variance estimates used in Taylor series method. Although, strictly speaking, variance employed in the test-based method is an estimate of the variance under the null condition, the method has been found to be useful over a wide range of departures from the null hypothesis. This is one reason that these intervals, on average, tend to be of shorter length than the intervals based on the Taylor series method. Its chief advantage is its computational simplicity and the fact that the results usually agree with the chi-square test of significance.

If the $p$-value is near 1/2 so that the point estimate is close to the null value, both these intervals are interchangeable; neither is a first principle interval due to the lack of homoscedasticity. If $p$ (one-sided) is equal to $\alpha$ (or $1 - \alpha$), the proximal limit (at $H_0$) based on the test-based method is a first principle limit, but not the one based on the Taylor series method. If $p \ll \alpha$, the Taylor series interval is closer to the first principle because it allows for the lack of homoscedasticity (Miettinen, personal communication, 1994).

Simulation studies showed rather poor performance of the test-based method for large departures of the OR from the null value (Brown, 1981; Gart and Thomas, 1982). The method is known to perform well for ORs between 0.2 and 5.0, and Greenland (1984) reported that the limits are unsatisfactory for ORs of <0.1 or >10.0. Greenland also points out that the test-based limits are better suited to the OR estimates than to RD estimates. In general, the procedure gives results nearly comparable to that obtained from the Taylor series method for large samples, and none seems to perform well for small samples. Halperin (1977) found that for ORs between 0.25 and 4, the asymptotic coverage probability of the test-based method for the nominal 95% CI is between 0.93 and 0.95 and the asymptotic confidence coefficient approaches zero as the underlying true OR departs increasingly from the null value. Gart and Thomas (1982) reported that at the 95% level, under the two-sample binomial model, the modified logit method for the OR interval estimation (with 1/2 correction) typically has an actual confidence coefficient that is almost too large, while the test-based method has an actual confidence coefficient that is uniformly less than nominal when the OR is different from unity. For the nominal 95% confidence level, the true coverage probability of the test-based method in the unconditional space may be as low as 0.86. For some further discussion on the pros and cons of this issue, refer to the papers by Halperin (1977), Miettinen (1977), Fleiss (1979), Gart (1979), Brown (1981), Gart and Thomas (1982), and Greenland (1984).

### 3.1.5 Risk Ratio vs. Odds Ratio: A Comparison of Properties

Risk ratio and odds ratio are two measures for comparing risks; the former relates the chance or risk of developing outcome for exposed vs. unexposed groups, the latter relates their odds. Because odds are not ordinarily used in common language as chance or probability or risk, many people find the concept of an OR a bit more difficult to interpret than that of a RR.

Estimates of the RR and the OR are both commonly used to measure the strength of the association between exposure and disease. Both ratios can assume a non-negative value between 0 and $\infty$, but never <0. A value >1 indicates that risks or odds are greater with exposure, a value of 1 indicates that risks or odds are the same for the two groups, and a value <1 indicates lower risk or odds of disease with exposure. There may be differences in the numerical values of the two results, but they always point in the same general direction. Although no strict rules exist for the interpretation of the degree of risk associated with the numerical values of these two measures, Table 3.3 provides some general guidelines for this purpose.

One desirable property of the OR over the RR is that the former is unaffected whether the outcome of interest is the event being counted or its complement.

**TABLE 3.3**
**Guidelines for the Interpretation of the Values of RR and OR**

| Value | Effect of exposure |
|---|---|
| 0–0.3 | Strong benefit |
| 0.4–0.5 | Moderate benefit |
| 0.6–0.8 | Weak benefit |
| 0.9–1.1 | No effect |
| 1.2–1.6 | Weak hazard |
| 1.7–2.5 | Moderate hazard |
| ≥2.6 | Strong hazard |

From Greenberg, R. S., (1986) "Prospective Studies", In: *Encyclopedia of Statistical Sciences,* Vol. 7, pp. 315–319 (Eds. S. Kotz and N. L. Johnson), John Wiley & Sons, New York. With Permission.

To illustrate this point, let $p_1$ and $p_2$ be the probabilities denoting risks for developing cases in the population for exposed and unexposed groups, respectively. Then the RR and OR for exposed vs. unexposed groups are

$$\text{RR} = \frac{p_1}{p_2} \quad \text{and} \quad \text{OR} = \frac{p_1(1-p_2)}{p_2(1-p_1)}.$$

Compare the two groups with respect to being a noncase rather than being a case. The RR and OR are now given by

$$\text{RR}' = \frac{1-p_1}{1-p_2} \quad \text{and} \quad \text{OR}' = \frac{p_2(1-p_1)}{p_1(1-p_2)}.$$

It is readily observed that OR′ = 1/OR, but RR′ ≠ 1/RR. Thus, the use of the RR leads to different results, depending upon whether the study is reported in terms of the outcome of interest or its complement. For example, let $p_1 = 0.02$ and $p_2 = 0.01$. Then, it follows that

$$\text{RR} = \frac{0.02}{0.01} = 2, \quad \text{OR} = \frac{0.02/0.98}{0.01/0.99} \approx 2,$$

$$\text{RR}' = \frac{0.98}{0.99} \approx 1, \quad \text{OR}' = \frac{0.98/0.02}{0.99/0.01} \approx 0.5.$$

Thus, the exposed group has twice the odds of the unexposed group with respect to being a case or about one half the odds with respect to being a noncase. However, using the RR, the exposed group has about twice the chance of being a case, but nearly the same chance of being a noncase. If a logarithmic scale is used, $\log_e(\mathrm{OR}') = -\log_e(\mathrm{OR})$. Thus, on a log scale, OR and OR′ represent equal but opposite effects. No effect is indicated corresponding to $\mathrm{OR}' = \mathrm{OR} = 1$.

# References


**Anbar, D.** (1983). "On Estimating the Difference Between Two Probabilities with Special Reference to Clinical Trials", *Biometrics,* 39, 257–262.

**Anscombe, F. J.** (1956). "On Estimating Binomial Response Relations", *Biometrika,* 43, 461–464.

**Beal, F. L.** (1987). "Asymptotic Confidence Intervals for the Difference Between Two Binomial Parameters for Use with Small Samples", *Biometrics,* 43, 941–950.

**Breslow, N. E. and Day, N. E.** (1980). *Statistical Methods in Cancer Research, Vol. 1, The Analysis of Case-Control Studies.* International Agency for Research on Cancer, Lyons, France.

**Breslow, N. E. and Day, N. E.** (1987). *Statistical Methods in Cancer Research, Vol. 2, The Design and Analysis of Cohort Studies.* International Agency for Research on Cancer, Lyons, France.

**Bross, I.** (1954). "A Confidence Interval for a Percentage Increase", *Biometrics,* 10, 245–250.

**Brown, C. C.** (1981). "The Validity of Approximation Methods for Interval Estimation of the Odds Ratio", *Am. J. Epidemiol.,* 113, 474–480.

**Cassels, J. C.** (1971). "Summary of Major Findings of the Evans County Heart Disease Studies", *Arch. Intern. Med.,* 128, 887–889.

**Coe, P. R.** (1989). "Exact Repeated Confidence Intervals for Bernoulli Parameters in Group Sequential Experiments", Ph.D. Thesis, Northwestern University, Evanston, IL.

**Coe, P. R. and Tamhane, A. C.** (1993). "Small Sample Confidence Intervals for the Difference, Ratio and Odds Ratio of 2 Success Probabilities", *Commun. Stat. Simulat. Comput.,* 22, 925–938.

**Cox, D. R. and Snell, E. J.** (1989). *The Analysis of Binary Data,* 2nd ed. Chapman & Hall, London.

**Fleiss, J. L.** (1979). "Confidence Intervals for the Odds Ratio in Case-Control Studies: The State of the Art", *J. Chronic Dis.,* 32, 69–77.

**Gart, J. J.** (1962). "On the Combination of Relative Risks", *Biometrics,* 18, 601–610.

**Gart, J. J.** (1979). "Statistical Analyses of the Relative Risk", *Environ. Health Perspect.,* 32, 157–167.

**Gart, J. J. and Nam, J.** (1988). "Approximate Interval Estimation of the Ratio of Binomial Parameters: A Review and Corrections for Skewness", *Biometrics,* 44, 323–328.

**Gart, J. J. and Nam, J.** (1990). "Approximate Interval Estimation of the Difference in Binomial Parameters: Correction for Skewness and Extension to Multiple Tables", *Biometrics,* 46, 637–643.

**Gart, J. J. and Thomas, D. G.** (1982). "The Performance of Three Approximate Confidence Limit Methods for the Odds Ratio", *Am. J. Epidemiol.,* 115, 453–470.

**Gart, J. J. and Zwiefel, J. R.** (1967). "On the Bias of Various Estimators of the Logit and Its Variance, with Application to Quantal Bioassay", *Biometrika,* 54, 181–187.

**Greenberg, R. S.** (1986). "Prospective Studies", In: *Encyclopedia of Statistical Sciences.* Vol. 7, pp. 315–319 (Eds. S. Kotz and N. L. Johnson). John Wiley & Sons, New York.

**Greenland, S.** (1984). "A Counter Example to the Test-Based Principle of Setting Confidence Limits", *Am. J. Epidemiol.,* 120, 4–7.

**Haldane, J. B. S.** (1955). "The Estimation and Significance of the Logarithm of a Ratio of Frequencies", *Ann. Human Gen.,* 20, 309–311.

**Halperin, M.** (1977). "Estimability and Estimation in Case-Referent Studies (Letter to the Editor)", *Am. J. Epidemiol.,* 105, 496–498.

**Katz, D., Baptista, J., Azen, S. P., and Pike, M. C.** (1978). "Obtaining Confidence Intervals for the Risk Ratios in Cohort Studies", *Biometrics,* 34, 469–474.

**Kleinbaum, D. G., Kupper, L. L., and Morgenstern, H.** (1982). *Epidemiologic Research: Principles and Quantitative Methods.* Lifetime Learning Publications, Belmont, CA.

**Mantel, N.** (1980). "Biased References in Tests for Average Partial Association", *Am. Stat.,* 34, 190–191.

**Mee, R.** (1984). "Letter to the Editor", *Biometrics,* 40, 1175–1176.

**Miettinen, O. S.** (1976). "Estimability and Estimation in Case-Referent Studies", *Am. J. Epidemiol.,* 103, 226–235.

**Miettinen, O. S.** (1977). "Author's Reply to Letter by M. Halperin", *Am. J. Epidemiol.,* 105, 498–502.

**Nurminen, M.** (1986). "Letter to the Editor", *Biometrics,* 42, 675–676.

**Peskun, P. H.** (1993). "A New Confidence Interval Method Based on the Normal Approximation for the Difference of Two Binomial Probabilities", *J. Am. Stat. Assoc.,* 88, 656–661.

**Sahai, H. and Khurshid, A.** (1993). "Confidence Intervals for the Ratio of Two Poisson Means", *Math. Sci.,* 18, 43–50.

**Santner, T. J. and Snell, M. K.** (1980). "Small Sample Confidence Intervals for $p_1 - p_2$ and $p_2/p_1$ in $2 \times 2$ Contingency Tables", *J. Am. Stat. Assoc.,* 75, 386–394.

**Santner, T. J. and Yamagani, S.** (1993). "Invariant Small Sample Confidence Intervals for the Difference of Two Success Probabilities", *Commun. Stat. Simulat. Comput.,* 22, 33–59.

**Soms, A. P.** (1989a). "Exact Confidence Intervals Based on the Z Statistic for the Difference Between Two Proportions", *Commun. Stat. Simulat. Comput.,* 18, 1325–1341.

**Soms, A. P.** (1989b). "Some Recent Results for Exact Confidence Intervals for the Difference Between Two Proportions", *Commun. Stat. Simulat. Comput.,* 18, 1343–1357.

**StatXact** (1995). A Statistical Package for Exact Nonparametric Inference, Version 3. Cytel Software Corporation, Cambridge, MA.

**Thomas, D. G. and Gart, J. J.** (1977). "A Table of Exact Confidence Limits for Differences and Ratios of Two Proportions and Their Odds Ratio", *J. Am. Stat. Assoc.,* 72, 73–76.

**Woolf, B.** (1955). "On Estimating the Relation Between Blood Group and Disease", *Ann. Human Gen.,* 19, 251–253.

# 4 Retrospective (Case-Control) Studies

In retrospective or case-control studies information is obtained for all cases that occur in the study population during a defined period of time. In addition, a comparison group of noncases ("controls") is selected as a representative sample of the study population. The history of prior exposure or exposure distribution is then obtained for both groups of subjects, comparing cases and noncases.

For example, suppose a sample of $m_1$ cases and $m_2$ noncases are studied, with the results shown in Table 4.1. Let $p_1$ and $p_2$ be the true underlying proportions of cases and noncases that were exposed to the risk.

## 4.1 MEASURES OF RISK

We consider risk ratio (RR) and odds ratio (OR) as measures of risk for retrospective studies.

### 4.1.1 RISK RATIO

The RR relating the risks of exposure for case vs. noncase groups is defined as

$$\mathrm{RR} = p_1/p_2\,. \tag{4.1}$$

This RR can be estimated as

$$\hat{\mathrm{RR}} = \left(\left(\frac{a}{m_1}\right) \div \left(\frac{c}{m_2}\right)\right). \tag{4.2}$$

In a retrospective study the RR (Equation 4.1) measures the risk of exposure to an etiologic antecedent, given the presence or absence of the disease, which does not make much biological sense (the disease does not cause the risk). Thus, this type of RR is not usually of much interest. Note that the other RR, relating risks of developing outcomes for exposed vs. unexposed groups, discussed earlier in a prospective study, cannot be estimated in a retrospective

**TABLE 4.1**
**A 2 × 2 Display of Sample Data in a Retrospective Study**

| | Exposed | Unexposed | Total |
|---|---|---|---|
| Cases | $a$ | $b$ | $m_1$ |
| Noncases | $c$ | $d$ | $m_2$ |
| Total | $n_1$ | $n_2$ | $n$ |

study because the random samples are of cases and noncases rather than those with risk factor and those without risk factor.*

### 4.1.2 Odds Ratio

The odds ratio relating the odds of exposure for the case vs. noncase groups is defined as

$$\mathrm{OR} = \frac{p_1/(1-p_1)}{p_2/(1-p_2)} = \frac{p_1(1-p_2)}{p_2(1-p_1)}. \tag{4.3}$$

It is interesting to note that the other OR, relating odds of developing an outcome for exposed vs. unexposed groups, discussed earlier in a prospective study, is algebraically equivalent to Equation 4.3. To see this, consider a 2 × 2 table (Table 4.2), which gives the distribution of the number of subjects in a reference population according to the risk of exposure and the status of disease.

The OR, relating the odds of exposure for cases vs. noncases, is

$$\mathrm{OR} = \frac{\{\mathrm{A}/(\mathrm{A}+\mathrm{B})\} \div \{\mathrm{B}/(\mathrm{A}+\mathrm{B})\}}{\{\mathrm{C}/(\mathrm{C}+\mathrm{D})\} \div \{\mathrm{D}/(\mathrm{C}+\mathrm{D})\}} = \frac{\mathrm{AD}}{\mathrm{BC}}. \tag{4.4}$$

The OR, relating the odds of developing the outcome for the exposed vs. unexposed groups, to be denoted as OR′, is

* Strictly speaking, it is not correct to say that the RR cannot be estimated because the cases are generally not selected by a random sample, but via a census of cases in the study population-time. In addition, Miettinen (1976, 1985) has provided the following interpretation of estimated RR for a retrospective study. In a cohort study involving person-time data one truly obtains incidence rates as $a/\mathrm{PT}_1$ and $b/\mathrm{PT}_2$, respectively (see Section 9.1.2). In a case-control study instead of documenting $\mathrm{PT}_1$ and $\mathrm{PT}_2$ per se, a sample of size $c + d$ was taken from $\mathrm{PT}_1$ and $\mathrm{PT}_2$, leading to a "quasi" rate as $a/c$ and $b/d$, respectively. Thus, the empirical rate ratio is $(a/c)/(b/d) = ad/bc$.

**TABLE 4.2**
**A 2 × 2 Display of a Reference Population in an Epidemiologic Study**

| | Exposed | Unexposed | Total |
|---|---|---|---|
| Cases | A | B | A + B |
| Noncases | C | D | C + D |
| Total | A + C | B + D | A + B + C + D |

$$OR' = \frac{\{A/(A+C)\} \div \{C/(A+C)\}}{\{B/(B+D)\} \div \{D/(B+D)\}} = \frac{AD}{BC}. \quad (4.5)$$

Thus, the exposure OR and the risk OR′ are algebraically equivalent.

For rare conditions (in which the risk of developing the outcome is very low), the RR, relating risks of developing the outcome for exposed vs. unexposed groups, in the study population may be estimated from the OR in a case-control study* (see Appendix N). This result, as mentioned earlier, highlights the importance of the OR in case-control studies. It implies that a simple, small-group, short-term, inexpensive retrospective study can yield almost the same RR as that produced by a complicated, large-group, long-term, expensive prospective study. However, it should be borne in mind that the OR is generally only an approximation to the RR.

#### 4.1.2.1 Point Estimation

Table 4.1 shows that a sample estimate of the OR is obtained as

$$\hat{OR} = \frac{\hat{p}_1/(1-\hat{p}_1)}{\hat{p}_2/(1-\hat{p}_2)} = \frac{(a/m_1) \div (b/m_1)}{(c/m_2) \div (d/m_2)} = \frac{ad}{bc}. \quad (4.6)$$

Note that the estimator (Equation 4.6) estimates the relative odds of exposure in diseased individuals as compared to nondiseased individuals, which is equivalent to the relative odds of disease in exposed individuals as compared to unexposed individuals. This estimate of the OR is also a consistent estimator in that, assuming unbiased sampling methods for selecting cases and controls,

* Under certain, fairly general conditions the rare disease assumption is not necessary for the OR to provide a valid estimate of the RR. For example, in population-based case-control studies in which controls are selected to represent the total population (not only the noncases), the relative risk can be estimated without the assumption of the rarity of the disease. This follows from the fact that in this instance *a/b* and *c/d* would now estimate A/B and (A + C)/(B + D), respectively, and the ratio *(a/b)* ÷ *(c/d)* would then estimate (A/B) ÷ (A + C)/(B + D) = A/(A + C) ÷ B/(B + D). Also, in case-control studies involving incident cases, although we cannot estimate specific rates or risks, we can estimate the ratio of these rates or risks by OR (Miettinen, 1976; Greenland and Thomas, 1982; Greenland et al., 1986).

its value approaches the true value of the OR in the population as the number of cases and controls in the sample becomes large. It should, however, be noted that although Equation 4.6 defines a consistent estimator, it is not an unbiased one in the strict statistical sense.

*Maximum Likelihood Estimator*

The sample estimator (Equation 4.6) also represents the maximum likelihood solution for the OR, assuming two independent binomial samplings, as shown in Table 4.1. This is the so-called *unconditional maximum likelihood estimate,* which is conditional on only the row marginals of Table 4.1 being fixed (see Appendix C). The estimator (Equation 4.6) is a maximum likelihood estimator provided simple random samples of fixed sizes $m_1$ and $m_2$ have been selected from theoretically infinite populations of cases and controls; or random samples with replacements have been selected from finite populations of cases and controls. The estimator is also a maximum likelihood estimator under the assumption of a cross-sectional design involving a total sample of fixed size $n$, where the cell entries follow a multinomial distribution.

*Conditional Maximum Likelihood Estimator*

The so-called conditional maximum likelihood estimate of the OR is obtained by assuming that all the marginal totals of Table 4.1 are fixed. The notations for such a table are shown in Table 4.4, in which the only cell entry that can vary is the number of exposed cases $(x)$. Conditional on all marginal totals being fixed, the maximum likelihood estimate of the OR is obtained by maximizing the function (Equation 4.11) with respect to the parameter OR. However, the maximum of the conditional likelihood (Equation 4.11) is not determined so easily and has no explicit solution. Birch (1964), using the results of Cox (1958), showed that the conditional maximum likelihood estimate of the OR, say $\widehat{\text{OR}}_{\text{CML}}$, is the appropriate solution to the equation (see Appendix F)

$$x - E\left(X \mid \text{OR}\right) = 0, \tag{4.7}$$

where

$$E\left(X \mid \text{OR}\right) = \frac{\sum_{\delta_1 \le x \le \delta_2} x \binom{n_1}{x}\binom{n_2}{m_1 - x}(\text{OR})^x}{\sum_{\delta_1 \le k \le \delta_2} \binom{n_1}{k}\binom{n_2}{m_1 - k}(\text{OR})^k}$$

$$\delta_1 = \max\left(0, m_1 - n_2\right) \tag{4.8}$$

$$\delta_2 = \min\left(n_1, m_1\right)$$

represents the mean of the noncentral hypergeometric distribution defined in Equation 4.11. The estimator $\hat{\text{OR}}_{\text{CML}}$ is generally *not equal* to the unconditional maximum likelihood estimator $\hat{\text{OR}}$ given by Equation 4.6 (see, e.g., Mantel and Hankey, 1975).

The conditional maximum likelihood estimate of the OR may involve a polynomial of degree min $(n_1, m_1)$ in the OR and thus requires an iterative solution of Equation 4.7 coupled with Equation 4.8, using the trial and error values for the OR until Equation 4.7 is satisfied. The exact solution to $\hat{\text{OR}}_{\text{CML}}$ is available using the computer program of Thomas (1975) and Thomas and Gart (1992).

An asymptotic solution to the conditional maximum likelihood estimate of the OR, which is much simpler than using Equation 4.8, can be obtained by noting that for large $n$

$$\hat{E}\left(X \mid \text{OR}\right) = \hat{x},$$

where $\hat{x}$ is the solution to the quadratic equation

$$\frac{\hat{x}\left(n_2 - m_1 + \hat{x}\right)}{\left(m_1 - \hat{x}\right)\left(n_1 - \hat{x}\right)} = \hat{\text{OR}}, \tag{4.9}$$

such that all the factors and divisors on the left side of Equation 4.9 are positive. Solving Equation 4.9 explicitly, one obtains

$$\hat{x} = \left\| \left[ |Q| - \sqrt{Q^2 - \frac{m_1 n_1 \hat{\text{OR}}}{\hat{\text{OR}} - 1}} \right] \right\|, \tag{4.10}$$

where

$$Q = \frac{1}{2}\left(n_1 + m_1 + \frac{n}{\hat{\text{OR}} - 1}\right).$$

Thus, the asymptotic conditional maximum likelihood estimator can be obtained as the iterative solution to Equation 4.7 coupled with Equation 4.10, using the trial and error values of the OR, until Equation 4.7 is satisfied.

#### 4.1.2.2 Confidence Intervals

The formulas for calculating approximate confidence intervals (CIs) are the same as those discussed in Section 3.1.3.2 and are not presented here. However, this section does describe an exact method, which is somewhat tedious and time consuming, and an approximate procedure due to Cornfield (1956), which can calculate the confidence limits accurately. First is an example of a

**TABLE 4.3**
**Hypothetical Data of a Case-Control Study**

| | Exposed | Unexposed | Total |
|---|---|---|---|
| Cases | 20 | 30 | 50 |
| Controls | 10 | 40 | 50 |
| Total | 30 | 70 | 100 |

From Fleiss, J. L. (1979). *J. Chronic Dis.* 32, 69–77. With permission.

retrospective case-control study illustrating the computation of point estimates and the approximate CIs described in Section 3.1.3.2.

*Example 4.1*

Consider the hypothetical data of a case-control study, as shown in Table 4.3. The sample OR estimate (the unconditional maximum likelihood) is $\hat{OR} = (20 \times 40)/(10 \times 30) = 2.667$. Using a computer program, the conditional maximum likelihood estimate is obtained as 2.640. The exact 95% CI for the OR (using a computer program) is $1.005 \le OR \le 7.317$.

Now compare the results of the approximate methods with this result. The sample estimates of the standard errors for $\hat{OR}$ and $\log_e(\hat{OR})$ are given by

$$\hat{SE}\left\{\log_e\left(\hat{OR}\right)\right\} = \left(\frac{1}{20} + \frac{1}{10} + \frac{1}{30} + \frac{1}{40}\right)^{0.5} = 0.456,$$

and

$$\hat{SE}\left(\hat{OR}\right) = 2.667 \times 0.456 = 1.217.$$

**Taylor series method** — Using the direct approach without logarithmic transformation, a 95% CI for the OR is obtained as

$$2.667 \pm 1.96 \times 1.217 = (0.282, 5.052).$$

It can be verified that by adding 0.5 to each cell entry, an improved CI estimate for the OR is (0.312, 4.874). When comparing this result to the exact CI, note that the approximation is rather poor. Among other shortcomings, it includes the value of 1, contradicting the evidence from the exact CI. Using the logarithmic transformation, a 95% CI for $\log_e$(OR) is obtained as

$$\log_e(2.667) \pm 1.96 \times 0.456 = (0.087, 1.875),$$

which yields a 95% CI for the OR as (1.090, 6.521). It can be verified further that by adding 0.5 to each cell entry, an improved CI estimate for the OR is (1.076, 6.246). Comparing this result to the exact CI, note that the use of the logarithmic transformation yields much better accuracy than using the direct approach.

**Test-based method** — To obtain a CI for the OR using this method, note that

$$\chi^2_{\text{MH}} = \frac{(100-1)(20\times 40 - 10\times 30)^2}{30\times 70\times 50\times 50} = 4.714.$$

Thus, a 95% CI for the OR, using the direct approach, is

$$= 2.667 \pm 1.96\sqrt{(2.667-1)^2/4.714} = (1.162, 4.172).$$

Comparing this result to the exact CI, again note that the test-based limits using the direct approach are too narrow. Using the logarithmic transformation, a 95% CI for $\log_e$ (OR) is

$$\log_e(2.667) \pm 1.96\sqrt{\{\log_e(2.667)\}^2/4.714} = (0.095, 1.866),$$

which yields a 95% CI for the OR of (1.100, 6.462). Comparing this result to that of the exact CI, note that this interval is much closer to the exact interval. The lower limit of the interval agrees more closely with the exact interval, but its upper limit is still too low.

The following describe two additional methods of computing CIs for the OR, which, although computationally cumbersome, provide accurate limits, especially for moderate to small sample sizes.

*An Exact Method*

Given a 2 × 2 table, the marginal totals for all three sampling designs usually provide no information concerning the magnitude of association between the risk and outcome variables.* Thus, one would not incur any serious bias by assuming all the marginal totals are fixed. For a detailed discussion of the theoretical principles supporting the use of the conditional distribution of data assuming all the marginals as fixed, see Cox and Hinkley (1974) and Cox and Snell (1989).

An exact inference for the OR can be made in the 2 × 2 table with fixed marginals because the specification of any single cell frequency automatically determines the value in other cells. Thus, it suffices to consider a single cell

* It has been shown that the marginal totals do contain information on the association between row and column factors of the table. However, the amount of information conveyed is sufficiently small, therefore, conditioning on marginals is still considered appropriate.

**TABLE 4.4**
**A 2 × 2 Display of Sample Data in an Epidemiologic Study with All Marginals Fixed**

| | Exposed | Unexposed | Total |
|---|---|---|---|
| Cases | $x$ | $m_1 - x$ | $m_1$ |
| Noncases | $n_1 - x$ | $n_2 - m_1 + x$ | $m_2$ |
| Total | $n_1$ | $n_2$ | $n$ |

*Note:* $\max(0, m_1 - n_2) \le x \le \min(n_1, m_1)$.

frequency as variable, which is usually taken as the number of exposed cases, for example, $x$, as shown in Table 4.4.

Let $X$ be the random variable representing the number of exposed cases. For any arbitrary value of the OR, the distribution of the random variable $X$, assuming fixed marginals, is a *noncentral hypergeometric distribution* (see, e.g., Fisher, 1935; Cornfield, 1956; Lehmann, 1986):

$$P\left(X = x \mid \mathrm{OR}\right) = \frac{\binom{n_1}{x}\binom{n_2}{m_1 - x}(\mathrm{OR})^x}{\sum_{\delta_1 \le k \le \delta_2} \binom{n_1}{k}\binom{n_2}{m_1 - k}(\mathrm{OR})^k}, \tag{4.11}$$

where $\delta_1 = \max(0, m_1 - n_2) \le x \le \min(n_1, m_1) = \delta_2$. For the special case of OR = 1, the above distribution reduces to

$$P(X = x) = \frac{\binom{n_1}{x}\binom{n_2}{m_1 - x}}{\binom{n}{m_1}}, \tag{4.12}$$

which is known as the (central) hypergeometric distribution (see Appendix H).

As seen above, the probability model that defines the distribution of exposed cases $(x)$ in a 2 × 2 table with fixed marginals is hypergeometric, but its non-null form (OR ≠ 1) involves the noncentral hypergeometric distribution. The probability function of the noncentral hypergeometric distribution is mathematically much more complicated than its null version because it involves the OR as the measure of strength of association between the risk factor and the disease state. Noncentral hypergeometric distribution is the name given by Wallenius (1963) in his Ph.D. thesis, which may be referred to for additional details.

An exact CI for the OR is readily obtained by using an argument tied to hypothesis testing. To provide a general idea of how this procedure works, we first discuss the method of obtaining an exact CI for the binomial parameter $p$. For a binomial random variable $X$, we have

$$\boldsymbol{P}(X = x) = \binom{n}{x} p^x (1-p)^{n-x}; \quad x = 0, 1, 2, \ldots, n$$

To construct an exact CI for $p$, find an interval consisting of all the values of $p$ such that the data obtained in the sample would result in acceptance of the null hypothesis

$$H_0: p = p^*,$$

if one were using a two-tailed binomial test. More precisely, if we want to form a 100(1 – α)% CI for $p$, we observe the value of the random variable $X$ and then ask, For the given value of $X$, which values may we use for $p^*$ in the null hypothesis, such that a two-tailed binomial test would result in the acceptance of $H_0$? Those values of $p$ would be in our CI.

Because each tail of the binomial test has probability α/2, the value of the lower confidence limit ($p_L$) is selected as the value of $p$, that would barely result in the rejection of $H_0$ for a given value of $X$, for example $x$, or a larger value. Thus, $p_L$ is selected such that

$$\boldsymbol{P}(X \ge x \mid p = p_L) = \sum_{k=x}^{n} \binom{n}{k} (p_L)^k (1-p_L)^{n-k} = \alpha/2.$$

Next, the value of the upper confidence limit ($p_U$) is selected as the value of $p$ that would barely result in the rejection of $H_0$ for $x$ or a value smaller than $x$. Thus, $p_U$ is selected such that

$$\boldsymbol{P}(X \le x \mid p = p_U) = \sum_{k=0}^{x} \binom{n}{k} (p_U)^k (1-p_U)^{n-k} = \alpha/2.$$

Thus, an "exact"* 100(1 – α)% CI for $p$ is given by ($p_L$, $p_U$) where

* The use of the term "exact" is somewhat of a misnomer. Because of the discrete nature of the binomial distribution, the confidence limits determined by Equation 4.13 are usually conservative. Similarly, because the hypergeometric distribution is discrete, the limits determined by Equations 4.14 and 4.15 usually do not attain a prespecified confidence coefficient of exactly 1 – α, but rather 1 – α′, where α′ < α. The results are exact in the sense that the confidence coefficient is at least 1 – α. For a discussion of mid-$p$ CIs, which usually reduce the conservativeness, see Appendix I. Miettinen (1974) pointed out that the limits determined by Equations 4.14 and 4.15 are too wide; in particular with α = 1, the interval has nonzero width and recommended the use of the mid-$p$ method.

$$P(p_L \le p \le p_U) \ge 1 - \alpha. \quad (4.13)$$

Using arguments similar to those above, an exact $100(1 - \alpha)\%$ CI for the OR is given by ($OR_L$, $OR_U$), where $OR_L$ and $OR_U$ are determined by the equations (see, e.g., Cornfield, 1956; Fisher, 1962; Stenhouse, 1963; Mantel and Hankey, 1971; Thomas, 1971):

$$P(X \ge x \mid OR = OR_L) = \frac{\sum_{k=x}^{\delta_2} \binom{n_1}{k}\binom{n_2}{m_1 - k}(OR_L)^k}{\sum_{\delta_1 \le u \le \delta_2} \binom{n_1}{u}\binom{n_2}{m_1 - u}(OR_L)^u} = \alpha/2 \quad (4.14)$$

and

$$P(X \le x \mid OR = OR_U) = \frac{\sum_{k=\delta_1}^{x} \binom{n_1}{k}\binom{n_2}{m_1 - k}(OR_U)^k}{\sum_{\delta_1 \le u \le \delta_2} \binom{n_1}{u}\binom{n_2}{m_1 - u}(OR_U)^u} = \alpha/2. \quad (4.15)$$

Note that when $x = \max(0, m_1 - n_2)$ so that $\hat{OR} = 0$, only an upper limit need be determined; conversely, when $x = \min(n_1, m_1)$ so that $\hat{OR} = \infty$, only a lower limit need be determined. In these two situations, it is said that the data tables are degenerate and the method breaksdown. The determination of $OR_L$ and $OR_U$ from the above expressions is generally extremely tedious and time consuming, because each iteration in the process entails calculating a complicated sum of hypergeometric probabilities. Fortunately, numerical algorithms and computer programs are generally available that can be used for this purpose (Mantel and Hankey, 1971; Thomas, 1971, 1975; Baptista and Pike, 1977; Pagano and Tritchler, 1983). More efficient algorithms for obtaining this type of exact confidence limits are described in Mehta et al. (1985) and Vollset et al. (1991). The latter algorithms utilize a quadratic time network approach and its modifications and are shown to be a considerable improvement over the algorithm developed by Thomas (1971, 1975), which relies on exhaustive enumeration, and by Pagano and Tritchler (1983), which uses the fast Fourier transform. These algorithms are quite general and are applicable for the computation of exact CIs for the common OR in a series of $2 \times 2$ tables. Vollset et al. (1991) assessed these algorithms and provided an improved version of the network algorithm. Computer software on both mainframe and microcomputing systems implementing these algorithms are also available (see Vollset and Hirji, 1991; Thomas and Gart, 1992; EpiInfo, 1994; StatXact, 1995). Coe and

Tamhane (1993) proposed a new method and computational algorithm for constructing small sample CIs for the OR. A FORTRAN program for implementing their algorithm is given by Coe (1989).

*Cornfield's Method*

An approximate procedure, given by Cornfield (1956), is generally available which can calculate confidence limits fairly accurately. Fisher (1962) gives the simplest formulation of Cornfield's method.

Approximate Cornfield's limits may be determined using the asymptotic results for the noncentral hypergeometric distribution (Equation 4.11). The asymptotic theory, based on the results of Stevens (1951), was rigorously developed and described by Cornfield (1956) and Hannan and Harkness (1963). It can be shown that as $n$ becomes large, Equation 4.11 is asymptotically normally distributed with asymptotic mean and variance

$$\hat{E}(X \mid \text{OR}) = \hat{x} \tag{4.16}$$

$$\hat{\text{Var}}(X \mid \text{OR}) = \left[\frac{1}{\hat{x}} + \frac{1}{m_1 - \hat{x}} + \frac{1}{n_1 - \hat{x}} + \frac{1}{n_2 - m_1 + \hat{x}}\right]^{-1}, \tag{4.17}$$

where $\hat{x}$ is the appropriate solution to the quadratic equation

$$\frac{\hat{x}(n_2 - m_1 + \hat{x})}{(m_1 - \hat{x})(n_1 - \hat{x})} = \text{OR}, \tag{4.18}$$

determined such that it yields positive numbers for all the factors and divisors on the left side of Equation 4.18 (i.e., all the estimated entries in Table 4.1). If OR = 1, the quadratic equation reduces to a linear equation and the result on the expectation is exact. Otherwise it holds only asymptotically.

The approximate lower and upper confidence limits of the OR, for example, $\text{OR}_\text{L}$ and $\text{OR}_\text{U}$, are determined by solving the equations

$$\frac{x - \hat{E}(X \mid \text{OR}_\text{L}) - 0.5}{\sqrt{\hat{\text{Var}}(X \mid \text{OR}_\text{L})}} = Z_{\alpha/2} \tag{4.19}$$

and

$$\frac{x - \hat{E}(X \mid \text{OR}_\text{U}) + 0.5}{\sqrt{\hat{\text{Var}}(X \mid \text{OR}_\text{U})}} = -Z_{\alpha/2}, \tag{4.20}$$

where $Z_{\alpha/2}$ is the upper 100($\alpha$/2)th percentile of the standard normal distribution.

Substituting the values of $\hat{E}(X|\text{OR})$ and $\hat{\text{Var}}(X|\text{OR})$ for OR = $\text{OR}_\text{L}$ and OR = $\text{OR}_\text{U}$ from Equations 4.16 and 4.17 into Equations 4.19 and 4.20, one obtains

$$\frac{x - \hat{x}_\text{L} - 0.5}{\sqrt{\left[\frac{1}{\hat{x}_\text{L}} + \frac{1}{m_1 - \hat{x}_\text{L}} + \frac{1}{n_1 - \hat{x}_\text{L}} + \frac{1}{n_2 - m_1 + \hat{x}_\text{L}}\right]^{-1}}} = Z_{\alpha 2}$$

and

$$\frac{x - \hat{x}_\text{U} + 0.5}{\sqrt{\left[\frac{1}{\hat{x}_\text{U}} + \frac{1}{m_1 - \hat{x}_\text{U}} + \frac{1}{n_1 - \hat{x}_\text{U}} + \frac{1}{n_2 - m_1 + \hat{x}_\text{U}}\right]^{-1}}} = -Z_{\alpha 2},$$

where $\hat{x}_\text{L}$ and $\hat{x}_\text{U}$ represent the values of the solution to Equation 4.18 which correspond to the lower and upper confidence limits of the OR rather than to the point estimate.

To determine $\text{OR}_\text{L}$, first obtain $\hat{x}_\text{L}$ as the smallest real root of the quartic equation in $x_\text{L}$ given by

$$\left(x - x_\text{L} - 0.5\right)^2 \left[\frac{1}{x_\text{L}} + \frac{1}{m_1 - x_\text{L}} + \frac{1}{n_1 - x_\text{L}} + \frac{1}{n_2 - m_1 + x_\text{L}}\right] = Z_{\alpha/2}^2 \quad (4.21)$$

subject to the condition

$$\max\left(0, m_1 - n_2\right) \le \hat{x}_\text{L} \le \min\left(n_1, m_1\right).$$

Then $\text{OR}_\text{L}$ is calculated from the equation

$$\text{OR}_\text{L} = \frac{\hat{x}_\text{L}\left(n_2 - m_1 + \hat{x}_\text{L}\right)}{\left(m_1 - \hat{x}_\text{L}\right)\left(n_1 - \hat{x}_\text{L}\right)}. \quad (4.22)$$

Similarly,

$$\text{OR}_\text{U} = \frac{\hat{x}_\text{U}\left(n_2 - m_1 + \hat{x}_\text{U}\right)}{\left(m_1 - \hat{x}_\text{U}\right)\left(n_1 - \hat{x}_\text{U}\right)}, \quad (4.23)$$

where $\hat{x}_\text{U}$ is obtained as the largest real root of the quartic equation in $x_\text{U}$ given by

$$\left(x - x_U + 0.5\right)^2 \left[ \frac{1}{x_U} + \frac{1}{m_1 - x_U} + \frac{1}{n_1 - x_U} + \frac{1}{n_2 - m_1 + x_U} \right] = Z^2_{\alpha/2} \tag{4.24}$$

subject to the condition

$$\max\left(0, m_1 - n_2\right) \le \hat{x}_U \le \min\left(n_1, m_1\right).$$

Note that, in principle, Cornfield's method has the advantage of approximating the mean and variance using the cell frequencies that correspond to the confidence limit value of the OR rather than that of point estimate.

Mantel and Fleiss (1980) proposed a simple rule to determine whether Cornfield's method provides a reasonable approximation of the exact interval, which is quite complex and tedious to calculate. For a 95% CI, one simply determines whether the intervals

$$\hat{x}_L \pm 1.96 \left[ \frac{1}{\hat{x}_L} + \frac{1}{m_1 - \hat{x}_L} + \frac{1}{n_1 - \hat{x}_L} + \frac{1}{n_2 - m_1 + \hat{x}_L} \right]^{-0.5} \tag{4.25}$$

and

$$\hat{x}_U \pm 1.96 \left[ \frac{1}{\hat{x}_U} + \frac{1}{m_1 - \hat{x}_U} + \frac{1}{n_1 - \hat{x}_U} + \frac{1}{n_2 - m_1 + \hat{x}_U} \right]^{-0.5} \tag{4.26}$$

are both contained within the range of possible values for $x$ under the assumption that all the marginals are fixed, i.e.,

$$\max\left(0, m_1 - n_2\right) \le x \le \min\left(n_1, m_1\right).$$

Solving quadratic Equations 4.21 and 4.24 for $\hat{x}_L$ and $\hat{x}_U$ is rather tedious and usually requires the use of a computer program. Following Cornfield (1956), Gart (1971) recommended a relatively easy iterative procedure that can be readily implemented using a hand calculator. The method uses the iterative relation

$$\hat{x}_i = x \pm \frac{1}{2} \pm Z_{\alpha/2} \left[ \frac{1}{\hat{x}_{i-1}} + \frac{1}{m_1 - \hat{x}_{i-1}} + \frac{1}{n_1 - \hat{x}_{i-1}} + \frac{1}{n_2 - m_1 + \hat{x}_{i-1}} \right]^{-0.5},$$

where $\hat{x}_0 = x$, the plus signs correspond to the upper limit, and the minus signs correspond to the lower limit. Thus, the values of $\hat{x}_i$ converge to $\hat{x}_U$ by using the plus signs and to $\hat{x}_L$ by using the minus signs. When the numbers are rather small, the iterative procedure may break down because it is possible that $\hat{x}_i$

may be negative or greater than $\min(n_1,m_1)$. A different starting value of $\hat{x}_0$ is then recommended.

Gart (1971) also suggested an accelerated iterative procedure that employs the relation

$$\hat{x}_i' = x \pm \frac{1}{2} \pm Z_{\alpha/2}\left[\frac{1}{\hat{x}_{i-1}^*} + \frac{1}{m_1 - \hat{x}_{i-1}^*} + \frac{1}{n_1 - \hat{x}_{i-1}^*} + \frac{1}{n_2 - m_1 + \hat{x}_{i-1}^*}\right]^{-0.5},$$

where $\hat{x}_i^* = [i\ \hat{x}_i' + (i-1)\ \hat{x}_{i-1}^*]/(2i-1)$ and $\hat{x}_0^* = x$. This procedure may sometimes converge about twice as rapidly as the previous one. If $x = 0$ or any one of the other cell entries is zero, then only one limit may be determined. In that case let $\hat{x}_0$ or $\hat{x}_0^* = 1/2$.

Gart and Thomas (1982) investigated the accuracy of Cornfield's limits using the iterative procedure when sampling from two independent binomials (the unconditional space). They found that the procedure yielded reasonably accurate solutions when the smallest cell entry, consistent with the limit, exceeds 2 [i.e., $\min(x, m_1 - x, n_1 - x, n_2 - m_1 + x) \geq 2$]. Gart (1971) pointed out that when the iterative procedure fails, the solution usually will not be accurate. In addition, Gart and Thomas (1982) compared the accuracy of Cornfield's limits to those determined by the Taylor series and test-based methods when sampling from two independent binomials. They found that Cornfield's limits, without continuity correction, were generally more accurate than the limits obtained by other two methods. Similarly, using a simulation study for the case when all the marginals are assumed fixed (the conditional space), Brown (1981) reported that Cornfield's limits with continuity correction were more accurate than those determined by either logit or test-based methods for various sample sizes and OR values included in the study. Among computer software to determine Cornfield's limits are Thomas (1975), Thomas and Gart (1992), and EpiInfo (1994). A calculator program for determining Cornfield's limits is given by Guess (1982).

*Example 4.2*

Consider a subset of the data from a case-control study on smoking and lung cancer described by Wynder and Cornfield (1953) and discussed further by Cornfield (1956) and Kleinbaum et al. (1982). The data are shown in Table 4.5

For the data of Table 4.5, the sample OR estimate (unconditional maximum likelihood) is $\hat{\text{OR}} = (60 \times 11)/(32 \times 3) = 6.875$. The conditional maximum likelihood estimate, using a computer program, is obtained as 6.747.

The following illustrates the computation of CIs using an "exact" method and the Cornfield's method.

**Exact method** — An exact CI of the OR, for example, $(\text{OR}_\text{L}, \text{OR}_\text{U})$, with 95% confidence coefficient, is determined by solving the following equations for $\text{OR}_\text{L}$ and $\text{OR}_\text{U}$:

**TABLE 4.5**
**Data on Smoking and Lung Cancer from a Case-Control Study**

| | Smoker | Nonsmoker | Total |
|---|---|---|---|
| Lung cancer | 60 | 3 | 63 |
| Without lung cancer | 32 | 11 | 43 |
| Total | 92 | 14 | 106 |

From Wynder, E.L. and Cornfield, J. (1953). *N. Engl. J. Med.*, 248, 411–444. With permission.

$$\frac{\sum_{k=60}^{\delta_2}\binom{92}{k}\binom{14}{63-k}(\text{OR}_\text{L})^k}{\sum_{\delta_1\le u\le\delta_2}\binom{92}{u}\binom{14}{63-u}(\text{OR}_\text{L})^u}=0.025$$

and

$$\frac{\sum_{k=\delta_1}^{60}\binom{92}{k}\binom{14}{63-k}(\text{OR}_\text{U})^k}{\sum_{\delta_1\le u\le\delta_2}\binom{92}{u}\binom{14}{63-u}(\text{OR}_\text{U})^u}=0.025,$$

where $\delta_1$ = max (0, 63–14) = 49, $\delta_2$ = min (92, 63) = 63. These equations are rather cumbersome to solve. Using a computer program, the confidence limits are $\text{OR}_\text{L}$ = 1.626 and $\text{OR}_\text{U}$ = 40.358.

**Cornfield's method** — To compute the 95% CI using Cornfield's approximation, first obtain $\hat{x}_\text{L}$ as the smallest real root of the quartic equation in $x_\text{L}$ of the form

$$(60-x_\text{L}-0.5)^2\left(\frac{1}{x_\text{L}}+\frac{1}{63-x_\text{L}}+\frac{1}{92-x_\text{L}}+\frac{1}{14-63+x_\text{L}}\right)=(1.96)^2,$$

subject to the condition that $49 \le \hat{x}_\text{L} \le 63$. With the assistance of an electronic calculator, it can be shown that the smallest real root within the above range is $\hat{x}_\text{L}$ = 56.0956. Similarly, obtain $\hat{x}_\text{U}$ as the largest real root of the quartic equation in $x_\text{U}$ of the form

$$(60 - x_U + 0.5)^2 \left( \frac{1}{x_U} + \frac{1}{63 - x_U} + \frac{1}{92 - x_U} + \frac{1}{14 - 63 + x_U} \right) = (1.96)^2,$$

subject to the condition that $49 \leq \hat{x}_U \leq 63$. Again, with the assistance of an electronic calculator, it can be shown that the largest real root within the above range is $\hat{x}_U = 62.1859$.

Using Equations 4.22 and 4.23, one obtains

$$\mathrm{OR}_L = \frac{(56.0956)(14 - 63 + 56.0956)}{(63 - 56.0956)(92 - 56.0956)} = 1.606$$

and

$$\mathrm{OR}_U = \frac{(62.1859)(14 - 63 + 62.1859)}{(63 - 62.1859)(92 - 62.1859)} = 33.783.$$

For comparison purposes, one can show that the 95% CI for the OR by the Taylor series method, via the logarithm transformation, is (1.788, 26.442) and that by using the test-based method it is (2.027, 23.318). As seen earlier, the exact 95% CI using a computer program is (1.626, 40.358). Thus, Cornfield's limits are much more accurate than the other two approximate limits. To check the validity of Cornfield's approximation, the intervals determined by Mantel-Fleiss conditions (Equations 4.25 and 4.26) are (52.360, 59.832) and (59.148, 65.224), respectively. Because max $(0, m_1 - n_2) = 49$ and min $(n_1, m_1) = 63$, the interval (59.15, 65.22) does not satisfy the requisite conditions, but it is probably close enough to consider Cornfield's limits adequate.

### *Other Methods*

Several other approaches to asymptotic intervals for the OR have appeared in the literature. Refer to the first principles intervals, notably those based on the score statistic (Miettinen, 1985; Miettinen and Nurminen, 1985). For a discussion of an exact confidence interval which incorporates the mid-$p$ adjustment, see Appendix I.

# References

**Baptista, J. and Pike, M. C.** (1977). "Exact Two-Sided Confidence Limits for the Odds Ratio in a 2 × 2 Table", *Appl. Stat.,* 26, 216–220.

**Birch, M. W.** (1964). "The Detection of Partial Association, I: The 2 × 2 Case", *J. R. Stat. Soc.,* B, 26, 313–324.

**Brown, C. C.** (1981). "The Validity of Approximation Methods for Interval Estimation of the Odds Ratio", *Am. J. Epidemiol.,* 113, 474–480.

**Coe, P. R.** (1989). "Exact Repeated Confidence Intervals for Bernoulli Parameters in Group Sequential Experiments", Ph.D. Thesis, Northwestern University, Evanston, IL.

**Coe, P. R. and Tamhane, A. C.** (1993). "Small Sample Confidence Intervals for the Difference, Ratio and Odds Ratio of 2 Success Probabilities", *Commun. Stat. Simulat. Comput.,* 22, 925–938.

**Cornfield, J.** (1956). "A Statistical Problem Arising from Retrospective Studies", In: *Proc. 3rd Berkeley Symp. Mathematical Statistics and Probability* (Ed. J. Neyman). pp. 135–148. University of California Press, Berkeley.

**Cox, D. R.** (1958). "Two Further Applications of a Model for Binary Regression", *Biometrika,* 45, 562–565.

**Cox, D. R. and Hinkley, D. V.** (1974). *Theoretical Statistics.* Chapman & Hall, London.

**Cox, D. R. and Snell, E. J.** (1989). *The Analysis of Binary Data,* 2nd ed. Chapman & Hall, New York.

**EpiInfo** (1994). EpiInfo, Version 6. USD, Inc., Stone Mountain, GA.

**Fisher, R. A.** (1935). "The Logic of Inductive Inference", *J. R. Stat. Soc.,* A, 98, 39–54.

**Fisher, R. A.** (1962). "Confidence Limits for a Cross-Product Ratio", *Aust. J. Stat.,* 4, 41–45.

**Fleiss, J. L.** (1979). "Confidence Intervals for the Odds Ratio in Case-Control Studies: The State of the Art", *J. Chronic Dis.,* 32, 69–77.

**Gart, J. J.** (1971). "The Comparison of Proportions: A Review of Significance Tests, Confidence Intervals, and Adjustments for Stratification", *Rev. Int. Stat. Inst.,* 39, 148–169 (errata, *ibid.,* 1972, 40, 221).

**Gart, J. J. and Thomas, D. G.** (1982). "The Performance of Three Approximate Confidence Limit Methods for the Odds Ratio", *Am. J. Epidemiol.,* 115, 453–470.

**Greenland, S. and Thomas, D. C.** (1982). "On the Need for the Rare Disease Assumption in the Case-Control Studies", *Am. J. Epidemiol.,* 116, 547–553.

**Greenland, S., Thomas, D. C., and Morgenstern, H.** (1986). "The Rare Disease Assumption Revisited", *Am. J. Epidemiol.,* 124, 869–876.

**Guess, H. A.** (1982). "Confidence Intervals for the Odds Ratio in Case-Control Studies: A Calculator Program for Cornfield's Method", *Comput. Prog. Biomed.,* 4, 73–76.

**Hannan, J. and Harkness, W. L.** (1963). "Normal Approximation to the Distribution of Two Independent Binomials, Conditional on a Fixed Sum", *Ann. Math. Stat.,* 34, 1593–1995.

**Kleinbaum, D. G., Kupper, L. L., and Morgenstern, H.** (1982). *Epidemiologic Research: Principles and Quantitative Methods.* Lifetime Learning Publications, Belmont, CA.

**Lehmann, E. L.** (1959, 1986). *Testing Statistical Hypotheses,* 1st, 2nd eds. John Wiley & Sons, New York.

**Mantel, N. and Fleiss, J.** (1980). "Minimum Expected Cell Size Requirements for the Mantel-Haenszel One Degree of Freedom Chi-Square Test and a Related Rapid Procedure", *Am. J. Epidemiol.,* 112, 129–139.

**Mantel, N. and Hankey, B. F.** (1971). "Programmed Analysis of a 2 × 2 Contingency Table", *Am. Stat.,* 25, 40–44.

**Mantel, N. and Hankey, B. F.** (1975). "The Odds Ratio of a 2 × 2 Contingency Table", *Am. Stat.,* 29, 143–145.

**Mehta, C. R., Patel, N. R., and Gray, R.** (1985). "Computing an Exact Confidence Interval for the Common Odds Ratio in Several 2 × 2 Contingency Tables", *J. Am. Stat. Assoc.,* 80, 969–973.

**Miettinen, O. S.** (1974). "Comment on 'Some Reasons for Not Using the Yates' Continuity Correction on 2 × 2 Contingency Tables' by W. J. Conover", *J. Am. Stat. Assoc.,* 69, 380–382.

**Miettinen, O. S.** (1976). "Estimability and Estimation in Case-Referent Studies", *Am. J. Epidemiol.,* 103, 226–235.

**Miettinen, O. S.** (1985). *Theoretical Epidemiology: Principles of Occurrence Research in Medicine.* John Wiley & Sons, New York.

**Miettinen, O. S. and Nurminen, M.** (1985). "Comparative Analysis of Two Rates", *Stat. Med.,* 4, 213–226.

**Pagano, M. and Tritchler, D.** (1983). "Algorithm for the Analysis of Several 2 × 2 Contingency Tables", *SIAM J. Sci. Stat. Comput.,* 4, 302–309.

**StatXact**, (1995). *A Statistical Package for Exact Nonparametric Inference,* Version 3. Cytel Software Corporation, Cambridge, MA.

**Stenhouse, N. S.** (1963). "Correction to 'Confidence Limits for a Cross-Product Ratio'", *Aust. J. Statistics,* 5, 125–126.

**Stevens, W. L.** (1951). "Mean and Variance of an Entry in a Contingency Table", *Biometrika,* 38, 468–470.

**Thomas, D. G.** (1971). "Exact Limits for the Odds Ratio in a 2 × 2 Table", *Appl. Stat.,* 20, 105–110.

**Thomas, D. G.** (1975). "Exact and Asymptotic Methods for the Combination of 2 × 2 Tables", *Comput. Biomed. Res.,* 8, 423–446.

**Thomas, D. G. and Gart, J. J.** (1992). "Improved and Extended Exact and Asymptotic Methods for the Combination of 2 × 2 Tables, Version 2", *Comput. Biomed. Res.,* 25, 75–84.

**Vollset, S. E. and Hirji, K. F.** (1991). "A Micro-Computer Program for Exact and Asymptotic Analysis of Several 2 × 2 Tables", *Epidemiology,* 2, 217–220.

**Vollset, S. E., Hirji, K. F., and Elashoff, R. M.** (1991). "Fast Computation of Exact Confidence Limits for the Common Odds Ratio in a Series of 2 × 2 Tables", *J. Am. Stat. Assoc.,* 86, 404–409.

**Wallenius, K. J.** (1963). "Biased Sampling: the Noncentral Hypergeometric Probability Distribution", Ph.D. Thesis, Stanford University, Stanford, CA.

**Wynder, E. L. and Cornfield, J.** (1953). "Cancer of the Lung in Physicians", *N. Engl. J. Med.,* 248, 441–444.

# 5 Cross-Sectional Studies

The statistical inference for the risk difference (RD), risk ratio (RR), and odds ratio (OR) for a cross-sectional study follows that for the prospective study. It can be shown that the parameters and their sample properties obtained from prospective studies are identical with those from cross-sectional studies. Thus, no differences exist between these two studies with regard to the formulas for tests of hypothesis and confidence intervals (CIs) for the RD, RR, and the OR. The principal difference arises in the interpretation of the results in view of the higher bias potential of a cross-sectional study relative to the prospective study. In addition, the feature common to all cross-sectional studies is that the disease state is the number of cases of disease in the population at a point in time. Thus, cross-sectional studies involve measures of disease prevalence rather than incidence, and the measures of risk discussed in Chapters 3 and 4 are measures of prevalence.

For example, suppose that a sample of $n$ subjects is classified according to the exposure status and the disease state. The results are shown in Table 5.1. Let $p_1$ and $p_2$ be the proportions denoting prevalence of disease in the population for exposed and unexposed groups, respectively. The sample estimates of $p_1$ and $p_2$ are obtained as

$$\hat{p}_1 = \frac{a}{n_1} \quad \text{and} \quad \hat{p}_2 = \frac{b}{n_2}.$$

## 5.1 MEASURES OF PREVALENCE

Consider prevalence difference (PD), prevalence ratio (PR), and prevalence odds ratio (POR) as the measures of prevalence for cross-sectional studies.

### 5.1.1 Prevalence Difference

The PD for exposed vs. unexposed groups is defined as

$$\text{PD} = p_1 - p_2.$$

**TABLE 5.1**
**A 2 × 2 Display of Sample Data in a Cross-Sectional Study**

| | Exposed | Unexposed | Total |
|---|---|---|---|
| Cases | $a$ | $b$ | $m_1$ |
| Noncases | $c$ | $d$ | $m_2$ |
| Total | $n_1$ | $n_2$ | $n$ |

### 5.1.2 Prevalence Ratio

The PR is the quotient of two prevalences defined as

$$\text{PR} = \frac{p_1}{p_2}.$$

### 5.1.3 Prevalence Odds Ratio

The POR is the ratio of the prevalence odds for exposed vs. unexposed groups, defined as

$$\text{POR} = \frac{p_1/(1-p_1)}{p_2/(1-p_2)}.$$

If we denote the prevalence of a particular disease in the population by $p$, then it can be shown that when the incidence rate *(I)* is constant over time, the prevalence odds is equal to incidence rate times average disease duration *(d)* (Rothman, 1986); in other words,

$$\frac{p}{(1-p)} = Id.$$

In cross-sectional studies the logarithm of the OR serves an important and useful role as a measure of the degree of association between the two variables under examination. For a discussion of the use of the log OR in the context of cross-sectional studies, see Fleiss (1981).

## 5.2 POINT AND INTERVAL ESTIMATION

The methods of point and interval estimation for the measures of risk discussed in Chapters 3 and 4 are equally applicable in a cross-sectional study. The

**TABLE 5.2**
**Data on Chronic Bronchitis Among Welders and Unexposed Workers from a Cross-Sectional Study**

| | Exposed | Unexposed | Total |
|---|---|---|---|
| Disease | 15 | 5 | 20 |
| No disease | 237 | 175 | 412 |
| Total | 252 | 180 | 432 |

From Sjogren, B. and Ulfvarson, V. (1985). *Scand. J. Work Environ. Health,* 11, 27–32. With permission.

discussion of all the formulas parallels the discussion presented in these chapters and is not presented here.

*Example 5.1*

Consider the following data from a cross-sectional study reported by Sjogren and Ulfvarson (1985) of the prevalence of respiratory disease symptoms among welders exposed to aluminum, stainless steel, or chromium. The study included a total of 252 welders and 180 unexposed workers, having similar distributions of age and smoking habits, with the prevalence of reported chronic bronchitis by exposure category shown in Table 5.2.

The data in Table 5.2 provide prevalence rates for exposed and unexposed groups:

$$\hat{p}_1 = \frac{15}{252} = 0.060$$

and

$$\hat{p}_2 = \frac{5}{180} = 0.028.$$

An estimate of the PD is

$$\hat{\text{PD}} = \hat{p}_1 - \hat{p}_2 = 0.032,$$

and a 95% CI for the PD using the Taylor series method is obtained as

$$0.032 \pm 1.96\sqrt{\frac{0.060(1-0.060)}{252} + \frac{0.028(1-0.028)}{180}} = (-0.006, 0.070).$$

To obtain a CI for the PD using the test-based method, note that

$$\chi^2_{\text{MH}} = \frac{(432-1)(15\times175-5\times237)^2}{252\times180\times20\times412} = 2.391.$$

Therefore, a 95% CI for the PD using this method is given by

$$0.032 \pm 1.96\sqrt{\frac{(0.032)^2}{2.391}} = (-0.009, 0.073).$$

An estimate of the PR is obtained as

$$\hat{\text{PR}} = \hat{p}_1/\hat{p}_2 = 2.143.$$

A 95% CI for $\log_e$(PR) using the Taylor series method is obtained as

$$\log_e(2.143) \pm 1.96\sqrt{\frac{(1-0.060)}{252(0.060)} + \frac{(1-0.028)}{180(0.028)}} = (-0.228, 1.752),$$

from which a 95% CI for the PR is given by (0.796, 5.766). As before, to obtain a CI for the PR using the test-based method, we have $\chi^2_{\text{MH}}$ = 2.391. Thus, a 95% CI for $\log_e$(PR) using this method is obtained as

$$\log_e(2.143) \pm 1.96\sqrt{\frac{\{\log_e(2.143)\}^2}{2.391}} = (-0.204, 1.728),$$

from which a 95% CI for the PR is given by (0.815, 5.629).

Finally, point estimates and the associated confidence intervals for the prevalence odds ratio, using the formulas described in Chapters 3 and 4, can be determined similarly.

# References

**Fleiss, J. L.** (1981). *Statistical Methods for Rates and Proportions,* 2nd ed. John Wiley & Sons, New York.

**Rothman, K. J.** (1986). *Modern Epidemiology.* Little, Brown, Boston.

**Sjogren, B. and Ulfvarson, V.** (1985). "Respiratory Systems and Pulmonary Function Among Welders Working with Aluminum, Stainless Steel and Railroad Tracks", *Scand. J. Work Environ. Health,* 11, 27–32.

# 6 Stratified Analysis

In analyzing epidemiologic data the researcher often wishes to adjust for the effects of certain extraneous variables so that the effects of the variables of interest can be estimated and understood more clearly. An epidemiologic study is frequently designed to investigate the association of a particular risk factor or exposure variable with a disease. Any extraneous variable that is an independent risk factor for the study disease and is also related to the exposure variable is called a *confounding factor*. Such variables may partially or completely account for any apparent association between an exposure variable and disease. Thus, a confounding factor tends to mask an underlying true association and may bias any estimation of the association between the disease and the risk factor. Any extraneous factor that may change the strength of the relationship between disease and exposure is known as an *effect modifying factor* or variable. The risk ratio and the odds ratio, which associate exposure and disease, would vary with the level of an effect-modifying variable. Confounding factors, and to a lesser degree, effect modifying factors, are treated somewhat differently than risk factors, which are of direct interest to the investigator because the former tends to be factors that are known to be related to both risk factors and disease. Therefore, it is necessary to adjust for confounding and effect modifiers in any study involving new risk factors. The purpose of a stratified analysis is to evaluate and remove confounding factors and to evaluate and describe effect modification. In addition, in randomized studies, a stratified analysis may be used to increase the precision of inferences particularly if stratified randomization had been used. A similar problem arises in a somewhat different context when a number of independent studies exist and the interest focuses on combining the results to give an overall picture of the studies.

## 6.1 CONFOUNDING AND INTERACTION

Confounding and interaction are two methodological concepts relevant to understanding the relationship of one or more independent variables (risk factors) to a dependent variable (response outcome). Confounding exists when the association between two variables is altered after accounting or controlling for the effect of a third variable. The third variable is referred to as a confounding variable or confounder.* Interaction exists when the association between two variables is different at different levels of a third variable. The third variable is referred to as an interaction variable.** Although they are two somewhat distinct concepts, they both entail the determination of an association between two or more variables so that additional variables that may affect this association have been accounted for or controlled.

For example, consider an association between the risk of myocardial infraction (MI) and systolic blood pressure (SBP). It is known that gender is an independent risk factor for MI and it is also associated with SBP. If an estimate of the association between MI and SBP is significantly different, depending on whether we ignore the proportion of males and females in the study sample or control it by studying the association separately for males and females, then gender is an example of a confounding variable. On the other hand, if an estimate of the association between MI and SBP is significantly different for males and females, then gender is an example of an interaction variable.

As another example, consider an association between alcohol consumption and heart disease with drinkers tending to have a higher risk of disease. It is known that cigarette smoking is an independent risk factor for heart disease and it is also known to be associated with alcohol consumption. Thus, if in a case-control study the case group contained a higher proportion of smokers than the control group, any apparent increased risk found to be associated with drinking may in fact be attributed to smoking. We could remove the effect of smoking (i.e., control for smoking) by studying the association between drinking and heart disease separately for smokers and nonsmokers. However, if an estimate of the association between drinking and heart disease is different between smokers and nonsmokers, then smoking is an example of an interaction variable.

No interaction is said to exist when the association between two variables is the same at every level of the third variable. For example, to assess interaction due to gender in studying the association between MI and SBP, the question is whether some estimate of this association, for example, the odds ratio (OR), changes with gender (e.g., whether the association is strong for males or is weak for females, or vice versa). If the OR varies with gender, we say that there is a gender × SBP interaction.

When both confounding and interaction are present for the same data, the use of an adjusted estimate of the association of interest, after controlling for confounding, would tend to disguise any interaction effects that may be present. For example, if an interaction exists between gender and SBP, the use of an adjusted OR, after controlling for gender, would disguise this interaction.

---

* The discussion of confounding presented here follows that of Kleinbaum et al. (1982, 1988). For an alternate definition of confounding, see Schlesselman (1982) and Miettinen (1985).

** An epidemiologist usually speaks and writes about effect modification, not interaction. The interaction variable is then referred to as an effect modifier.

**TABLE 6.1**
**A 2 × 2 Display of Sample Data in an Unstratified Analysis**

| Disease | Risk factor + | Risk factor − | Total |
|---|---|---|---|
| Cases | $a$ | $b$ | $m_1$ |
| Noncases | $c$ | $d$ | $m_2$ |
| Total | $n_1$ | $n_2$ | $n$ |

Thus, interaction normally should be assessed before confounding. The use of an adjusted estimate that controls for confounding is generally recommended when no meaningful interaction takes place. An adjustment for confounding is inappropriate in the presence of interaction.

Confounding and interaction are somewhat complex concepts and their complete treatment is beyond the scope of this volume. For further details and discussion, the reader is referred to Kleinbaum et al. (1982, 1988) and Schlesselman (1982).

## 6.2 ADJUSTMENT FOR CONFOUNDING IN A 2 × 2 TABLE

Consider a 2 × 2 table (Table 6.1) which relates the prevalence of a condition to a risk factor. Suppose the data of Table 6.1 were stratified into the $k$ 2 × 2 tables of Table 6.2 according to the $k$ levels of a confounding factor. Note that

$$\sum_{i=1}^{k} a_i = a,\ \sum_{i=1}^{k} b_i = b,\ \sum_{i=1}^{k} c_i = c,\ \sum_{i=1}^{k} d_i = d,\ \sum_{i=1}^{k} n_i = n.$$

The analysis of the relationship between the risk factor and the condition in separate subgroups, in which the subgroups are defined by levels of a confounding factor or combination of confounding factors, is referred to as stratified analysis and the subgroups are referred to as strata.

## 6.3 MEASURES OF RISK

As in the case of a single 2 × 2 table, consider RD, RR, and the OR as the measures of risk in a stratified analysis. From the outset, all stratified estimation is a matter of pooling comparative information over the strata.

**TABLE 6.2**
**A 2 × 2 Display of Sample Data in a Stratified Analysis:**

**Levels of a Confounding Factor**

**First Level**

| Condition | Risk Factor + | Risk Factor – | Total |
|---|---|---|---|
| Cases | $a_1$ | $b_1$ | $m_{11}$ |
| Noncases | $c_1$ | $d_1$ | $m_{21}$ |
| Total | $n_{11}$ | $n_{21}$ | $n_1$ |

***i*th Level**

| Condition | Risk Factor + | Risk Factor – | Total |
|---|---|---|---|
| Cases | $a_i$ | $b_i$ | $m_{1i}$ |
| Noncases | $c_i$ | $d_i$ | $m_{2i}$ |
| Total | $n_{1i}$ | $n_{2i}$ | $n_i$ |

***k*th Level**

| Condition | Risk Factor + | Risk Factor – | Total |
|---|---|---|---|
| Cases | $a_k$ | $b_k$ | $m_{1k}$ |
| Noncases | $c_k$ | $d_k$ | $m_{2k}$ |
| Total | $n_{1k}$ | $n_{2k}$ | $n_k$ |

### 6.3.1 Risk Difference

Consider various methods of point and interval estimation for the common RD in a stratified analysis.*

* Properly, for the RD, mutually standardized rates are computed with weights $n_{1i}n_{2i}/n_i$ and the differences are compared (see Section 10.2.1.1).

#### 6.3.1.1 Point Estimation

Consider a pooled (weighted) estimator, the Mantel-Haenszel estimator, and the maximum likelihood estimator as point estimates of the common RD.

*Pooled Estimator*

An estimate of the RD for the *i*th level of the confounding factor is

$$\hat{\text{RD}}_i = \frac{a_i}{n_{1i}} - \frac{b_i}{n_{2i}}. \tag{6.1}$$

An estimated variance for the $\hat{\text{RD}}_i$ is derived as the sum of two binomial variances and is given by

$$\hat{\text{Var}}\left(\hat{\text{RD}}_i\right) = \frac{a_i c_i}{n_{1i}^3} + \frac{b_i d_i}{n_{2i}^3} = \frac{n_{2i}^3\, a_i c_i + n_{1i}^3\, b_i d_i}{n_{1i}^3\, n_{2i}^3}. \tag{6.2}$$

A pooled (weighted) estimator of the common risk difference (RD) can be obtained as the weighted average of the $\hat{\text{RD}}_i$ with stratum-specific weight $W_i$ being the inverse of the stratum variance;* in other words,

$$\hat{\text{RD}}_w = \frac{\sum_{i=1}^{k} W_i \hat{\text{RD}}_i}{\sum_{i=1}^{k} W_i}, \tag{6.3}$$

where

$$W_i = \frac{n_{1i}^3\, n_{2i}^3}{n_{2i}^3\, a_i c_i + n_{1i}^3\, b_i d_i}. \tag{6.4}$$

*Mantel-Haenszel Estimator***

Greenland and Robins (1985) used the Mantel-Haenszel approach for estimating the measures of RD. The statistical properties of the Mantel-Haenszel estimators for the measures of RD are superior to any other procedure for very sparse data within strata, but the variance of the Mantel-Haenszel estimator is much greater than the variance of either the directly weighted or the maximum

* Miettinen (1985) pointed out that these weights are correlated with the stratum-specific values of the rate differences, just as are weights with marginal (null) estimates of variance, and may lead to biased results. The correct weights proposed are $n_{1i}n_{2i}/n_i$.

** The term *Mantel-Haenszel (MH) estimator* is used here in analogy with the MH estimator for the OR and in no way refers to the authors of the procedure.

likelihood estimate when the data are abundant. (Refer to the original paper for further details.)

*Maximum Likelihood Estimator*

The maximum likelihood estimator of the common RD ($\hat{\text{RD}}_{\text{ML}}$) is the solution to the equations (Miettinen, 1975; Rothman and Boice, 1982; Rothman, 1986)

$$\sum_{i=1}^{k} \frac{a_i}{\hat{R}_{ui} + \hat{\text{RD}}_{\text{ML}}} - \sum_{i=1}^{k} \frac{c_i}{1 - \hat{R}_{ui} - \hat{\text{RD}}_{\text{ML}}} = 0, \tag{6.5}$$

and, for each stratum $i$ ($i = 1,2,...,k$),

$$\frac{a_i}{\hat{R}_{ui} + \hat{\text{RD}}_{\text{ML}}} + \frac{b_i}{\hat{R}_{ui}} - \frac{c_i}{1 - \hat{R}_{ui} - \hat{\text{RD}}_{\text{ML}}} - \frac{d_i}{1 - \hat{R}_{ui}} = 0, \tag{6.6}$$

where $\hat{R}_{ui}$ is the maximum likelihood estimate of the cumulative incidence risk among the unexposed group in the $i$th stratum.* Note that there are $k + 1$ equations, one more than the number of strata to be solved. In addition to solving for $\hat{\text{RD}}_{\text{ML}}$, it is necessary to solve for $\hat{R}_{ui}$, the estimate for the cumulative incidence risk among the unexposed group in each stratum.

In order to solve for Equations 6.5 and 6.6, begin with the initial values as the observed incidence risk for each stratum. Note, however, that the value of $\hat{R}_{ui}$ that satisfies Equations 6.5 and 6.6 can be best achieved by starting with a trial value of $\hat{\text{RD}}_{\text{ML}}$, solving iteratively for each $\hat{R}_{ui}$, and then evaluating the left side of Equations 6.5 and 6.6. Each trial value for $\hat{\text{RD}}_{\text{ML}}$ requires an iterative solution for Equation 6.6 in each stratum. The procedure in general becomes very tedious and generally requires a computer program.

Under large sample conditions, an initial approximation of the value of $\hat{\text{RD}}_{\text{ML}}$ in the iterative solution to Equations 6.5 and 6.6 may be obtained by taking a weighted average of the stratum-specific RDs ($\hat{\text{RD}}_i$) given by (Miettinen, 1975)

$$\hat{\text{RD}}_{\text{ML}} = \frac{\sum_{i=1}^{k} W_i \hat{\text{RD}}_i}{\sum_{i=1}^{k} W_i},$$

where the weights $W_i$ are inversely proportional to the variance of the effect estimate in each stratum and are obtained as

* For a closed form solution to the likelihood equations (of the third degree) for the RD, see Miettinen (1985) and Miettinen and Nuriminen (1985).

$$W_i = \frac{n_{1i}\, n_{2i}\, n_i}{m_{1i}\, m_{2i}}.$$

The above estimate is useful as the first approximation or trial value of $\hat{\text{RD}}_{\text{ML}}$ in the iterative solution to Equations 6.5 and 6.6.

#### 6.3.1.2 Confidence Intervals

No viable approach exists for obtaining an exact confidence interval (CI) for the RD. Three commonly used approximate methods are described below.

*Pooling Method*

An approximate $100(1 - \alpha)\%$ CI can be obtained from an estimate of the variance of the pooled estimator (Equation 6.3) and then

$$\hat{\text{RD}}_w \pm Z_{\alpha/2}\sqrt{\hat{\text{Var}}\left(\hat{\text{RD}}_w\right)}, \tag{6.7}$$

where $\hat{\text{Var}}\left(\hat{\text{RD}}_w\right)$ can be obtained as

$$\begin{aligned}
\hat{\text{Var}}\left(\hat{\text{RD}}_w\right) &= \hat{\text{Var}}\left[\frac{\sum_{i=1}^{k} W_i \hat{\text{RD}}_i}{\sum_{i=1}^{k} W_i}\right] = \frac{\sum_{i=1}^{k} W_i^2 \hat{\text{Var}}\left(\hat{\text{RD}}_i\right)}{\left(\sum_{i=1}^{k} W_i\right)^2} \\
&= \frac{\left[\sum_{i=1}^{k} W_i^2 \frac{1}{W_i}\right]}{\left(\sum_{i=1}^{k} W_i\right)^2} = \frac{\sum_{i=1}^{k} W_i}{\left(\sum_{i=1}^{k} W_i\right)^2} \\
&= \frac{1}{\sum_{i=1}^{k} W_i}.
\end{aligned} \tag{6.8}$$

*Maximum Likelihood Method*

Maximum likelihood estimates $\hat{\text{RD}}_{\text{ML}}$ and $\hat{R}_{ui}$, obtained from Equations 6.5 and 6.6, can be used to derive an improved estimate of the variance of the rate difference ($\hat{\text{RD}}_i$) in each stratum. The improved estimates can be obtained by substituting $\hat{R}_{ui}$ for $b_i/n_{2i}$ and $\hat{R}_{ui} + \hat{\text{RD}}_{\text{ML}}$ for $a_i/n_{1i}$ into the variance formula

(Equation 6.2). The resulting weights (Equation 6.4), using the improved estimates, are

$$W_i = \frac{n_{1i}\, n_{2i}}{n_{1i}\hat{R}_{ui}\left(1-\hat{R}_{ui}\right) + n_{2i}\left(\hat{R}_{ui} + \hat{\mathrm{RD}}_{\mathrm{ML}}\right)\left(1-\hat{R}_{ui} - \hat{\mathrm{RD}}_{\mathrm{ML}}\right)}. \quad (6.9)$$

The new weights can then be used to obtain an estimate of the variance of the maximum likelihood estimator ( $\hat{\mathrm{RD}}_{\mathrm{ML}}$) using Equation 6.8. Using this method, an approximate 100(1 – α)% CI for the RD is then given by

$$\hat{\mathrm{RD}}_{\mathrm{ML}} \pm Z_{\alpha/2}\sqrt{\hat{\mathrm{Var}}\left(\hat{\mathrm{RD}}_{\mathrm{ML}}\right)}. \quad (6.10)$$

*Test-Based Method*

An alternative is to use the test-based method. As discussed earlier, a 100(1 – α)% CI for the RD using this method is

$$\hat{\mathrm{RD}}_w \pm Z_{\alpha/2}\sqrt{\left(\hat{\mathrm{RD}}_w\right)^2 / \chi^2_{\mathrm{MH}}}, \quad (6.11)$$

where $\chi^2_{\mathrm{MH}}$ is the Mantel-Haenszel chi-square statistic given by (see Appendix J)

$$\chi^2_{\mathrm{MH}} = \frac{\left[\sum_{i=1}^{k} a_i - \sum_{i=1}^{k} \frac{m_{1i}\, n_{1i}}{n_i}\right]^2}{\sum_{i=1}^{k} \frac{m_{1i}\, m_{2i}\, n_{1i}\, n_{2i}}{n_i^2\left(n_i - 1\right)}}. \quad (6.12)$$

Equation 6.11 can be rewritten more simply in terms of the standard normal statistic $\chi$ as

$$\hat{\mathrm{RD}}_w\left(1 \pm Z_{\alpha/2}/\chi\right).$$

*Example 6.1*

Consider the Evans County Heart Disease Study described in Chapter 3. Recall that the study assessed the putative association between catecholamine level (CAT) and the subsequent 7-year incidence of coronary heart disease (CHD) among a cohort of 609 males. Confidence intervals for risk measures were calculated for an unstratified crude analysis. To illustrate stratified analysis, we consider the control of age and electrocardiogram (ECG) in evaluating the CAT–CHD association, which were among several potentially confounding

**TABLE 6.3**
**Prevalence of CHD by CAT: Data Stratified by Age and ECG**

| Age <55, ECG = 0 | High CAT | Low CAT | Total |
|---|---|---|---|
| CHD | 1 | 17 | 18 |
| No CHD | 7 | 257 | 264 |
| Total | 8 | 274 | 282 |

| Age <55, ECG = 1 | High CAT | Low CAT | Total |
|---|---|---|---|
| CHD | 3 | 7 | 10 |
| No CHD | 14 | 52 | 66 |
| Total | 17 | 59 | 76 |

| Age ≥55, ECG = 0 | High CAT | Low CAT | Total |
|---|---|---|---|
| CHD | 9 | 15 | 24 |
| No CHD | 30 | 107 | 137 |
| Total | 39 | 122 | 161 |

| Age ≥55, ECG = 1 | High CAT | Low CAT | Total |
|---|---|---|---|
| CHD | 14 | 5 | 19 |
| No CHD | 44 | 27 | 71 |
| Total | 58 | 32 | 90 |

From Kleinbaum D. G., Kupper, L. L., and Morgenstern, H. (1982). *Epidemiologic Research: Principles and Quantitative Methods.* p. 334, Lifetime Learning Publications, Belmont, CA. With permission.

factors included in the study. The four strata resulting from using dichotomous categories of both AGE and ECG are shown in Table 6.3.

First, obtain point estimates of the RD using pooled and maximum likelihood estimates.

**Pooled estimate** — From the four stratified tables of Table 6.3, we have

$$\hat{RD}_1 = \frac{1}{8} - \frac{17}{274} = 0.063,$$

$$\hat{RD}_2 = \frac{3}{17} - \frac{7}{59} = 0.058,$$

$$\hat{RD}_3 = \frac{9}{39} - \frac{15}{122} = 0.108,$$

$$\hat{RD}_4 = \frac{14}{58} - \frac{5}{32} = 0.085.$$

In order to obtain a pooled estimate of the RD, first find

$$W_1 = \frac{n_{11}^3 n_{21}^3}{n_{21}^3 a_1 c_1 + n_{11}^3 b_1 d_1} = \frac{(8)^3 (274)^3}{(274)^3 \times 1 \times 7 + (8)^3 \times 17 \times 257} = 72.024,$$

$$W_2 = \frac{n_{12}^3 n_{22}^3}{n_{22}^3 a_2 c_2 + n_{12}^3 b_2 d_2} = \frac{(17)^3 (59)^3}{(59)^3 \times 3 \times 14 + (17)^3 \times 7 \times 52} = 96.889,$$

$$W_3 = \frac{n_{13}^3 n_{23}^3}{n_{23}^3 a_3 c_3 + n_{13}^3 b_3 d_3} = \frac{(39)^3 (122)^3}{(122)^3 \times 9 \times 30 + (39)^3 \times 15 \times 107} = 183.974,$$

$$W_4 = \frac{n_{14}^3 n_{24}^3}{n_{24}^3 a_4 c_4 + n_{14}^3 b_4 d_4} = \frac{(58)^3 (32)^3}{(32)^3 \times 14 \times 44 + (58)^3 \times 5 \times 27} = 137.419.$$

The results of the above computations can be summarized in a tabular form:

| $i$ | $W_i$ | $\hat{\text{RD}}_i$ | $W_i\hat{\text{RD}}_i$ |
|---|---|---|---|
| 1 | 72.024 | 0.063 | 4.538 |
| 2 | 96.889 | 0.058 | 5.620 |
| 3 | 183.974 | 0.108 | 19.869 |
| 4 | 137.419 | 0.085 | 11.681 |
| Total | 490.306 | — | 41.708 |

Using Equation 6.3, the pooled estimate of the RD is given by

$$\hat{\text{RD}}_w = \frac{41.708}{490.306} = 0.085.$$

**Maximum likelihood estimate** — In order to obtain the maximum likelihood estimate of the RD, note that likelihood Equations 6.5 and 6.6 are given by

$$\left[\frac{1}{\hat{R}_{u1} + \hat{\text{RD}}_{\text{ML}}} + \frac{3}{\hat{R}_{u2} + \hat{\text{RD}}_{\text{ML}}} + \frac{9}{\hat{R}_{u3} + \hat{\text{RD}}_{\text{ML}}} + \frac{14}{\hat{R}_{u4} + \hat{\text{RD}}_{\text{ML}}}\right]$$

$$-\left[\frac{7}{1 - \hat{R}_{u1} - \hat{\text{RD}}_{\text{ML}}} + \frac{14}{1 - \hat{R}_{u2} - \hat{\text{RD}}_{\text{ML}}} + \frac{30}{1 - \hat{R}_{u3} - \hat{\text{RD}}_{\text{ML}}} + \frac{44}{1 - \hat{R}_{u4} - \hat{\text{RD}}_{\text{ML}}}\right] = 0,$$

$$\left[\frac{1}{\hat{R}_{u1}+\hat{\text{RD}}_{\text{ML}}}+\frac{17}{\hat{R}_{u1}}\right]-\left[\frac{7}{1-\hat{R}_{u1}-\hat{\text{RD}}_{\text{ML}}}+\frac{257}{1-\hat{R}_{u1}}\right]=0,$$

$$\left[\frac{3}{\hat{R}_{u2}+\hat{\text{RD}}_{\text{ML}}}+\frac{7}{\hat{R}_{u2}}\right]-\left[\frac{14}{1-\hat{R}_{u2}-\hat{\text{RD}}_{\text{ML}}}+\frac{52}{1-\hat{R}_{u2}}\right]=0,$$

$$\left[\frac{9}{\hat{R}_{u3}+\hat{\text{RD}}_{\text{ML}}}+\frac{15}{\hat{R}_{u3}}\right]-\left[\frac{30}{1-\hat{R}_{u3}-\hat{\text{RD}}_{\text{ML}}}+\frac{107}{1-\hat{R}_{u3}}\right]=0,$$

$$\left[\frac{14}{\hat{R}_{u4}+\hat{\text{RD}}_{\text{ML}}}+\frac{5}{\hat{R}_{u4}}\right]-\left[\frac{44}{1-\hat{R}_{u4}-\hat{\text{RD}}_{\text{ML}}}+\frac{27}{1-\hat{R}_{u4}}\right]=0.$$

The maximum likelihood solution for the $\hat{\text{RD}}_{\text{ML}}$ using a computer program (Wolfram, 1991) is obtained as 0.086, which is in close agreement with the pooled estimate of 0.085.

Confidence intervals must be constructed next for the RD using the methods of pooling, maximum likelihood, and the test-based approach.

**Pooling method** — As before, $\hat{\text{RD}}_w = 0.085$, and using Equation 6.8, we have

$$\hat{\text{Var}}\left(\hat{\text{RD}}_w\right)=\frac{1}{490.306}=0.002.$$

Thus, a 95% CI for the RD is given by

$$0.085 \pm 1.96\sqrt{0.002}=(-0.003,\ 0.173).$$

**Maximum likelihood method** — To obtain a CI for the RD using this method, note that, using a computer program (Wolfram, 1991), the maximum likelihood estimates of the parameters of interest are

$$\hat{\text{RD}}_{\text{ML}}=0.0862,\ \hat{R}_{u1}=0.0617,\ \hat{R}_{u2}=0.1143,\ \hat{R}_{u3}=0.1267,\ \hat{R}_{u4}=0.1556.$$

Now, using Equation 6.9, the new weights are obtained as

$$W_1=\frac{(8)(274)}{274(0.0617+0.0862)(1-0.0617-0.0862)+8(0.0617)(1-0.0617)}$$

$$=62.639,$$

$$W_2 = \frac{(17)(59)}{59(0.1143+0.0862)(1-0.1143-0.0862)+17(0.1143)(1-0.1143)}$$

$$= 89.724,$$

$$W_3 = \frac{(39)(122)}{122(0.1267+0.0862)(1-0.1267-0.0862)+39(0.1267)(1-0.1267)}$$

$$= 192.171,$$

$$W_4 = \frac{(58)(32)}{32(0.1556+0.0862)(1-0.1556-0.0862)+58(0.1556)(1-0.1556)}$$

$$= 137.612.$$

Thus, a 95% CI for the RD using Equation 6.10 is given by

$$0.086 \pm 1.96\sqrt{\frac{1}{62.639+89.724+192.171+137.612}}$$

$$= 0.086 \pm 1.96\sqrt{0.002}$$

$$= (-0.003, 0.174).$$

**Test-based method** — To obtain a CI for the RD via the test-based method, first compute the value of the Mantel-Haenszel chi-square statistic using Equation 6.12. Thus,

$$\sum_{i=1}^{4} a_i = 1+3+9+14 = 27,$$

$$\frac{m_{11}n_{11}}{n_1} = \frac{18\times 8}{282} = 0.511,$$

$$\frac{m_{12}n_{12}}{n_2} = \frac{10\times 17}{76} = 2.237,$$

$$\frac{m_{13}n_{13}}{n_3} = \frac{24\times 39}{161} = 5.814,$$

$$\frac{m_{14}n_{14}}{n_4} = \frac{19 \times 58}{90} = 12.244,$$

$$\sum_{i=1}^{4} \frac{m_{1i}n_{1i}}{n_i} = 20.806.$$

We further obtain

$$\frac{m_{11}m_{21}n_{11}n_{21}}{n_1^2(n_1-1)} = \frac{18 \times 264 \times 8 \times 274}{(282)^2(281)} = 0.466,$$

$$\frac{m_{12}m_{22}n_{12}n_{22}}{n_2^2(n_2-1)} = \frac{10 \times 66 \times 17 \times 59}{(76)^2(75)} = 1.528,$$

$$\frac{m_{13}m_{23}n_{13}n_{23}}{n_3^2(n_3-1)} = \frac{24 \times 137 \times 39 \times 122}{(161)^2(160)} = 3.772,$$

$$\frac{m_{14}m_{24}n_{14}n_{24}}{n_4^2(n_4-1)} = \frac{19 \times 71 \times 58 \times 32}{(90)^2(89)} = 3.473.$$

Hence,

$$\sum_{i=1}^{4} \frac{m_{1i}m_{2i}n_{1i}n_{2i}}{n_i^2(n_i-1)} = 9.239,$$

and, using Equation 6.12, the value of the Mantel-Haenszel chi-square statistic is

$$\chi^2_{\text{MH}} = \frac{(27-20.806)^2}{9.239} = 4.153.$$

Therefore, a 95% CI for the RD using the test-based method is obtained as

$$(0.085) \pm 1.96\sqrt{\frac{(0.085)^2}{4.153}} = (0.003, 0.167).$$

Note that the test-based limits are too narrow and do not include the value of zero, in contrast to the earlier evidence.*

* It can be verified that an application of the continuity correction for $\chi^2_{\text{MH}}$ yields test-based limits which are similar to earlier results.

#### 6.3.1.3 Test for Homogeneity of Risk Differences

A test for homogeneity of effect over strata in terms of a uniform risk difference can be carried out by the statistic

$$\sum_{i=1}^{k}\left[\frac{\left(\hat{\text{RD}}_i - \hat{\text{RD}}_w\right)^2}{\hat{\text{Var}}\left(\hat{\text{RD}}_i\right)}\right], \tag{6.13}$$

which asymptotically has a chi-square distribution with $k - 1$ degrees of freedom. Note that $\hat{\text{RD}}_i$, $\hat{\text{Var}}(\hat{\text{RD}}_i)$, and $\hat{\text{RD}}_w$ are defined by Equations 6.1, 6.2, and 6.3, respectively. The validity assumption of the test statistic (Equation 6.13) requires that each stratum-specific estimate has normal sampling distribution and may not be satisfied for strata with relatively small data.

For the data in Example 6.1, test statistic 6.13 is calculated as

$$\frac{(0.063-0.085)^2}{0.0139}+\frac{(0.058-0.085)^2}{0.0103}+\frac{(0.108-0.085)^2}{0.0054}+\frac{(0.085-0.085)^2}{0.0073}$$
$$=0.204$$

and from the chi-square table

$$P\left(\chi_3^2 > 0.204\right) = 0.977.$$

Thus, the hypothesis of the homogeneity of the RDs for age and ECG strata cannot be rejected. Hence, evidence that the RDs are different for four strata under consideration is lacking.

### 6.3.2 Risk Ratio

Various methods of point and interval estimation of the common RR are considered in a stratified analysis.

#### 6.3.2.1 Point Estimation

A pooled (weighted) estimator, the Mantel-Haenszel estimator, and the maximum likelihood estimator are considered as point estimates of the common risk ratio.*

*Pooled Estimator*

An estimate of the risk ratio for the *i*th level of the confounding factor is

* Properly, for the RR mutually standardized rates are computed with weights $n_{1i}n_{2i}/n_i$ and then the ratios are compared (see Section 10.2.2.2).

$$\hat{RR}_i = \frac{a_i/n_{1i}}{b_i/n_{2i}}. \tag{6.14}$$

An approximate variance estimate for $\log_e(\hat{RR}_i)$ can be obtained, using the result in Appendix B, as

$$\hat{Var}\left\{\log_e\left(\hat{RR}_i\right)\right\} = \frac{c_i}{a_i n_{1i}} + \frac{d_i}{b_i n_{2i}}. \tag{6.15}$$

A pooled estimator of the logarithm of the common RR can be obtained as the weighted average of $\log_e(\hat{RR}_i)$, with stratum-specific weight being the inverse of the variance estimate*:

$$\log_e\left(\hat{RR}_w\right) = \frac{\sum_{i=1}^{k} W_i \log_e\left(\hat{RR}_i\right)}{\sum_{i=1}^{k} W_i} \tag{6.16}$$

and

$$\hat{RR}_w = \exp\left[\log_e\left(\hat{RR}_w\right)\right], \tag{6.17}$$

where

$$W_i = \frac{a_i b_i n_{1i} n_{2i}}{a_i d_i n_{1i} + b_i c_i n_{2i}}. \tag{6.18}$$

*Mantel-Haenszel Estimator***

In analogy with the Mantel-Haenszel estimator for the common OR, given by Equation 6.32, one can obtain the Mantel-Haenszel estimator for the common RR as the weighted average of $\hat{RR}_i$, with stratum-specific weight $W_i$ being equal to $(n_{1i}/n_i)b_i$. This approximates the inverse of $\hat{Var}(\hat{RR}_i)$ when the true common RR is near 1. Thus, the Mantel-Haenszel estimator of the common RR is obtained as (see, e.g., Nurminen, 1981; Tarone, 1981)

* Miettinen (1985) has pointed out that these weights are correlated with the stratum-specific values of the rate differences, just as are weights with marginal (null) estimates of variance, and may lead to biased results. The correct weights proposed are $n_{1i}n_{2i}/n_i$.

** The term Mantel-Haenszel (MH) is used here in analogy with the MH estimator for the OR and in no way refers to the authors of the procedure.

$$\hat{RR}_{MH} = \frac{\sum_{i=1}^{k}\left(\frac{n_{1i}}{n_i}\right)b_i\left(\frac{a_i n_{2i}}{b_i n_{1i}}\right)}{\sum_{i=1}^{k}\left(\frac{n_{1i}}{n_i}\right)b_i} = \frac{\sum_{i=1}^{k}\left(\frac{n_{2i}}{n_i}\right)a_i}{\sum_{i=1}^{k}\left(\frac{n_{1i}}{n_i}\right)b_i}. \tag{6.19}$$

The estimator (Equation 6.19) also can be looked upon as the ratio of the mutually standardized rates with weights $n_{1i}n_{2i}/n_i$. Rothman and Boice (1982) stated that Equation 6.19 provides a good approximation to the maximum likelihood estimator. Tarone (1981) pointed out that the equation can be obtained as the value of the first iteration in the calculation of the maximum likelihood estimate for the common RR, assuming a Poisson distribution model.

*Maximum Likelihood Estimator*

The maximum likelihood estimate of the overall RR ( $\hat{RR}_{ML}$) can be obtained as the solution to the equations (Miettinen, 1975; Rothman and Boice, 1982; Rothman, 1986)

$$\sum_{i=1}^{k}\left\{\frac{a_i - (n_{1i})(\hat{RR}_{ML})(\hat{R}_{ui})}{1-(\hat{RR}_{ML})(\hat{R}_{ui})}\right\} = 0, \tag{6.20}$$

where, for each stratum $i$ ($i$ = 1,2,...,$k$)

$$(\hat{R}_{ui}) = \frac{a_i + n_{2i} + (b_i + n_{1i})(\hat{RR}_{ML})}{2(n_i)(\hat{RR}_{ML})} - \left\{\left[\frac{a_i + n_{2i} + (b_i + n_{1i})(\hat{RR}_{ML})}{2(n_i)(\hat{RR}_{ML})}\right]^2 - \frac{m_{1i}}{(n_i)(\hat{RR}_{ML})}\right\}^{0.5}. \tag{6.21}$$

Thus, unlike the case of the RD, the maximum likelihood solution for each $\hat{R}_{ui}$ has a closed-form expression conditional on $\hat{RR}_{ML}$. The above equations can be solved iteratively.

Under large sample conditions, an initial approximation to the value of $\hat{RR}_{ML}$ in the solutions to Equations 6.20 and 6.21 can be obtained by taking a weighted average of the stratum-specific log RR (Miettinen, 1975):

$$\hat{RR}_{ML} = \exp\left[\frac{\sum_{i=1}^{k} W_i \log_e\left(\hat{RR}_i\right)}{\sum_{i=1}^{k} W_i}\right],$$

where $\hat{RR}_i$ is defined as it was in Equation 6.14, and the weight $W_i$ is inversely proportional to the variance of the logarithm of the effect estimate in each stratum and is obtained as

$$W_i = \frac{m_{1i} n_{1i} n_{2i}}{m_{2i} n_i}.$$

The above estimate is useful as the first approximation or initial value of $\hat{RR}_{ML}$ in the iterative solution to Equations 6.20 and 6.21. Miettinen (1985) pointed out that the simpler and more appropriate initial estimate for the maximum likelihood equation is given by the estimator (Equation 6.19).

#### 6.3.2.2 Confidence Intervals

As for the individual RR, an exact CI for the common RR in a stratified analysis is not available. If risks are small, however, the odds ratio may be used to estimate the RR. Because an exact CI for the common OR can be determined conditionally on all the marginals of the 2 × 2 table, this value can be used as a surrogate for the RR.

Approximate CIs can be determined by the use of the methods of pooling, maximum likelihood, Mantel-Haenszel, and the test-based approach.

*Pooling Method*

An approximate 100(1 – α)% CI can be obtained by first determining an estimate of the variance of the pooled estimator (Equation 6.16) and then using the formula

$$\log_e\left(\hat{RR}_w\right) \pm Z_{\alpha/2}\sqrt{\hat{Var}\left\{\log_e\left(\hat{RR}_w\right)\right\}},$$

where, as in Equation 6.8, $\hat{\text{Var}}\{\log_e(\hat{\text{RR}}_w)\}$ is given by

$$\hat{\text{Var}}\left\{\log_e\left(\hat{\text{RR}}_w\right)\right\} = \frac{1}{\sum_{i=1}^{k} W_i}, \tag{6.22}$$

with $W_i$ being given in Equation 6.18. The CI for the RR follows by taking the antilogarithms of the corresponding endpoints.

*Maximum Likelihood Method*

Again, the maximum likelihood estimates $\hat{\text{RR}}_{\text{ML}}$ and $\hat{R}_{ui}$, obtained from Equations 6.20 and 6.21, can be used to derive an improved estimate of the variance of the logarithm of the RR estimate in each stratum. The improved estimates can be obtained by substituting $n_{1i}\hat{R}_{ui}\hat{\text{RR}}_{\text{ML}}$ for $a_i$ and $n_{2i}\hat{R}_{ui}$ for $b_i$ into the variance formula (Equation 6.15). The resulting weights (Equation 6.18), using the improved estimates, are

$$W_i = \frac{n_{1i}n_{2i}\hat{R}_{ui}\hat{\text{RR}}_{\text{ML}}}{n_{1i}\left(1-\hat{R}_{ui}\right)\hat{\text{RR}}_{\text{ML}} + n_{2i}\left(1-\hat{R}_{ui}\hat{\text{RR}}_{\text{ML}}\right)}. \tag{6.23}$$

The new weights can be used to obtain a variance estimate of the logarithm of the maximum likelihood estimator ($\hat{\text{RR}}_{\text{ML}}$) similar to Equation 6.8. An approximate 100(1 – α)% CI for $\log_e$(RR) using this method is then given by

$$\log_e\left(\hat{\text{RR}}_{\text{ML}}\right) \pm Z_{\alpha/2}\sqrt{\hat{\text{Var}}\left\{\log_e\left(\hat{\text{RR}}_{\text{ML}}\right)\right\}}. \tag{6.24}$$

*Mantel-Haenszel Method*

Using this method, an approximate 100(1 – α)% CI can be obtained by first determining an estimate of the variance of the logarithm of the Mantel-Haenszel estimator (Equation 6.19) and then using the formula

$$\log_e\left(\hat{\text{RR}}_{\text{MH}}\right) \pm Z_{\alpha/2}\sqrt{\hat{\text{Var}}\left\{\log_e\left(\hat{\text{RR}}_{\text{MH}}\right)\right\}}. \tag{6.25}$$

An estimate of the variance of the logarithm of $\hat{\text{RR}}_{\text{MH}}$ is obtained approximately as (Greenland and Robins, 1985)

$$\hat{\text{Var}}\left\{\log_e\left(\hat{\text{RR}}_w\right)\right\} = \frac{\sum_{i=1}^{k}\left(m_{1i}n_{1i}n_{2i} - a_ib_in_i\right)/n_i^2}{\left[\sum_{i=1}^{k}\left(\frac{n_{2i}}{n_i}\right)a_i\right]\left[\sum_{i=1}^{k}\left(\frac{n_{1i}}{n_i}\right)b_i\right]}. \tag{6.26}$$

The STATCALC procedure of EpiInfo (1994) calculates the Mantel-Haenszel limits determined by Equation 6.25 using the variance estimate given by Equation 6.26.

*Test-Based Method*

A fourth alternative is to use the test-based limits. As discussed earlier, a $100(1-\alpha)\%$ approximate CI for $\log_e(\text{RR})$ using this method is

$$\log_e\left(\hat{\text{RR}}_{\text{MH}}\right) \pm Z_{\alpha/2}\sqrt{\left\{\log_e\left(\hat{\text{RR}}_{\text{MH}}\right)\right\}^2 / \chi^2_{\text{MH}}}, \tag{6.27}$$

where $\chi^2_{\text{MH}}$ is the Mantel-Haenszel chi-square statistic given in Equation 6.12. From this, a $100(1-\alpha)\%$ CI for the RR can be written more simply in terms of the standard normal statistic $\chi$ as

$$\left(\hat{\text{RR}}_{\text{MH}}\right)^{\left(1 \pm Z_{\alpha/2}/\chi\right)}.$$

*Example 6.2*

Consider the Evans County Heart Disease Study described in Chapter 3. First obtain point estimates of the RR using the pooled, Mantel-Haenszel, and the maximum likelihood estimates.

**Pooled estimate** — From the stratified data of Table 6.3,

$$\hat{\text{RR}}_1 = \frac{1/8}{17/274} = 2.015,$$

$$\hat{\text{RR}}_2 = \frac{3/17}{7/59} = 1.487,$$

$$\hat{\text{RR}}_3 = \frac{9/39}{15/122} = 1.877,$$

$$\hat{\text{RR}}_4 = \frac{14/58}{5/32} = 1.545.$$

In order to obtain $\log_e(\hat{\text{RR}}_w)$, we need to determine the stratum-specific weight $W_i$, i.e.,

$$W_1 = \frac{a_1 b_1 n_{11} n_{21}}{b_1 c_1 n_{21} + a_1 d_1 n_{11}} = \frac{(1)(17)(8)(274)}{(17)(7)(274)+(1)(257)(8)} = 1.075,$$

$$W_2 = \frac{a_2 b_2 n_{12} n_{22}}{b_2 c_2 n_{22} + a_2 d_2 n_{12}} = \frac{(3)(7)(17)(59)}{(7)(14)(59)+(3)(52)(17)} = 2.497,$$

$$W_3 = \frac{a_3 b_3 n_{13} n_{23}}{b_3 c_3 n_{23} + a_3 d_3 n_{13}} = \frac{(9)(15)(39)(122)}{(15)(30)(122)+(9)(107)(39)} = 6.947,$$

$$W_4 = \frac{a_4 b_4 n_{14} n_{24}}{b_4 c_4 n_{24} + a_4 d_4 n_{14}} = \frac{(14)(5)(58)(32)}{(5)(44)(32)+(14)(27)(58)} = 4.486.$$

The results of the above computations can be summarized in a tabular form:

| $i$ | $W_i$ | $\hat{RR}_i$ | $\log_e(\hat{RR}_i)$ | $W_i \log_e(\hat{RR}_i)$ |
|---|---|---|---|---|
| 1 | 1.075 | 2.015 | 0.701 | 0.753 |
| 2 | 2.497 | 1.487 | 0.397 | 0.991 |
| 3 | 6.947 | 1.877 | 0.630 | 4.374 |
| 4 | 4.486 | 1.545 | 0.435 | 1.952 |
| Total | 15.005 | — | — | 8.070 |

Thus, using Equations 6.16, 6.17, and 6.22,

$$\log_e\left(\hat{RR}_w\right) = \frac{8.070}{15.005} = 0.538, \quad \hat{RR}_w = 1.713$$

$$\hat{Var}\left\{\log_e\left(\hat{RR}_w\right)\right\} = \frac{1}{15.005} = 0.067.$$

**Maximum likelihood estimate** — In order to obtain the maximum likelihood estimate of the RR, the likelihood Equations 6.20 and 6.21 are

$$\frac{1-8\hat{RR}_{ML}\hat{R}_{u1}}{1-\hat{RR}_{ML}\hat{R}_{u1}} + \frac{3-17\hat{RR}_{ML}\hat{R}_{u2}}{1-\hat{RR}_{ML}\hat{R}_{u2}} + \frac{9-39\hat{RR}_{ML}\hat{R}_{u3}}{1-\hat{RR}_{ML}\hat{R}_{u3}} + \frac{14-58\hat{RR}_{ML}\hat{R}_{u4}}{1-\hat{RR}_{ML}\hat{R}_{u4}} = 0$$

$$\hat{R}_{u1} = \frac{(1+274)+(17+8)\hat{RR}_{ML}}{2(282)\hat{RR}_{ML}} - \left(\left[\frac{(1+274)+(17+8)\hat{RR}_{ML}}{2(282)\hat{RR}_{ML}}\right]^2 - \frac{18}{(282)\hat{RR}_{ML}}\right)^{0.5},$$

$$\hat{R}_{u2} = \frac{(3+59)+(7+17)\hat{RR}_{ML}}{2(76)\hat{RR}_{ML}} - \left(\left[\frac{(3+59)+(7+17)\hat{RR}_{ML}}{2(76)\hat{RR}_{ML}}\right]^2 - \frac{10}{(76)\hat{RR}_{ML}}\right)^{0.5},$$

$$\hat{R}_{u3} = \frac{(9+122)+(15+39)\hat{\text{RR}}_{\text{ML}}}{2(161)\hat{\text{RR}}_{\text{ML}}} - \left( \left[ \frac{(9+122)+(15+39)\hat{\text{RR}}_{\text{ML}}}{2(161)\hat{\text{RR}}_{\text{ML}}} \right]^2 - \frac{24}{(161)\hat{\text{RR}}_{\text{ML}}} \right)^{0.5},$$

$$\hat{R}_{u4} = \frac{(14+32)+(5+58)\hat{\text{RR}}_{\text{ML}}}{2(90)\hat{\text{RR}}_{\text{ML}}} - \left( \left[ \frac{(14+32)+(5+58)\hat{\text{RR}}_{\text{ML}}}{2(90)\hat{\text{RR}}_{\text{ML}}} \right]^2 - \frac{19}{(90)\hat{\text{RR}}_{\text{ML}}} \right)^{0.5}.$$

The maximum likelihood solution for $\hat{\text{RR}}_{\text{ML}}$ using a computer program (Wolfram, 1991) is obtained as 1.710, which is in close agreement with the pooled estimate of 1.713.

**Mantel-Haenszel estimate** — Next, obtain the Mantel-Haenszel estimate of the RR and an estimate of the variance of its logarithm. The quantities needed for the computation are summarized in tabular form:

| $i$ | $a_i$ | $b_i$ | $m_{1i}$ | $n_{1i}$ | $n_{2i}$ | $n_i$ | $(n_{2i}/n_i)a_i$ | $(n_{1i}/n_i)b_i$ |
|---|---|---|---|---|---|---|---|---|
| 1 | 1 | 17 | 18 | 8 | 274 | 282 | 0.972 | 0.482 |
| 2 | 3 | 7 | 10 | 17 | 59 | 76 | 2.329 | 1.566 |
| 3 | 9 | 15 | 24 | 39 | 122 | 161 | 6.820 | 3.634 |
| 4 | 14 | 5 | 19 | 58 | 32 | 90 | 4.978 | 3.222 |
| Total | | | | | | | 15.099 | 8.904 |

Using Equations 6.19 and 6.26,

$$\hat{\text{RR}}_{\text{MH}} = \frac{15.099}{8.904} = 1.696$$

and

$$\hat{\text{Var}}\left\{\log_e\left(\hat{\text{RR}}_{\text{MH}}\right)\right\} =$$

$$\left[ \frac{(18)(8)(274)-(1)(17)(282)}{(282)^2} + \frac{(10)(17)(59)-(3)(7)(76)}{(76)^2} \right.$$

$$\left. + \frac{(24)(39)(122)-(9)(15)(161)}{(161)^2} + \frac{(19)(58)(32)-(14)(5)(90)}{(90)^2} \right]$$

$$\div (15.099)(8.904) = \frac{9.039}{134.442} = 0.067.$$

Next, construct CIs for the RR using pooling, maximum likelihood, Mantel-Haenszel, and test-based methods.

**Pooling method** — As obtained previously, $\log_e(\hat{RR}_w) = 0.538$ and $\hat{Var}\{\log_e(\hat{RR}_w)\} = 0.067$. Thus, a 95% CI for $\log_e$(RR), using this method, is obtained as

$$0.538 \pm 1.96\sqrt{0.067} = (0.031, 1.045),$$

from which a 95% CI for the RR is given by (1.032, 2.843).

**Maximum likelihood method** — To obtain a CI for the RR using this method, note that the maximum likelihood estimates of the parameters of interest using a computer program (Wolfram, 1991) are

$$\hat{RR}_{ML} = 1.7097,\ \hat{R}_{u1} = 0.0626,\ \hat{R}_{u2} = 0.1132,\ \hat{R}_{u3} = 0.1275,\ \hat{R}_{u4} = 0.1445.$$

Using Equation 6.23, the new weights are obtained:

$$W_1 = \frac{(8)(274)(0.0626)(1.7097)}{1.7097(1-0.0626)8 + (1-0.0626\times 1.7097)274} = 0.911,$$

$$W_2 = \frac{(17)(59)(0.1132)(1.7097)}{1.7097(1-0.1132)17 + (1-0.1132\times 1.7097)59} = 2.646,$$

$$W_3 = \frac{(39)(122)(0.1275)(1.7097)}{1.7097(1-0.1275)39 + (1-0.1275\times 1.7097)122} = 6.753,$$

$$W_4 = \frac{(58)(32)(0.1445)(1.7097)}{1.7097(1-0.1445)58 + (1-0.1445\times 1.7097)32} = 4.210.$$

Thus, a 95% CI for $\log_e$(RR), using this method, is obtained as

$$\begin{aligned} &\log_e(1.710) \pm 1.96\sqrt{\frac{1}{0.911 + 2.646 + 6.753 + 4.210}} \\ &= 0.536 \pm 1.96\sqrt{0.069} \\ &= (0.021, 1.051), \end{aligned}$$

from which a 95% CI for the RR is given by (1.021, 2.861).

**Mantel-Haenszel method** — As obtained previously, $\hat{\text{RR}}_{\text{MH}} = 1.696$ and $\hat{\text{Var}}\{\log_e(\hat{\text{RR}}_{\text{MH}})\} = 0.067$. Thus, a 95% CI for $\log_e(\text{RR})$, using this method, is obtained as

$$\log_e(1.696) \pm 1.96\sqrt{0.067} = (0.021, 1.036),$$

from which a 95% CI for the RR is given by (1.021, 2.818).

**Test-based method** — To obtain a CI for the RR using the test-based procedure, note that as obtained in Example 6.1, $\chi^2_{\text{MH}} = 4.153$. Therefore, a 95% CI for $\log_e(\text{RR})$ is obtained as

$$\log_e(1.696) \pm 1.96\sqrt{\{\log_e(1.696)\}^2 / 4.153} = (0.021, 1.036),$$

from which a 95% CI for the RR is given by (1.021, 2.818).

### 6.3.2.3 Test for Homogeneity of Risk Ratios

A test for homogeneity of effect over strata in terms of a uniform RR can be carried out by the statistic

$$\sum_{i=1}^{k}\left[\frac{\left[\log_e\left(\hat{\text{RR}}_i\right) - \log_e\left(\hat{\text{RR}}_w\right)\right]^2}{\hat{\text{Var}}\left\{\log_e\left(\hat{\text{RR}}_i\right)\right\}}\right], \tag{6.28}$$

which asymptotically has a chi-square distribution with $k - 1$ degrees of freedom. Note that $\hat{\text{RR}}_i$, $\hat{\text{Var}}\{\log_e(\hat{\text{RR}}_i)\}$, and $\log_e(\hat{\text{RR}}_w)$ are defined by Equations 6.14, 6.15, and 6.16, respectively.

For the data in Example 6.2, test statistic (6.28) is calculated as

$$\frac{(0.701-0.538)^2}{0.9302} + \frac{(0.397-0.538)^2}{0.4005} + \frac{(0.630-0.538)^2}{0.1439} + \frac{(0.435-0.538)^2}{0.2229}$$
$$= 0.185,$$

and from the chi-square table

$$P\left(\chi^2_3 > 0.185\right) = 0.980.$$

Thus, the hypothesis of the homogeneity of RRs for different age and ECG strata cannot be rejected. Hence, we lack evidence that the RRs are different for four strata under consideration.

## 6.3.3. Odds Ratio

Now consider various methods of point and interval estimation of the common OR in a stratified analysis.

### 6.3.3.1 Point Estimation

Consider three methods of point estimation of the common OR in a stratified analysis: logit, Mantel-Haenszel, and the maximum likelihood estimators. In addition, an estimator due to Birch (1964), and its improvement due to Goodman (1969) and some other estimates, are mentioned briefly.

*Logit Estimator*

According to this procedure, the adjusted OR is obtained as the antilog of the pooled (weighted) estimate of the logarithms of the individual ORs calculated at different levels of the confounding factor. The weights are chosen as the inverses of the sampling variances of the logarithms of the ORs. Thus, for the *i*th level of the confounding factor

$$\hat{\mathrm{OR}}_i = \frac{a_i d_i}{b_i c_i} \tag{6.29}$$

and

$$\hat{\mathrm{Var}}\left\{\log_e\left(\hat{\mathrm{OR}}_i\right)\right\} = \frac{1}{a_i} + \frac{1}{b_i} + \frac{1}{c_i} + \frac{1}{d_i}. \tag{6.30}$$

The weighted average of $\log_e(\hat{\mathrm{OR}}_i)$, with the weight $W_i$ determined as the inverse of Equation 6.30, is

$$\log_e\left(\hat{\mathrm{OR}}_{\mathrm{w}}\right) = \frac{\sum_{i=1}^{k} W_i \log_e\left(\hat{\mathrm{OR}}_i\right)}{\sum_{i=1}^{k} W_i}, \tag{6.31}$$

from which the estimated common OR will be obtained as $\exp\{\log_e(\hat{\mathrm{OR}}_{\mathrm{w}})\}$.

Notice that the rationale for the weight $W_i$ is that estimates with small variance have relatively large weight and estimates with large variance have relatively small weight in determining the overall summary OR. As indicated previously, we use the logarithms of the ORs because they introduce approximate normality into the otherwise extremely skewed distribution of the OR. The estimator (Equation 6.31) is also known as Woolf's estimator, following Woolf (1955), who first presented it.

Equation 6.31 makes it clear that the logit estimator cannot be calculated if any cell entry into any one of the strata is zero. As mentioned earlier in the case of a single $2 \times 2$ table, a modification that avoids this problem is based on the work of Haldane (1955) and Anscombe (1956), who showed that a least-biased estimator of the log OR from the $i$th stratum is

$$\log_e\left(\hat{\mathrm{OR}}_i'\right) = \log_e\left[\frac{(a_i + 0.5)(d_i + 0.5)}{(b_i + 0.5)(c_i + 0.5)}\right],$$

which is obtained simply by adding 0.5 to each cell entry in the sample OR formula. Gart (1966) and Gart and Zweifel (1967) suggested a modified logit estimator of the form

$$\log_e\left(\hat{\mathrm{OR}}_{\mathrm{MW}}\right) = \frac{\sum_{i=1}^{k} W_i' \log_e\left(\hat{\mathrm{OR}}_i'\right)}{\sum_{i=1}^{k} W_i'},$$

where

$$W_i' = \left[\frac{1}{(a_i + 0.5)} + \frac{1}{(b_i + 0.5)} + \frac{1}{(c_i + 0.5)} + \frac{1}{(d_i + 0.5)}\right]^{-1}.$$

The modified logit estimator is also known as the empirical logit estimator.

The results of Gart and Zweifel (1967), who studied various estimators of the log odds ratio and estimators of the variance of the log odds ratio estimators, suggested that $(W_i')^{-1}$ is the least-biased estimator of the variance of $\log_e(\hat{\mathrm{OR}}_i')$. Similarly, Walter (1985) pointed out that the addition of 0.5 in all possible tables gives better bias and mean square error properties than if added only as necessary when a zero cell occurs. For the asymptotic case of large sample sizes in each stratum, the logit and the modified logit estimators have the same large sample distribution as the maximum likelihood estimator. In practice the large sample variances are equal, so the logit estimators and the maximum likelihood estimator are equally efficient. However, for the stratified data involving large numbers of strata, each containing only a few cases or controls, the modified logit estimate may be subject to excessive bias and is not recommended for general use (Gart, 1970; McKinlay, 1978).

Finally, a natural method for estimating an overall summary relative risk may be to add the corresponding cell entries of the $k$ tables, obtaining a pooled estimator

$$\hat{\text{OR}}_{\text{P}} = \frac{\left(\sum_{i=1}^{k} a_i\right)\left(\sum_{i=1}^{k} d_i\right)}{\left(\sum_{i=1}^{k} b_i\right)\left(\sum_{i=1}^{k} c_i\right)}.$$

The estimator $\hat{\text{OR}}_{\text{P}}$ is inconsistent, however, and may produce undesirable estimates. The speciousness of this estimator is well known and was illustrated by Cornfield (1956) and Gart (1962).* Note that the logit estimator defined by Equation 6.31 is essentially a weighted geometric mean of the individual OR obtained from each stratum. It is also possible to construct ordinary weighted arithmetic and harmonic means, leading to the estimators

$$\hat{\text{OR}}_{\text{A}} = \frac{\sum_{i=1}^{k} W_i \hat{\text{OR}}_i}{\sum_{i=1}^{k} W_i}$$

and

$$\hat{\text{OR}}_{\text{H}} = \frac{\sum_{i=1}^{k} W_i}{\sum_{i=1}^{k} W_i \left(\frac{1}{\hat{\text{OR}}_i}\right)}.$$

Gart (1962) showed that both these estimators are also asymptotically efficient. Thus, on the basis of their asymptotic properties, one cannot designate any single estimator ($\hat{\text{OR}}_{\text{W}}$, $\hat{\text{OR}}_{\text{A}}$, $\hat{\text{OR}}_{\text{H}}$) as the best. However, the logit estimator has the desirable property of invariance. In other words, if the positives and negatives are interchanged and the corresponding OR is denoted by OR′, then $\hat{\text{OR}}_{\text{W}} = 1/\hat{\text{OR}}'_{\text{W}}$. The same invariance property also holds on their confidence limits.

* This phenomenon is often referred to as *Simpson's paradox*. This occurs when either the magnitude or direction of the association between two variables is influenced by a third factor, which may act as a confounder. By failing to control for its effect, the value of the observed association may appear to be greater than the reality.

*Mantel-Haenszel Estimator*

The most widely used estimator of the common OR, based on stratified $2 \times 2$ tables, is the Mantel-Haenszel (MH) estimator.* This estimator is the weighted average of individual $\hat{OR}_i$, with the weight $W_i$ being equal to $(b_i c_i / n_i)$, which approximates the inverse of $\hat{Var}\{(\hat{OR}_i)\}$ when the true common OR is near 1 (see, e.g., Mantel et al., 1977). Thus, the Mantel-Haenszel estimator of the common OR is obtained as

$$\hat{OR}_{MH} = \frac{\sum_{i=1}^{k}\left(\frac{b_i c_i}{n_i}\right)\left(\frac{a_i d_i}{b_i c_i}\right)}{\sum_{i=1}^{k}\left(\frac{b_i c_i}{n_i}\right)} = \frac{\sum_{i=1}^{k}\left(\frac{a_i d_i}{n_i}\right)}{\sum_{i=1}^{k}\left(\frac{b_i c_i}{n_i}\right)}. \quad (6.32)$$

As indicated above, it can be verified readily that the weights employed in the Mantel-Haenszel estimator are inversely proportional to the variance of the stratum-specific OR under the null condition.** Consequently, $\hat{OR}_{MH}$ is optimally weighted for each stratum-specific OR estimate near 1. The estimator (Equation 6.32) also can be considered as the weighted average of the cross-products upon adjustment for their expectations. The null information divided by null expectation yields $1/n_i$ as the required weight (Miettinen, unpublished). Another interesting property of this estimator, as pointed out by Mantel and Haenszel (1959), is that $\hat{OR}_{MH}$ equals unity only when the Mantel-Haenszel chi-square statistic ($\chi^2_{MH}$), given by Equation 6.12, is zero. This provides a

* Mantel and Haenszel, in their classic 1959 paper, proposed several other summary estimators of the adjusted OR for use in retrospective (case-control) studies.

** It follows that

$$\hat{Var}\left(\hat{OR}_i\right) \simeq \left(\frac{a_i d_i}{b_i c_i}\right)^2 \left(\frac{1}{a_i} + \frac{1}{b_i} + \frac{1}{c_i} + \frac{1}{d_i}\right).$$

If $\hat{OR}_i \simeq 1$, $a_i d_i \simeq b_i c_i$ so that

$$\hat{Var}\left(\hat{OR}_i\right) \simeq \left(\frac{a_i + d_i}{b_i c_i} + \frac{b_i + c_i}{b_i c_i}\right) = \frac{n_i}{b_i c_i}.$$

direct mathematical relationship between the $\hat{OR}_{MH}$ and the $\chi^2_{MH}$ that is not true for other estimators.

Theoretical investigation of the Mantel-Haenszel estimator, with regard to bias and variance, has shown that the estimator compares favorably with the maximum likelihood estimator under a variety of conditions (Breslow and Liang, 1982). In particular, for matched-pair data, $\hat{OR}_{MH}$ is the conditional maximum likelihood estimator of the OR; however, $\hat{OR}_{MH}$ and both conditional and unconditional maximum likelihood estimators of the OR generally differ. In addition, research has shown that the statistical properties of the estimator are similar to those that are based on logistic regression models. Furthermore, whereas the directly pooled estimator requires reasonably large data within each stratum, the Mantel-Haenszel estimator is appropriate even if the data within strata are small. Finally, it may be observed that the estimator is extremely simple to compute and is not affected by the zeroes in the tables.

*Maximum Likelihood Estimator*

The unconditional likelihood (L) function can be written as (Gart, 1962)

$$L = \prod_{i=1}^{k} (p_{1i})^{a_i} (1 - p_{1i})^{b_i} (p_{2i})^{c_i} (1 - p_{2i})^{d_i}, \tag{6.33}$$

where $p_{1i}$ and $p_{2i}$ are probabilities denoting the risk of being positives in the two samples for the $i$th stratum. To obtain the maximum likelihood (ML) estimate of the common OR, the likelihood function L (Equation 6.33) must be maximized with respect to $p_{1i}$ and $p_{2i}$ subject to the condition that $OR_i = OR_j$ for all $i$ and $j$. By the invariance property of the maximum likelihood estimation, the ML estimator of the common OR is then given by

$$\hat{OR}_{ML} = \frac{\hat{p}_{1i}(1 - \hat{p}_{2i})}{\hat{p}_{2i}(1 - \hat{p}_{1i})}, \tag{6.34}$$

where $\hat{p}_{1i}$ and $\hat{p}_{2i}$ are the ML estimators of $p_{1i}$ and $p_{2i}$ for any pairs of stratified samples under the restriction.

The solution to the likelihood equations, however, is quite complicated and leads to a system of $k - 1$ simultaneous third degree equations. Gart (1962) indicates that these equations are the same as those determined by Bartlett (1935) and Norton (1945) in finding the expected values of the entries in the tables prior to computing the chi-square statistics of their tests. Computing software are now generally available to carry out the requisite computation (Thomas, 1975; Martin and Austin, 1991; Thomas and Gart, 1992). Furthermore, the unconditional maximum likelihood approach corresponds to log-linear or logistic regression analysis and any of the standard programs for these models can also be used.

*Conditional Maximum Likelihood Estimator*

Conditional on all marginal totals being fixed for each 2 × 2 table, the maximum likelihood estimate of the OR is obtained by maximizing the joint conditional distribution of the cell entries ($a_1, a_2, \ldots, a_k$) given by Equation 6.50, with respect to the parameter OR. Again, the direct determination of the maximum of the conditional likelihood (Equation 6.50) is quite complex. However, the conditional maximum likelihood estimator of the common OR can be shown to be the solution to the equation (Birch, 1964)

$$\sum_{i=1}^{k} a_i - \sum_{i=1}^{k} E(a_i), \tag{6.35}$$

where

$$E(a_i) = \frac{\sum_{\delta_{1i} \le a_i \le \delta_{2i}} a_i \binom{n_{1i}}{a_i}\binom{n_{2i}}{b_i}(\mathrm{OR})^{a_i}}{\sum_{\delta_{1i} \le j \le \delta_{2i}} \binom{n_{1i}}{j}\binom{n_{2i}}{m_{1i}-j}(\mathrm{OR})^{j}}$$

$$\delta_{1i} = \max(0, m_{1i} - n_{2i}) \tag{6.36}$$

$$\delta_{2i} = \min(n_{1i}, m_{1i})$$

represents the mean of the noncentral hypergeometric distribution.

Thus, the conditional maximum likelihood estimate of the OR requires an iterative solution of Equation 6.35 coupled with Equation 6.36, using the trial and error values for the OR, until Equation 6.35 is satisfied. The computer programs developed by Thomas (1975), Martin and Austin (1991), and Thomas and Gart (1992) can be employed to perform the requisite computations.

An asymptotic solution to the conditional maximum likelihood estimator of the OR, which is much simpler to compute than to use Equation 6.35, can be obtained by noting that for large $n$

$$\hat{E}(a_i) = \hat{a}_i,$$

where $\hat{a}_i$ is the solution to the quadratic equation

$$\frac{\hat{a}_i(n_{2i} - m_{1i} + \hat{a}_i)}{(m_{1i} - \hat{a}_i)(n_{1i} - \hat{a}_i)} = \hat{\mathrm{OR}}, \tag{6.37}$$

such that all the factors and divisors on the left side of Equation 6.37 are positive. Note that Equation 6.37 represents the (unconditional) maximum likelihood solution for the common OR based on 2 × 2 tables (compare to Equation 6.34). Solving Equation 6.37 explicitly for $\hat{a}_i$, one obtains

$$\hat{a}_i = \left|\left[|Q_i| - \sqrt{Q_i^2 - \frac{m_{1i} n_{1i} \hat{\text{OR}}}{\hat{\text{OR}} - 1}}\right]\right|, \quad (6.38)$$

where

$$Q_i = \frac{1}{2}\left(n_{1i} + m_{1i} + \frac{n_i}{\hat{\text{OR}} - 1}\right).$$

The asymptotic conditional maximum likelihood estimate of the common OR is obtained as the solution to the equation

$$\sum_{i=1}^{k} a_i - \sum_{i=1}^{k} \hat{a}_i = 0. \quad (6.39)$$

Thus, the asymptotic conditional maximum likelihood estimate can be obtained as the iterative solution to Equation 6.39 coupled with Equation 6.38, using the trial and error values of the OR, until Equation 6.39 is satisfied. Gart (1971) also gives an iterative procedure (Cornfield, 1956) for obtaining an asymptotic solution to Equation 6.39. The computer programs by Thomas (1975) and Thomas and Gart (1992) also perform these calculations. (The use of Equation 6.39 generally gives similar results, as opposed to the more complex Equation 6.35, except when the average number of subjects per stratum is fairly small.)

*Birch-Goodman Estimators*

For an OR value near unity, a locally good approximation, suggested by Birch (1964) using a method proposed by Cox (1958), to the maximum likelihood estimate is

$$\hat{\text{OR}}_{\text{BH}} = \exp\left[\frac{\sum_{i=1}^{k} \{(a_i d_i) - (b_i c_i)\}/n_i}{\sum_{i=1}^{k} \hat{\text{Var}}(a_i \mid \text{OR} = 1)}\right], \quad (6.40)$$

where

$$\hat{\text{Var}}(a_i \mid \text{OR} = 1) = \frac{m_{1i} m_{2i} n_{1i} n_{2i}}{n_i^2 (n_i - 1)}. \tag{6.41}$$

The estimator (Equation 6.40), however, is not consistent. An improvement of $\hat{\text{OR}}_{\text{BH}}$, which is appropriate when the OR is not close to 1, was discussed by Goodman (1969), but involves complex numerical computations.

*Other Estimators*

Yusuf et al. (1985) and Berlin et al. (1989) discuss a variant of the Mantel-Haenszel estimator of the common odds ratio determined by

$$\exp\left[\frac{\sum_{i=1}^{k} \left(a_i - E(a_i)\right)}{\sum_{i=1}^{k} \text{Var}(a_i)}\right],$$

where $E(a_i)$ and $\text{Var}(a_i)$ are the mean and variance of the hypergeometric distribution obtained under the assumption of the fixed marginals and the null value of the odds ratio (see Appendix J). The estimator should perform well for balanced designs when the odds ratio is near unity. However, the procedure is found to perform rather poorly in case of some unbalanced designs when the odds ratio departs markedly from the null value, and is also shown to be inconsistent (Greenland and Salvan, 1990). Davis (1985) considered a generalization of the Mantel-Haenszel estimator to the situation involving nonconstant odds ratio with covariates. Gastwirth and Greenhouse (1987) developed some analogs of the Mantel-Haenszel and the maximum likelihood estimators of a common odds ratio to analyze hiring data in equal employment cases. Laird and Mosteller (1990) discussed some statistical methods for combining results involving random effects models of odds ratio parameters. Pigeot (1990) proposed a new class of noniterative estimators of a common odds ratio, which, under the usual assumption of independence and homogeity of the odds ratio, leads to asymptotically optimal estimators, that is, estimators which are consistent, asymptotically normal and asymptotically efficient. Similarly, some estimators based on jackknife principle proposed by Quenouille (1949, 1956) and Miller (1974) have been considered by Breslow and Liang (1982) and Pigeot (1991a,b,c). For a comprehensive and theoretical review of various point estimators of a common odds ratio, see Hauck (1987, 1989) and Emerson (1994).

### 6.3.3.2 Confidence Intervals

We now consider methods for constructing CIs using the point estimates based on the logit, Mantel-Haenszel, and maximum likelihood estimators, as well as the test-based method, Cornfield's method, and an exact method. Birch's procedure (1964) and its improvement by Goodman (1969) and some other methods are also briefly outlined.

*Logit Method*

The logit estimator of the logarithm of the common OR is

$$\log_e\left(\hat{\text{OR}}_w\right) = \frac{\sum_{i=1}^{k} W_i \log_e \hat{\text{OR}}_i}{\sum_{i=1}^{k} W_i}.$$

An estimate of the variance of this estimator is

$$\begin{aligned}
\hat{\text{Var}}\left\{\log_e\left(\hat{\text{OR}}_w\right)\right\} &= \frac{\sum_{i=1}^{k} (W_i)^2 \hat{\text{Var}}\left\{\log_e\left(\hat{\text{OR}}_i\right)\right\}}{\left(\sum_{i=1}^{k} W_i\right)^2} \\
&= \frac{\sum_{i=1}^{k} (W_i)^2 \times \frac{1}{W_i}}{\left(\sum_{i=1}^{k} W_i\right)^2} = \frac{\sum_{i=1}^{k} W_i}{\left(\sum_{i=1}^{k} W_i\right)^2} \qquad (6.42) \\
&= \frac{1}{\sum_{i=1}^{k} W_i}.
\end{aligned}$$

Therefore, a $100(1-\alpha)\%$ CI for $\log_e(\text{OR})$ is given by

$$\log_e\left(\hat{\text{OR}}_w\right) \pm Z_{\alpha/2}\sqrt{\left(1\Big/\sum_{i=1}^{k} W_i\right)}, \qquad (6.43)$$

from which a $100(1-\alpha)\%$ CI for the common OR can be obtained by taking antilogarithms of the endpoints of the confidence limits determined by Equation 6.43. The logit method with 1/2 correction factor has been implemented on BMDP Software package (Dixon, 1992).

*Mantel-Haenszel Method*

The Mantel-Haenszel estimator of the common OR is

$$\hat{\text{OR}}_{\text{MH}} = \frac{\sum_{i=1}^{k}\left(\frac{a_i d_i}{n_i}\right)}{\sum_{i=1}^{k}\left(\frac{b_i c_i}{n_i}\right)}. \tag{6.44}$$

Despite the computational simplicity of the $\hat{\text{OR}}_{\text{MH}}$, noted earlier, this estimator has one serious drawback: It has no convenient, simple, and generally useful estimate of its variance.* The most simple estimate, which is still not at all simple, is

$$\hat{\text{Var}}_{\text{MH}}\left\{\log_e\left(\hat{\text{OR}}_{\text{MH}}\right)\right\} = \frac{\sum_{i=1}^{k}\left(\frac{a_i d_i}{n_i}\right)^2\left(\frac{1}{a_i}+\frac{1}{b_i}+\frac{1}{c_i}+\frac{1}{d_i}\right)}{\left(\sum_{i=1}^{k}\frac{a_i d_i}{n_i}\right)^2}. \tag{6.45}$$

This formula was developed under the limiting condition that the number of subjects per stratum becomes large, involving very few strata (Hauck, 1979; Guilbaud, 1983). Ury (1982) proposed a modification of Equation 6.45 that he attributes to Gart, which seems to perform better in small samples. Because $\hat{\text{OR}}_{\text{MH}}$ is consistent as $k$ increases, and the sample size in each table remains constant (Breslow, 1981), this method may be expected to be superior to others with sparse data. Breslow (1981) elaborated another formula assuming fixed marginals and under the limiting condition that the number of strata becomes large, with few subjects per stratum but it is not consistent when the number of strata is fixed. In addition, Breslow and Liang (1982) proposed a symmetric version of Equation 6.45 by weighting the two formulas to derive a combined formula given by

$$\hat{\text{Var}}_{\text{BL}}\left\{\log_e\left(\hat{\text{OR}}_{\text{MH}}\right)\right\} = \tag{6.46}$$

$$\left[\frac{\sum_{i=1}^{k}\left(\frac{a_i d_i}{n_i}\right)^2\left(\frac{1}{a_i}+\frac{1}{b_i}+\frac{1}{c_i}+\frac{1}{d_i}\right)\sum_{i=1}^{k}\left(\frac{b_i c_i}{n_i}\right)^2\left(\frac{1}{a_i}+\frac{1}{b_i}+\frac{1}{c_i}+\frac{1}{d_i}\right)}{\left(\sum_{i=1}^{k}\frac{a_i d_i}{n_i}\right)^2\left(\sum_{i=1}^{k}\frac{b_i c_i}{n_i}\right)^2}\right]^{0.5}.$$

* Mantel and Haenszel (1959) did not give an estimate of the variance.

Equation 6.46 is generally applicable; however, it is not suitable for the case in which a large data set is subdivided into many strata, some containing small frequencies. A method proposed by Robins, Breslow and Greenland (1986) and Robins, Greenland and Breslow (1986) is satisfactory for the above case, as well as cases in which only a few strata exist, none containing small frequencies. The proposed estimator is

$$\hat{\mathrm{Var}}_{\mathrm{RBG}}\left\{\log_e\left(\hat{\mathrm{OR}}_{\mathrm{MH}}\right)\right\} = \frac{\sum_{i=1}^{k} P_i R_i}{2\left(\sum_{i=1}^{k} R_i\right)^2} + \frac{\sum_{i=1}^{k} (P_i S_i + Q_i R_i)}{2\left(\sum_{i=1}^{k} R_i\right)\left(\sum_{i=1}^{k} S_i\right)} + \frac{\sum_{i=1}^{k} Q_i S_i}{2\left(\sum_{i=1}^{k} S_i\right)^2}, \quad (6.47)$$

where

$$P_i = (a_i + d_i)/n_i,$$

$$Q_i = (b_i + c_i)/n_i,$$

$$R_i = (a_i d_i)/n_i,$$

$$S_i = (b_i c_i)/n_i.$$

Using the variance estimators Equations 6.45, 6.46, or 6.47, a 100(1 – α)% CI for $\log_e$(OR) can be obtained as

$$\log_e\left(\hat{\mathrm{OR}}_{\mathrm{MH}}\right) \pm Z_{\alpha/2}\sqrt{\hat{\mathrm{Var}}\left\{\log_e\left(\hat{\mathrm{OR}}_{\mathrm{MH}}\right)\right\}}. \quad (6.48)$$

Mantel-Haenszel confidence limits (Equation 6.48) using the variance formula (Equation 6.47) can be determined by the STATCALC procedure from EpiInfo (1994) and the program EXACT by Martin and Austin (1991). Some recent Monte Carlo work by Mehta and Walsh (1992) indicates that the interval based on variance formula (Equation 6.47) performs well even for very sparse data sets provided the method does not degenerate due to many empty cells.

#### *Maximum Likelihood Method*

Maximum likelihood estimates of the cell entries in the 2 × 2 table can be used to derive an improved estimate of the variance of the logarithm of the OR estimator in each stratum. The improved estimates can be obtained by substituting the estimated values of the cell entries that satisfy Equations 6.36 or 6.38 into the variance formula, Equation 6.30. The new weights can then be used to obtain a variance of the logarithm of the maximum likelihood estimator ($\hat{OR}_{ML}$) using Equation 6.42. An approximate 100(1 – α)% CI for $\log_e$(OR) using this method is given by

$$\log_e\left(\hat{OR}_{ML}\right) \pm Z_{\alpha/2}\sqrt{\hat{Var}\left\{\log_e\left(\hat{OR}_{ML}\right)\right\}}.$$

*Test-Based Method*

As discussed earlier, a 100(1 – α)% CI for $\log_e$(OR) using this method can be obtained as

$$\log_e\left(\hat{OR}_{MH}\right) \pm Z_{\alpha/2}\sqrt{\left\{\log_e\left(\hat{OR}_{MH}\right)\right\}^2 / \chi^2_{MH}}, \tag{6.49}$$

where $\chi^2_{MH}$ is the value of the Mantel-Haenszel chi-square statistic as given by Equation 6.12. A 100(1 – α)% CI for the OR can be written in terms of the standard normal statistic $\chi$ as

$$\left(\hat{OR}_{MH}\right)^{\left(1 \pm Z_{\alpha/2}/\chi\right)}.$$

*Birch-Goodman Methods*

For OR values near unity, Birch (1964) suggested a simple numerical method for calculating the confidence limits:

$$\hat{OR}_{BH} \exp\left\{\pm Z_{\alpha/2}\sqrt{\sum_{i=1}^{k} \hat{Var}\left(a_i \mid OR = 1\right)}\right\},$$

where $\hat{OR}_{BH}$ and $\hat{Var}(a_i | OR = 1)$ are given as in Equations 6.40 and 6.41. Goodman (1969) also suggested similar limits, which require considerably more computation.

*Example 6.3*

Consider the unpublished data from the Israeli Ischemic Heart Disease Study, relating the prevalence of MI and SBP, as given in Kahn and Sempos (1989). The study also was described and discussed by Groen et al. (1968) and Kahn et al. (1971). The relevant data are summarized in Table 6.4.

Suppose Table 6.4 is stratified into two 2 × 2 tables corresponding to two levels of the confounding factor age (≥60, <60), as shown in Table 6.5. The unadjusted OR, without controlling for age, is

**TABLE 6.4**
**Data Showing Relationship between SBP and MI: Unstratified Sample**

| | SBP | | |
|---|---|---|---|
| **MI** | **≥140** | **<140** | **Total** |
| Yes | 29 | 27 | 56 |
| No | 711 | 1244 | 1955 |
| Total | 740 | 1271 | 2011 |

From Kahn, H. A. and Sempos, C. T. (1989). *Statistical Methods in Epidemiology.* Oxford University Press, New York, p. 105. With permission.

$$\hat{OR} = \frac{29 \times 1244}{27 \times 711} = 1.879.$$

We now calculate the adjusted OR using the logit, Mantel-Haenszel, and maximum likelihood estimates.

**Logit estimate** — From the two stratified tables of Table 6.5, we have

$$\hat{OR}_1 = \frac{9 \times 73}{6 \times 115} = 0.952,$$

$$\hat{OR}_2 = \frac{20 \times 1171}{21 \times 596} = 1.871,$$

$$\log_e\left(\hat{OR}_1\right) = -0.049,$$

$$\log_e\left(\hat{OR}_2\right) = 0.627,$$

$$\hat{Var}\left\{\log_e\left(\hat{OR}_1\right)\right\} = \frac{1}{9} + \frac{1}{6} + \frac{1}{115} + \frac{1}{73} = 0.3002,$$

$$\hat{Var}\left\{\log_e\left(\hat{OR}_2\right)\right\} = \frac{1}{20} + \frac{1}{21} + \frac{1}{596} + \frac{1}{1171} = 0.1002,$$

$$W_1 = \frac{1}{0.3002} = 3.331,$$

$$W_2 = \frac{1}{0.1002} = 9.980.$$

**TABLE 6.5**
**Data Showing Relationship between SBP and MI: Stratified by Age**

**Age ≥60**

| MI | SBP ≥140 | SBP <140 | Total |
|---|---|---|---|
| Yes | 9 | 6 | 15 |
| No | 115 | 73 | 188 |
| Total | 124 | 79 | 203 |

**Age <60**

| MI | SBP ≥140 | SBP <140 | Total |
|---|---|---|---|
| Yes | 20 | 21 | 41 |
| No | 596 | 1171 | 1767 |
| Total | 616 | 1192 | 1808 |

From Kahn, H. A. and Sempos, C. T. (1989). *Statistical Methods in Epidemiology*. Oxford University Press, New York, p. 106. With permission.

The adjusted estimate of the logarithm of the common OR, using Equation 6.31, is

$$\log_e\left(\hat{OR}_w\right) = \frac{(3.331)(-0.049) + (9.980)(0.627)}{3.331 + 9.980} = 0.458,$$

from which the estimate of the common OR is

$$\hat{OR}_w = \exp(0.458) = 1.581.$$

**Mantel-Haenszel estimate** — The Mantel-Haenszel estimate of the common OR, using Equation 6.32, is

$$\hat{OR}_{MH} = \frac{\{(9 \times 73)/203\} + \{(20 \times 1171)/1808\}}{\{(115 \times 6)/203\} + \{(596 \times 21)/1808\}} = 1.569.$$

**Maximum likelihood estimate** — The conditional maximum likelihood estimate using a computer program (Thomas and Gart, 1992) is obtained as 1.577.

Thus, instead of estimating the OR relating SBP to MI as 1.879, we estimate it as 1.581 (logit), 1.569 (Mantel-Haenszel), or 1.577 (maximum likelihood) after removing the part of the confounding due to age.

We now compute CIs of the common OR using the logit, Mantel-Haenszel, and test-based methods.

**Logit method** — As determined earlier, $\log_e(\hat{OR}_w) = 0.458$. Using Equation 6.42, one obtains

$$\hat{Var}\left\{\log_e\left(\hat{OR}_w\right)\right\} = \frac{1}{3.331 + 9.980} = 0.075.$$

Thus, a 95% CI for $\log_e(\text{OR})$ using this method is

$$0.458 \pm 1.96\sqrt{0.075} = (-0.079, 0.995),$$

from which a 95% CI for the OR is given by (0.924, 2.705).

**Mantel-Haenszel method** — As determined earlier, $\hat{OR}_{MH} = 1.569$. Using Equation 6.45,

$$\hat{Var}_{MH}\left\{\log_e\left(\hat{OR}_{MH}\right)\right\} = \frac{\left(\frac{9\times 73}{203}\right)^2 (0.3002) + \left(\frac{20\times 1171}{1808}\right)^2 (0.1002)}{\left(\frac{9\times 73}{203} + \frac{20\times 1171}{1808}\right)^2}$$

$$= 0.0761.$$

Thus, a 95% CI for $\log_e(\text{OR})$ is

$$\log_e(1.569) \pm 1.96\sqrt{0.0761} = (-0.090, 0.991),$$

from which a 95% CI for the OR is given by (0.914, 2.694).

Similarly, using Equation 6.46,

$$\hat{\text{Var}}_{\text{BL}}\left\{\log_e\left(\hat{\text{OR}}_{\text{MH}}\right)\right\} = \left[\left\{\frac{\left(\frac{9\times 73}{203}\right)^2(0.3002)+\left(\frac{20\times 1171}{1808}\right)^2(0.1002)}{\left(\frac{9\times 73}{203}+\frac{20\times 1171}{1808}\right)^2}\right\}\right.$$

$$\left.\times\left\{\frac{\left(\frac{6\times 115}{203}\right)^2(0.3002)+\left(\frac{21\times 596}{1808}\right)^2(0.1002)}{\left(\frac{6\times 115}{203}+\frac{21\times 596}{1808}\right)^2}\right\}\right]^{0.5}$$

$$= (0.0761\times 0.0776)^{0.5}$$

$$= 0.0769,$$

which yields a 95% CI for the OR of (0.910, 2:702). Finally, in order to use Equation 6.47, the various terms needed to calculate this variance are

$$P_1 = 0.4039,\ R_1 = 3.2365,\ Q_1 = 0.5961,\ S_1 = 3.3990$$

$$P_2 = 0.6587,\ R_2 = 12.9535,\ Q_2 = 0.3413,\ S_2 = 6.9226$$

leading to

$$\hat{\text{Var}}_{\text{RBG}}\left\{\log_e\left(\hat{\text{OR}}_{\text{MH}}\right)\right\} = \frac{9.8397}{2(16.1900)^2}+\frac{12.2831}{2(16.1900)(10.3216)}+\frac{4.3888}{2(10.3216)^2}$$

$$= 0.0762,$$

which yields a 95% CI for the OR of (0.913, 2.695). Note that for this example, all the variance formulas lead to nearly the same result.

**Test-based method** — To determine the CI via the test-based method, note that by using Equation 6.12 for the stratified data in Table 6.5, one obtains

$$\chi^2_{\text{MH}} = \frac{\left[(9+20)-\left\{\left(\frac{15\times 124}{203}\right)+\left(\frac{41\times 616}{1808}\right)\right\}\right]^2}{\frac{124\times 79\times 15\times 188}{(203)^2(203-1)}+\frac{616\times 1192\times 41\times 1767}{(1808)^2(1808-1)}}$$

$$= 2.794.$$

Thus, a 95% CI for $\log_e(\text{OR})$ is

$$\log_e(1.569) \pm 1.96\sqrt{\{\log_e(1.569)\}^2/2.794} = (-0.078, 0.979),$$

from which a 95% CI for the OR is given by (0.925, 2.662).

Note that in this example, the logit, the Mantel-Haenszel, and the test-based methods give CIs which are quite close. Note also that these values were calculated for strata containing cell frequencies as small as 6 and 9. For large data sets, one would expect much closer agreement.

We now describe two additional methods of computing CIs which, although computationally complex, provide accurate limits, especially in small to moderately sized samples.

*An Exact Method*

Similar to the case of the single 2 × 2 table considered in Section 4.1.2.2, the probability of obtaining the cell entries $(a_1, a_2, ..., a_k)$ in a set of $k$ 2 × 2 tables, which is conditional on the marginal totals for each of the $k$ 2 × 2 tables and the common OR, is given by (see, e.g., Cox, 1966; Gart, 1970; Lehmann, 1986; Santner and Duffy, 1989)

$$\boldsymbol{P}(a_1, a_2, ..., a_k \mid \text{OR}) = \prod_{i=1}^{k} \frac{\binom{n_{1i}}{a_i}\binom{n_{2i}}{b_i}(\text{OR})^{a_i}}{\sum_{\delta_{1i} \le j \le \delta_{2i}} \binom{n_{1i}}{j}\binom{n_{2i}}{m_{1i} - j}(\text{OR})^j},$$

$$\delta_{1i} = \max(0, m_{1i} - n_{2i}) \qquad (6.50)$$

$$\delta_{2i} = \min(n_{1i}, m_{1i})$$

where $a_i = 0, 1, ..., \min(n_{1i}, m_{1i})$ $(i = 1, ..., k)$. As originally noted by Fisher (1935), this distribution is known as extended (noncentral) hypergeometric distribution (see e.g., Harkness, 1965). When OR = 1, the probability expression (Equation 6.50) reduces to the product of $k$ hypergeometric distributions (Cox, 1966; Gart, 1970) and forms the basis for the Fisher's exact test of the hypothesis of no association in k 2 × 2 tables.

The tail probabilities for exact confidence limits can be obtained by evaluating the sum of the probabilities determined in Equation 6.50 for all possible values of $\sum_{i=1}^{k} a_i$ equal to or greater than the actual value observed, and for all possible combination of cell frequencies that yield a given value of $\sum_{i=1}^{k} a_i$. Thus, the lower confidence limit of a $100(1 - \alpha)\%$ CI is the value of the OR ($\text{OR}_\text{L}$) such that it yields an upper tail probability of $\alpha/2$:

$$\sum_{\substack{\text{all combinations} \\ \sum_{i=1}^{k} a_i \geq \text{observed}}} P\left(a_1, a_2, \ldots, a_k \mid \text{OR} = \text{OR}_\text{L}\right) = \alpha/2. \tag{6.51}$$

Similarly, the upper confidence limit is obtained by summing over all values of $\sum_{i=1}^{k} a_i$ that are less than or equal to the observed value, and for all combinations of cell frequencies that yield a given value for $\sum_{i=1}^{k} a_i$. Thus, the upper confidence limit is the value of the OR ($\text{OR}_\text{U}$) such that it yields a lower tailed probability of $\alpha/2$:

$$\sum_{\substack{\text{all combinations} \\ \sum_{i=1}^{k} a_i \leq \text{observed}}} P\left(a_1, a_2, \ldots, a_k \mid \text{OR} = \text{OR}_\text{U}\right) = \alpha/2. \tag{6.52}$$

Note in Equations 6.51 and 6.52 that the summation extends to the set of all $k$-fold partitions of $\sum_{i=1}^{k} a_i$ such that $\sum_{i=1}^{k} a_i \geq a$ ($\leq a$), where $a$ is the observed value.

Equations 6.51 and 6.52 are solved through trial and error for $\text{OR}_\text{L}$ and $\text{OR}_\text{U}$.* As remarked earlier, the task of solving these equations numerically is exceedingly complex. For details on numerical algorithms and computer programs, see Thomas (1975), Pagano and Tritchler (1983), Mehta et al. (1985), EGRET (1991), Martin and Austin (1991), Vollset and Hirji (1991), Vollset et al. (1991), Thomas and Gart (1992), Granville and Schifflers (1993), EpiInfo (1994), Hirji and Vollset (1994), and StatXact (1995).

When $n_{1i} = n_{2i} = 1$, the matched pair case, the exact confidence limits can be found from tables of the binomial distribution (see Section 7.1.1.3). Similarly, when $n_{1i} = 1$ and $n_{2i} = M$, the multiple controls matched per case, both exact and approximate confidence limits can be developed as in Section 7.2.2.2.

### *Cornfield's Method*

Approximate confidence limits, analogous to Cornfield's method for a single $2 \times 2$ table, may be determined from the asymptotic results (Gart, 1970, 1971). As in the case of a single $2 \times 2$ table, for large $n_i$, $a_i$ is normally distributed with asymptotic mean and variance given by

$$\hat{E}\left(a_i \mid \text{OR}\right) = \hat{a}_i \tag{6.53}$$

* The use of the term *exact* is a misnomer. Because of the discrete nature of the noncentral hypergeometric distribution, the actual confidence level of $1 - \alpha'$, where $\alpha' < \alpha$, is obtained rather than a prespecified confidence coefficient of exactly $1 - \alpha$. The results are *exact* in the sense that the confidence coefficient is at least $1 - \alpha$. Thus, these intervals are usually very conservative. For a discussion of mid-*p* CIs, which usually reduce the conservativeness, see Appendix I.

and

$$\hat{\text{Var}}(a_i \mid \text{OR}) = \left[\frac{1}{\hat{a}_i} + \frac{1}{m_{1i} - \hat{a}_i} + \frac{1}{n_{1i} - \hat{a}_i} + \frac{1}{n_{2i} - m_{1i} + \hat{a}_i}\right]^{-1}, \tag{6.54}$$

where $\hat{a}_i$ is the appropriate solution to the quadratic equation

$$\frac{\hat{a}_i(n_{2i} - m_{1i} + \hat{a}_i)}{(m_{1i} - \hat{a}_i)(n_{1i} - \hat{a}_i)} = \text{OR}, \tag{6.55}$$

determined in such a way that they yield positive numbers for all the factors and divisors on the left side of Equation 6.55, in other words, all the estimated entries in the $2 \times 2$ tables in Table 6.2. It follows *a fortori* that the distribution of $\sum_{i=1}^{k} a_i$ is asymptotically normal with asymptotic mean and variance given by

$$\hat{E}\left(\sum_{i=1}^{k} a_i \mid \text{OR}\right) = \sum_{i=1}^{k} \hat{E}(a_i \mid \text{OR}) \tag{6.56}$$

and

$$\hat{\text{Var}}\left(\sum_{i=1}^{k} a_i \mid \text{OR}\right) = \sum_{i=1}^{k} \hat{\text{Var}}(a_i \mid \text{OR}). \tag{6.57}$$

Thus, for any positive value of the OR, one can determine the asymptotic mean and variance of $\sum_{i=1}^{k} a_i$ by solving a set of $k$ quadratic equations such as Equation 6.55. For a large value of $k$ and small values of $n_{1i}$ and $n_{2i}$, the asymptotic normality of $\sum_{i=1}^{k} a_i$, follows from Liapounov's form of the central limit theorem (see Cramér, 1946); however, in such a case the exact mean and variance must be determined (see Gart, 1970).

The approximate lower and upper limits of the OR, $\text{OR}_\text{L}$ and $\text{OR}_\text{U}$, are determined as solutions to the equations

$$\frac{\sum_{i=1}^{k} a_i - \hat{E}\left(\sum_{i=1}^{k} a_i \mid \text{OR}_\text{L}\right) - 0.5}{\sqrt{\hat{\text{Var}}\left(\sum_{i=1}^{k} a_i \mid \text{OR}_\text{L}\right)}} = Z_{\alpha/2} \tag{6.58}$$

and

$$\frac{\sum_{i=1}^{k} a_i - \hat{E}\left(\sum_{i=1}^{k} a_i \,\middle|\, \mathrm{OR_U}\right) + 0.5}{\sqrt{\hat{\mathrm{Var}}\left(\sum_{i=1}^{k} a_i \,\middle|\, \mathrm{OR_U}\right)}} = -Z_{\alpha/2}, \tag{6.59}$$

where $Z_{\alpha/2}$ is the upper $100(\alpha/2)$th percentile of the standard normal distribution. Substituting the values of $\hat{E}(\sum_{i=1}^{k} a_i \mid \mathrm{OR})$ and $\hat{\mathrm{Var}}(\sum_{i=1}^{k} a_i \mid \mathrm{OR})$ for OR = $\mathrm{OR_L}$ and OR = $\mathrm{OR_U}$, from Equations 6.56 and 6.57, into Equations 6.58 and 6.59, one obtains

$$\frac{\sum_{i=1}^{k} a_i - \sum_{i=1}^{k} \hat{a}_{\mathrm{L}i} - 0.5}{\sqrt{\sum_{i=1}^{k}\left[\frac{1}{\hat{a}_{\mathrm{L}i}} + \frac{1}{m_{1i} - \hat{a}_{\mathrm{L}i}} + \frac{1}{n_{1i} - \hat{a}_{\mathrm{L}i}} + \frac{1}{n_{2i} - m_{1i} + \hat{a}_{\mathrm{L}i}}\right]^{-1}}} = Z_{\alpha\,2} \tag{6.60}$$

and

$$\frac{\sum_{i=1}^{k} a_i - \sum_{i=1}^{k} \hat{a}_{\mathrm{U}i} + 0.5}{\sqrt{\sum_{i=1}^{k}\left[\frac{1}{\hat{a}_{\mathrm{U}i}} + \frac{1}{m_{1i} - \hat{a}_{\mathrm{U}i}} + \frac{1}{n_{1i} - \hat{a}_{\mathrm{U}i}} + \frac{1}{n_{2i} - m_{1i} + \hat{a}_{\mathrm{U}i}}\right]^{-1}}} = -Z_{\alpha\,2}, \tag{6.61}$$

where $\hat{a}_{\mathrm{L}i}$ and $\hat{a}_{\mathrm{U}i}$ represent the values of the solution to Equation 6.55, which correspond to the lower and upper confidence limits of the OR rather than of the point estimate.

Equations 6.60 and 6.61 must be solved iteratively coupled with Equation 6.55, using the trial and error values, until the equations are satisfied. For each limit, it is necessary to solve $k$ quadratic equations of the form of Equation 6.55 by trial and error. Cornfield's limits may be determined using the STATCALC procedure from EpiInfo (1994) and the programs of Thomas (1975), Martin and Austin (1991), and Thomas and Gart (1992).

*Example 6.4*

Consider the case-control study reported by Rothman (1982) and discussed further by Rothman (1986) in examining the association between spermicide

**TABLE 6.6**
**Data Showing the Distribution of Infants with CHD and DS, and Healthy Controls According to MSUBC: Stratified by Maternal Age**

| | Maternal age | | | | | | | | |
|---|---|---|---|---|---|---|---|---|---|
| | <35 | | | ≥35 | | | Totals | | |
| | MSUBC | | | MSUBC | | | MSUBC | | |
| | + | – | Total | + | – | Total | + | – | Total |
| DS | 3 | 9 | 12 | 1 | 3 | 4 | 4 | 12 | 16 |
| Controls | 104 | 1059 | 1163 | 5 | 86 | 91 | 109 | 1145 | 1254 |
| Total | 107 | 1068 | 1175 | 6 | 89 | 95 | 113 | 1157 | 1270 |

From Rothman, K. J. (1982). *Am. J. Pub. Health,* 72, 399–401. With permission.

use near the time of conception and the risk of Down's syndrome. The data in Table 6.6 show the distribution of infants with congenital heart disease (CHD) and Down's syndrome (DS) and healthy controls according to maternal spermicide use before conception (MSUBC) and by maternal age at the time of delivery. We outline the computation of the common OR using an exact method and Cornfield's method.

**Exact method** — Note that Table 6.6 contains four exposed cases, three in the age group <35 and one in the age group ≥35. In the first age group the number of exposed cases can vary from 0 to 12, assuming fixed marginals. In the second age group the number of exposed cases can vary from 0 to 4. Thus, a total of 13 × 5 = 65 exposure outcomes exist for the two strata. Of a total of 65 possible outcomes, we have 50 outcomes with $\sum_{i=1}^{2} a_i > 4$ and 5 outcomes with $\sum_{i=1}^{2} = 4$. These 55 equally or more extreme outcomes than that actually observed are shown in Table 6.7. The lower and upper 95% confidence limits for the OR ($OR_L$, $OR_U$) are obtained by trial and error such that the contributions to the tail probabilities equal 0.025 in each tail via Equations 6.51 and 6.52. The resulting 95% confidence limits using a computer program (Thomas and Gart, 1992) are $OR_L = 0.863$ and $OR_U = 12.875$.

**Cornfield's method** — To obtain a 90% CI according to this method, we set up Equations 6.55, 6.60, and 6.61 for the data in Table 6.6 with $Z_{\alpha/2} = 1.64$. The trial and error solution to Equation 6.60, coupled with Equation 6.55, yields $a_{L1} = 1.542$ and $a_{L2} = 0.356$. Similarly, the trial and error solution to Equation 6.61, coupled with Equation 6.55, yields $a_{U1} = 5.772$ and $a_{U2} = 1.370$. The resulting 90% confidence limits for the OR are $OR_L = 1.480$ and $OR_U = 9.724$. The corresponding 95% confidence limits using a computer program (Thomas and Gart, 1992) are $OR_L = 0.999$ and $OR_U = 13.140$.

### *Other Methods*

Several other approaches to asymptotic intervals have appeared in the literature. Of particular interest is the score statistic and the first principle interval

**TABLE 6.7**
**Arrangement of All Possible Combinations of Exposed Cases by Age Group, with at Least 4 Exposed Cases, for the Data of Table 6.6**

| Total no. exposed Cases | Distrib. of exposed cases by age group | Total no. exposed cases | Distrib. of exposed cases by age group | Total no. exposed cases | Distrib. of exposed cases by age group |
|---|---|---|---|---|---|
| 16 | 12–4 | 10 | 10–0 | 6 | 6–0 |
| 15 | 12–3 | 10 | 9–1 | 6 | 5–1 |
| 15 | 11–4 | 10 | 8–2 | 6 | 4–2 |
| 14 | 12–2 | 10 | 7–3 | 6 | 3–3 |
| 14 | 11–3 | 10 | 6–4 | 6 | 2–4 |
| 14 | 10–4 | 9 | 9–0 | 5 | 5–0 |
| 13 | 12–1 | 9 | 8–1 | 5 | 4–1 |
| 13 | 11–2 | 9 | 7–2 | 5 | 3–2 |
| 13 | 10–3 | 9 | 6–3 | 5 | 2–3 |
| 13 | 9–4 | 9 | 5–4 | 5 | 1–4 |
| 12 | 12–0 | 8 | 8–0 | 4 | 4–0 |
| 12 | 11–1 | 8 | 7–1 | 4 | 3–1 |
| 12 | 10–2 | 8 | 6–2 | 4 | 2–2 |
| 12 | 9–3 | 8 | 5–3 | 4 | 1–3 |
| 12 | 8–4 | 8 | 4–4 | 4 | 0–4 |
| 11 | 11–0 | 7 | 7–0 | | |
| 11 | 10–1 | 7 | 6–1 | | |
| 11 | 9–2 | 7 | 5–2 | | |
| 11 | 8–3 | 7 | 4–3 | | |
| 11 | 7–4 | 7 | 3–4 | | |

From Rothman, K. J. (1986). *Modern Epidemiology.* Little, Brown, Boston, p. 206. With permission.

based on its chi-square function (see Miettinen, 1985; Miettinen and Nurminen, 1985). Similarly, Mantel (1977) and McKinlay (1978) proposed alternative approaches to determining approximate CIs which in large samples should give results equivalent to those obtained by the Mantel-Haenszel method.

The interval proposed by Mantel (1977) is similar to that of the Cornfield except that it uses the exact hypergeometric mean and variance instead of the asymptotic values as employed in the Cornfield's interval. Thus, Mantel's method is applicable in both asymptotic cases: fixed-number-of-strata as well as increasing-number-of-strata, while Cornfield's method is applicable in the fixed-number-of-strata case only. Similarly, Levin (1984) proposed some improvements to Cornfield's interval, which have been discussed further by Gart (1987). Flanders (1985) and Phillips and Hall (1987) discuss some alternative approaches to variance estimation of the Mantel-Haenszel odds ratio and log odds ratio estimators. Sato (1990) proposed a new method for confidence interval which is based on the asymptotic distribution of the Mantel-Haenszel estimator rather than its logarithmic transformation. The method has been shown to be valid for both sparse and abundant data situations, and compares favorably with the Robins, Breslow and Greenland procedure determined by (6.48). More recently, Pigeot (1991a) has described an approach based on a jackknife estimator of a common odds ratio. For a discussion of an 'exact' confidence interval which incorporates the mid-p adjustment, see Appendix I. For a comprehensive and theoretical review of various interval estimators for a common odds ratio, see Hauck (1987, 1989) and Emerson (1994).

#### 6.3.3.3 Test for Homogeneity of Odds Ratios

An estimate of the common OR in a series of $2 \times 2$ tables is generally valid only when the measures of association between risk factor and disease outcome are the same for all tables (no interaction). Then a single summary OR serves as an accurate estimate of that association. Thus, before computing the adjusted OR and its CI, it may be worthwhile to test for the presence of interaction. In general, in a stratified analysis, the hypothesis of no interaction is

$$H_0 : \mathrm{OR}_1 = \mathrm{OR}_2 = \cdots = \mathrm{OR}_k \text{ vs.}$$

$$H_1 : \mathrm{OR}_i \neq \mathrm{OR}_j \text{ (for at least one } (i, j), i \neq j),$$

which can be tested by

$$\sum_{i=1}^{k} \left[ \frac{\left\{\log_e\left(\hat{\mathrm{OR}}_i\right) - \log_e\left(\hat{\mathrm{OR}}_w\right)\right\}^2}{\hat{\mathrm{Var}}\left\{\log_e\left(\hat{\mathrm{OR}}_i\right)\right\}} \right]. \tag{6.62}$$

The statistic (6.62) asymptotically has a chi-square distribution with $k - 1$ degrees of freedom (Woolf, 1955). Note that $\log_e\left(\hat{\mathrm{OR}}_w\right)$ is the logit estimator, as defined in Equation 6.31.

For the data in Example 6.3, test statistic (6.62) is calculated as

$$\frac{(-0.049 - 0.458)^2}{0.3002} + \frac{(0.627 - 0.458)^2}{0.1002} = 1.141,$$

and, from the chi-square table,

$$P\left(\chi_1^2 > 1.141\right) = 0.285.$$

Thus, the hypothesis of the homogeneity of the ORs for different age groups cannot be rejected. Hence, evidence that the ORs are different for two age groups under consideration is lacking.

The test described above is commonly known as the Woolf's test for homogeneity, which uses a large sample chi-square approximation. Because the exact test of homogeneity (Zelen, 1971) is computationally complex, the most common homogeneity tests use critical regions based on asymptotic distribution theory. The other homogeneity tests commonly encountered in the literature are the likelihood ratio test (Fienberg, 1985), Pearson chi-square test (Zelen, 1971; Halperin et al. 1977), Breslow-Day test (Breslow and Day, 1980), a modified Breslow-Day test (Tarone, 1985), and the two conditional score tests, especially designed for the "sparse data" situation (Liang and Self, 1985). More recently, Levin (1992) considered some tests of homogeneity with improved power in sparse tables. Below is a brief description of the Breslow-Day test, which has been recommended for general use and may be readily calculated with the assistance of a handheld calculator, although not as easily as with Woolf's test.

The Breslow-Day statistic is defined as

$$\sum_{i=1}^{k} \frac{(a_i - \hat{a}_i)^2}{\hat{\text{Var}}(\hat{a}_i)}, \tag{6.63}$$

where

$$\hat{a}_i = \left\| \left[ |Q_i| - \sqrt{Q_i^2 - \frac{m_{1i} n_{1i} \hat{\text{OR}}}{\hat{\text{OR}} - 1}} \right] \right\|^{-1}, \tag{6.64}$$

$$\hat{\text{Var}}(\hat{a}_i) = \left[ \frac{1}{\hat{a}_i} + \frac{1}{m_{1i} - \hat{a}_i} + \frac{1}{n_{1i} - \hat{a}_i} + \frac{1}{n_{2i} - m_{1i} - \hat{a}_i} \right],$$

$$Q_i = \frac{1}{2}\left( n_{1i} + m_{1i} + \frac{n_i}{\hat{\text{OR}} - 1} \right), \tag{6.65}$$

and $\hat{\text{OR}}$ is an estimate of the common OR obtained by any one of the estimation procedures described previously. The statistic (6.63) has asymptotically a chi-square distribution with $k - 1$ degrees of freedom. Using the logit estimator $\hat{\text{OR}}_W = 1.581$ in Equations 6.64 and 6.65, the resulting values of $\hat{a}_i$ and $\hat{\text{Var}}(\hat{a}_i)$ for the data in Example 6.3 are $\hat{a}_1 = 10.593$, $\hat{\text{Var}}(\hat{a}_1) = 2.911$, $\hat{a}_2 = 18.324$, and $\hat{\text{Var}}(\hat{a}_2) = 9.881$. Finally, the value of test statistic (6.63) is calculated as 1.156, which gives a value similar to that obtained by the Woolf's method.

Odoroff (1970) presented some Monte Carlo results on small sample properties of the Woolf's test, as well as comparisons with several alternative tests. Jones et al. (1989) studied the effect of increasing stratification on the size and power of the above-mentioned tests using Monte Carlo simulation. Five of the seven statistics studied by Jones et al. are for 'large-stratum' setting. One of the 'large-stratum' statistics is the Pearson chi-square test of the null hypothesis of homogeneity of odds ratios and one other is the score statistic by Breslow and Day. Jones et al. (1989) reported that for 'non-sparse' data setting the Pearson chi-square test performs best in terms of power, although, considering both size and power, they recommended Breslow-Day test for general use. In sparse data settings, when all tables regardless of the sample size have ORs generated from the same distribution, the first score test of Liang and Self seems to perform best. In sparse data settings, with a large table having an OR of 1 and many small tables with ORs >1, the second score test was found to work best. In general, the study found that all homogeneity tests have rather low power, especially when the data are sparse. Paul and Donner (1989) performed a simulation study to compare the performance of two likelihood ratio tests, six score tests and a test based on logit estimator of the common odds ratio. These tests also apply to the asymptotic situation in which the number of strata is fixed, but the sample size within each stratum becomes increasingly large. Based on their relative performance in terms of size and power, they recommended approximate score test by Tarone (1985) based on the Mantel-Haenszel estimator of the common odds ratio for general use. For very large samples in balanced or mildly unbalanced designs, they also recommended a noniterative test by Gart (1966) based on the modified logit estimator of the common odds ratio. In addition, Paul and Donner (1992) reported a simulation study to compare the small sample performance, in terms of size of the statistics applicable to 'large-stratum' setting. They found that as long as the stratum sample size is at least 10, all test statistics had similar performance in terms of maintaining the nominal level. They recommended the use of Breslow-Day test because of its computational simplicity. The exact test of homogeneity and some other asymptotic tests can be performed using EGRET (1994) and StatXact (1995) software. The Breslow-Day test was implemented in SAS-PC, and the program EXACT by Martin and Austin (1991) performs the likelihood ratio test. Tests of homogeneity of odds ratios under multiple matching have been considered by Ejigou and McHugh (1984), Liang and Self (1985), Zelterman and Le (1991) and Levin (1992).

One may want to compare ORs calculated from different strata in terms of their ratios. A large sample $100(1-\alpha)\%$ CI for $\log_e(\mathrm{OR}_i/\mathrm{OR}_j)$, $i,j = 1,2,\ldots,k$, can be determined by

$$\log_e\left(\hat{\mathrm{OR}}_i/\hat{\mathrm{OR}}_j\right) \pm Z_{\alpha/2}\sqrt{\hat{\mathrm{Var}}\left\{\log_e\left(\hat{\mathrm{OR}}_i\right)\right\} + \hat{\mathrm{Var}}\left\{\log_e\left(\hat{\mathrm{OR}}_j\right)\right\}}, \qquad (6.66)$$

where $\hat{\text{Var}}\{\log_e(\hat{\text{OR}}_i)\}$ and $\hat{\text{Var}}\{\log_e(\hat{\text{OR}}_j)\}$ are defined by Equation 6.30. The CI for the ratio $\text{OR}_i/\text{OR}_j$ is determined by taking the antilogarithms of the corresponding endpoints of Equation 6.66. Goodman (1964) proposed methods for determining simultaneous CIs for a set of ratios $\text{OR}_i/\text{OR}_j$, and Hilbron (1981) considered methods for adjusting for confounding.

#### 6.3.3.4 A Comparison of Estimators of Odds Ratios

Using a simulation study, McKinlay (1978) compared several estimators of the overall OR in a stratified analysis and found that all the estimators, other than the Mantel-Haenszel estimator, were sensitive to the assumption of uniformity of the OR across all strata. He noted further that the Mantel-Haenszel estimator was preferable even when the OR was constant across all strata. In terms of asymptotic properties, the logit, unconditional maximum likelihood, and the Birch estimators were found to have the same asymptotic variances. The asymptotic efficiency of the Mantel-Haenszel estimator under the null condition was demonstrated by Hauck (1979). The asymptotic results mentioned above were derived under the assumption that the number of strata remains fixed, but the number of observations within each stratum increases without bound. Breslow (1981) investigated the asymptotic behavior of the estimators under the assumption that the number of strata becomes large, but the number of observations within each stratum is small. The results of his study showed that the Mantel-Haenszel and the conditional maximum likelihood estimators were both consistent, but neither the logit (with 1/2 correction factor) nor the asymptotic unconditional ML estimates converged to the true OR. The unconditional ML produced considerably biased estimates when the number of subjects in each stratum was fairly small. For the extreme situation involving only one case and one control in each stratum, as the number of strata increased, the unconditional ML estimate approached the square of that value, rather than the true value of the OR. However, when the number of strata is small relative to the number of cases and controls, the bias is negligible. For a wide range of OR values and exposure probabilities among the control group, the MH estimator was found to be nearly fully efficient; its asymptotic variance was larger than that of the conditional ML by >10% only infrequently. In general, the conditional ML was found to be no less biased nor any more precise than the MH.

Some additional studies by Tarone et al. (1983) and Hauck and Donner (1988) corroborate the finding that the MH estimator is not fully asymptotically efficient when the odds ratio differs from the null value. However, the Monte Carlo results by Donner and Hauck (1986) and Hauck and Donner (1988) indicate that the MH estimator has very high asymptotic efficiency both for the case when the number of strata is fixed and when it becomes large. Further, the studies by Liang (1985) and Donald and Donner (1990) show that the MH estimator remains consistent and asymptotically normal even when the assumption of independent trials is violated. In addition, results by McKinlay

(1978), Breslow (1981) and Tarone, Gart and Hauck (1983) point out that although the logit estimator performs well for the small number of strata with large data counts, the estimator is not competitive with the MH estimator for the increasing strata situation. Additional theoretical and empirical work by Liang (1985) points out that although the conditional ML estimator is consistent and asymptotically normal, the estimator is sensitive to the assumption of independent trials. For this situation, the ML estimator remains consistent, but the conditional ML estimator fails to converge to the true odds ratio. For results of various finite sample simulation studies comparing the estimators with respect to bias and mean squared error (MSE) criterion, see Hitchcock (1962), McKinlay (1975), Breslow and Liang (1982), Hauck, Anderson and Leahy (1982) and O'Gorman et al. (1988). More recently, in a series of papers, Pigeot (1991a,b,c) has carried out simulation studies to compare some jackknife estimators with the logit and the MH estimators concerning their bias, variance, MSE, and the asymptotic relative efficiency (ARE). The results indicate that the logit estimator has better MSE properties whereas the MH estimator behaves better concerning the bias than the MSE. Further, the MH estimator showed very good results concerning ARE and the results are relatively insensitive to the increasing number of strata. In general, the results are similar to those obtained in earlier studies.

## 6.4 MEASURES OF PREVALENCE

For cross-sectional studies, it is usually of interest to compute a single prevalence difference (PD), prevalence ratio (PR), or prevalence odds ratio (POR) across strata of a confounding variate so as to simplify the presentation of results. Similar to the case of RD, RR, and OR, a combined estimate of summary measures of effect for prevalence and associated CIs can be obtained by computing a weighted average of the PDs, PRs, or PORs in which the weights are inverses of the variances of the stratum-specific prevalence estimates. Similarly, one can obtain Mantel-Haenszel and maximum likelihood type estimates and associated CIs of the summary PD, PR, or POR. The discussion of all the results parallels the discussion presented earlier and is not repeated here.

# References

**Anscombe, F. J.** (1956). "On Estimating Binomial Response Relations", *Biometrika,* 43, 461–464.

**Bartlett, M. S.** (1935). "Contingency Table Interactions", *J. R. Stat. Soc.,* B, 11, 248–252.

**Berlin, J. A., Laird, N. M., Sacks, H. S., and Chalmers, T. C.** (1989). "A Comparison of Statistical Methods for Combining Event Rates from Clinical Trials", *Stat. Med.,* 8, 141–151.

**Birch, M. W.** (1964). "The Detection of Partial Association, I: The 2 × 2 Case", *J. R. Stat. Soc.,* B, 26, 313–324.

**Breslow, N. E.** (1981). "Odds Ratio Estimators When the Data Are Sparse", *Biometrika,* 68, 73–84.

**Breslow, N. E. and Day, N. E.** (1980). *Statistical Methods in Cancer Research, Vol. 1: The Analysis of Case-Control Studies.* International Agency for Research on Cancer, Lyons, France.

**Breslow, N. E. and Liang, K. Y.** (1982). "The Variance of the Mantel-Haenszel Estimator", *Biometrics,* 38, 943–952 (errata, *ibid.,* 1984, 40, 1217).

**Cornfield, J.** (1956). "A Statistical Problem Arising from Retrospective Studies", In: *Proc. 3rd Berkeley Symp. Mathematical Statistics and Probability* (Ed. J. Neyman). pp. 135–148. University of California Press, Berkeley.

**Cox, D. R.** (1958). "The Regression Analysis of Binary Sequence (with Discussion)", *J. R. Stat. Soc.,* B, 20, 215–242.

**Cox, D. R.** (1966). "A Simple Example of a Comparison Involving Quantal Data", *Biometrika,* 53, 215–220.

**Cox, D. R. and Snell, E. J.** (1989). *The Analysis of Binary Data,* 2nd ed. Chapman & Hall, London.

**Cramér, H.** (1946). *Mathematical Methods of Statistics.* Princeton University Press, Princeton, NJ.

**Davis, L. J.** (1985). "Generalization of the Mantel-Haenzel Estimator to Nonconstant Odds Ratios", *Biometrics,* 41, 487–495.

**Dixon, W. J.** (1992). *BMDP Statistical Software,* Vol. 1. University of California Press, Los Angeles, pp. 281–282.

**Donald, A. and Donner A.** (1990). "A Stimulation Study of the Analysis of Sets of 2 × 2 Contingency Tables Under Cluster Sampling: Estimation of a Common Odds Ratio", *J. Am. Stat. Assoc.,* 85, 537–543.

**Donner, A. and Hauck, W. W.** (1986). "The Large Sample Relative Efficiency of the Mantel-Haenszel Estimator in the Fixed-Strata Case", *Biometrics,* 42, 537–545.

**EGRET** (1994). EGRET: State of the Art Epidemiologic Computing. Statistics and Epidemiology Research Corporation, Seattle, WA.

**Ejigou, A. and McHugh, R.** (1984). "Testing the Homogeneity of Relative Risk Under Multiple Matching", *Biometrika,* 71, 408–411.

**Emerson, J. D.** (1994). "Combining Estimates of the Odds Ratio: The State of the Art", *Stat. Methods Med. Res.,* 3, 135–156.

**EpiInfo** (1994). EpiInfo, Version 6. USD, Inc., Stone Mountain, GA.

**Fienberg, S. E.** (1985). *The Analysis of Cross-Classified Categorical Data,* 2nd ed. MIT Press, Cambridge, MA.

**Fisher, R. A.** (1935). "The Logic of Inductive Inference", *J. Roy. Stat. Soc.,* A, 98, 39–54.

**Flanders, W. D.** (1985). "A New Variance Estimator for the Mantel-Haenszel Odds Ratio", *Biometrics,* 41, 637–642.

**Gart, J. J.** (1962). "On the Combination of Relative Risks", *Biometrics,* 18, 601–610.

**Gart, J. J.** (1966). "Alternative Analyses of Contingency Tables", *J. R. Stat. Soc.,* B, 28, 164–169.

**Gart, J. J.** (1970). "Point and Interval Estimation of the Common Odds Ratio in the Combination of $2 \times 2$ Tables with Fixed Marginals", *Biometrika,* 57, 471–475.

**Gart, J. J.** (1971). "The Comparison of Proportions: A Review of Significance Tests, Confidence Intervals, and Adjustments for Stratification", *Rev. Int. Stat. Inst.,* 39, 148–169 (errata, *ibid.,* 1972, 40, 221).

**Gart, J. J.** (1987). "The Equivalence of Two Corrections to the Approximate Mean of an Entry in a Contingency Table", *Biometrika,* 74, 661–663.

**Gart, J. J. and Zwiefel, J. R.** (1967). "On the Bias of Various Estimators of the Logit and Its Variance, with Application to Quantal Bioassay", *Biometrika,* 54, 181–187.

**Gastwirth, J. L. and Greenhouse, S. W.** (1987). "Estimating a Common Relative Risk: Application in Equal Employment", *J. Am. Stat. Assoc.,* 82, 38–45.

**Goodman, L. A.** (1964). "Simple Methods for Analyzing Three-Factor Interaction in Contingency Tables", *J. Am. Stat. Assoc.,* 59, 319–332.

**Goodman, L. A.** (1969). "On Partitioning $\chi^2$ and Detecting Partial Association in Three-Way Contingency Tables", *J. R. Stat. Soc.,* B, 31, 486–498.

**Granville, V. and Schifflers, E.** (1993). "Efficient Algorithms for Exact Inference in $2 \times 2$ Contingency Tables", *Stat. Comput.,* 3, 83–87.

**Greenland, S. and Robins, J. M.** (1985). "Estimation of a Common Effect Parameter from Sparse Follow-Up Data", *Biometrics,* 41, 55–68.

**Greenland, S. and Salvan, A.** (1990). "Bias in the One-Step Method for Pooling Study Results", *Stat. Med.,* 9, 247–251.

**Groen, J. J., Medalie, J. H., Neufeld, H. N., Riss, E., Bachrach, C. A., Mount, F. W., and Smith, H.** (1968). "An Epidemiologic Investigation of Hypertension and Ischemic Heart Disease Within a Defined Segment of the Adult Male Population of Israel", *Isr. J. Med. Sci.,* 4, 177–194.

**Guilbaud, O.** (1983). "On the Large-Sample Distribution of the Mantel-Haenszel Odds-Ratio Estimator", *Biometrics,* 39, 523–525.

**Haldane, J. B. S.** (1955). "The Estimation and Significance of the Logarithm of a Ratio of Frequencies", *Ann. Human Gen.,* 20, 309–311.

**Halperin, M., Ware, J. H., Byar, D. P., Mantel, N., Brown, C. C., Koziol, J., Gail, M., and Green, S. B.** (1977). "Testing for Interaction in an $I \times J \times K$ Contingency Table", *Biometrika,* 64, 271–275.

**Harkness, W. L.** (1965). "Properties of the Extended Hypergeometric Distribution", *Ann. Math. Stat.,* 36, 938–945.

**Hauck, W. W.** (1979). "The Large-Sample Variance of the Mantel-Haenszel Estimator of a Common Odds Ratio", *Biometrics,* 35, 817–820.

**Hauck, W. W.** (1987). "Estimation of a Common Odds Ratio", In: *Biostatistics, Advances in the Statistical Sciences.* Vol. 5. pp. 125–150. (Eds. J. B. MacNeil and G. J. Umphrey). D. Reidel, Boston.

**Hauck, W. W.** (1989). "Odds Ratio Interference from Stratified Samples", *Comm. Stat. Theory Method,* 18, 767–800.

**Hauck, W. W. and Donner, A.** (1988). "The Asymptotic Relative Efficiency of the Mantel-Haenszel Estimator in the Increasing-Number-of-Strata Case", *Biometrics,* 44, 379–384.

**Hauck, W. W., Anderson, S., and Leahy, F. J., III** (1982). "Finite Sample Properties of Some Old and Some New Estimators of a Common Odds Ratio from Multiple 2 × 2 Tables", *J. Am. Stat. Assoc.,* 77, 145–152.

**Hilbron, D. C.** (1981). "The Analysis of Odds Ratios in Stratified Contingency Tables", *Biometrics,* 37, 55–66.

**Hirji, K. F. and Vollset, S. E.** (1994). "Computing Exact Distributions for Several 2 × 2 Tables", *Appl. Stat.,* 43, 270–274 (Algorithm AS 289).

**Hitchcock, S. E.** (1962). "A Note on the Estimation of the Parameters of the Logistic Function, Using the Minimum Logit $\chi^2$ Method", *Biometrika,* 49, 250–252.

**Jones, M. P., O'Gorman, T. W., Lemke, J. H., and Woolson, R. F.** (1989). "A Monte Carlo Investigation of Homogeneity Tests of the Odds Ratio Under Various Sample Size Configurations", *Biometrics,* 45, 171–181.

**Kahn, H. A. and Sempos, C. T.** (1989). *Statistical Methods in Epidemiology.* Oxford University Press, New York.

**Kahn, H. A., Herman, J. B., Medalie, M. D., Newfeld, H. N., Riss, E., and Goldboart, V.** (1971). "Factors Related to Diabetes Incidence: A Multivariate Analysis of Two Years Observation on 10,000 Men: The Israel Ischemic Heart Disease Study", *J. Chronic Dis.,* 23, 617–629.

**Kleinbaum, D. G., Kupper, L. L., and Morgenstern, H.** (1982). *Epidemiologic Research: Principles and Quantitative Methods.* Lifetime Learning Publications, Belmont, CA.

**Kleinbaum, D. G., Kupper, L. L., and Muller, K. E.** (1988). *Applied Regression Analysis and Other Multivariate Methods.* PWS-Kent Publishing Company, Boston.

**Laird, N. M. and Mosteller, F.** (1990). "Some Statistical Methods for Combining Experimental Results", *Int. J. Technol. Assessment Health Care,* 6, 5–30.

**Lehmann, E. L.** (1959, 1986). *Testing Statistical Hypotheses,* 1st and 2nd eds. John Wiley & Sons, New York.

**Levin, B.** (1984). "Simple Improvements of Cornfield's Approximation to the Mean of a Noncentral Hypergeometric Random Variable", *Biometrika,* 71, 630–642.

**Levin, B.** (1992). "Tests of Odds Ratio Homogeneity With Improved Power in Sparse Fourfold Tables", *Commun. Stat. Theory Method,* 21, 1469–1500.

**Liang, K. Y.** (1985). "Odds Ratio Inference with Dependent Data", *Biometrika,* 72, 678–682.

**Liang, K. Y. and Self, S. G.** (1985). "Tests for Homogeneity of Odds Ratio When the Data Are Sparse", *Biometrika,* 72, 353–358.

**Mantel, N.** (1977). "Tests and Limits for the Common Odds Ratio of Several 2 × 2 Contingency Tables: Methods in Analogy with the Mantel-Haenszel Procedure", *J. Stat. Planning Inference,* 1, 179–189.

**Mantel, N., Brown, C. C., and Byar, D. P.** (1977). "Tests for Homogeneity of Effect in an Epidemiologic Investigation", *Am. J. Epidemiol.,* 106, 125–129.

**Mantel, N. and Haenszel, W. M.** (1959). "Statistical Aspects of the Analysis of Data from Retrospective Studies of Disease", *J. Nat. Cancer Inst.*, 22, 719–748.

**Martin, D. and Austin, H.** (1991). "An Efficient Program for Computing Conditional Maximum-Likelihood Estimates and Exact Confidence Limits for a Common Odds Ratio", *Epidemiology,* 2, 359–362.

**McKinlay, S. M.** (1975). "The Effects of Bias on Estimators of Relative Risk for Pair-Matched and Stratified Samples", *J. Am. Stat. Assoc.,* 70, 859–864.

**McKinlay, S. M.** (1978). "The Effect of Nonzero Second-Order Interaction on Combined Estimators of the Odds Ratio", *Biometrika,* 65, 191–202.

**Mehta, C. R., Patel, N. R., and Gray, R.** (1985). "Computing an Exact Confidence Interval for the Common Odds Ratio in Several 2 × 2 Contingency Tables", *J. Am. Stat. Assoc.,* 80, 969–973.

**Mehta, C. R. and Walsh, S. J.** (1992). "Comparison of Exact, mid-*P,* and Mantel-Haenszel Confidence Intervals for the Common Odds Ratio Across Several 2 × 2 Contingency Tables", *Am. Stat.,* 46, 146–150.

**Miettinen, O. S.** (1975). Principles of Epidemiologic Research, unpublished course text, Department of Epidemiology and Biostatistics, School of Public Health, Harvard University, Cambridge, MA.

**Miettinen, O. S.** (1976). "Estimability and Estimation in Case-Referent Studies", *Am. J. Epidemiol.,* 103, 226–235.

**Miettinen, O. S.** (1985). *Theoretical Epidemiology: Principles of Occurrence Research in Medicine.* John Wiley & Sons, New York.

**Miettinen, O. S. and Nurminen, M.** (1985). "Comparative Analysis of Two Rates", *Stat. Med.,* 4, 213–226.

**Miller, R. G.** (1974). "The Jackknife — A Review", *Biometrika,* 61, 1–15.

**Norton, H. W.** (1945). "Calculation of Chi-Square for Complex Contingency Tables", *J. Am. Stat. Assoc.,* 40, 251–258.

**Nurminen, M.** (1981). "Asymptotic Efficiency of General Noniterative Estimators of Common Relative Risk", *Biometrika,* 68, 525–530.

**Odoroff, C. L.** (1970). "A Comparison of Minimum Logit Chi-Square Estimation and Maximum Likelihood Estimation in 2 × 2 × 2 and 3 × 2 × 2 Contingency Tables: Tests of Interaction", *J. Am. Stat. Assoc.,* 65, 1617–1631.

**O'Gorman, T. W., Woolson, R. F., Jones, M. P., and Lemke, J. H.** (1988). "A Monte Carlo Study of Three Odds Ratio Estimators and Four Tests of Association in Several 2 × 2 Tables when the Data Are Sparse", *Commun. Stat. Simulat. Comput.,* B, 17, 813–835.

**Pagano, M. and Tritchler, D.** (1983). "Algorithm for the Analysis of Several 2 × 2 Contingency Tables", *SIAM J. Sci. Stat. Comput.,* 4, 302–309.

**Paul, S. R. and Donner, A.** (1989). "A Comparison of Tests of Homogeneity of Odds Ratio in K 2 × 2 Tables", *Stat. Med.,* 11, 159–165.

**Paul, S. R. and Donner, A.** (1992). "Small Sample Performance of Tests of Homogeneity of Odds Ratio in K 2 × 2 Tables", *Stat. Med.,* 11, 159–165.

**Paul, S. R. and Donner, A.** (1989). "A Comparison of Tests of Homogeneity of Odds Ratio in K 2 × 2 Tables", *Stat. Med.,* 11, 159–165.

**Paul, S. R. and Donner, A.** (1992). "Small Sample Performance of Tests of Homogeneity of Odds Ratio in K 2 × 2 Tables", *Stat. Med.,* 11, 159–165.

**Phillips, A. and Holland, P. W.** (1987). "Estimators of the Variance of the Mantel-Haenszel Log-Odds-Ratio Estimate", *Biometrics,* 43, 425–431.

**Pigeot, I.** (1990). "A Class of Asymptotically Efficient Noniterative Estimators of a Common Odds Ratio", *Biometrika,* 77, 420–423.

**Pigeot, I.** (1991a). "A Jackknife Estimator of a Combined Odds Ratio", *Biometrics,* 47, 373–381.

**Pigeot, I.** (1991b). "A Simulation Study of Estimators of a Common Odds Ratio in Several 2 × 2 Tables", *J. Stat. Comut. Simul.,* 38, 65–82.

**Pigeot, I.** (1991c). "Asymptotic Relative Efficiency of Some Jackknife Estimators of a Common Odds Ratio", *Biometrical J.,* 33, 305–316.

**Quenouille, M. H.** (1949). "Approximate Tests of Correlation in Time Series", *J. Roy. Stat. Soc.* B, 11, 68–84.

**Quenouille, M. H.** (1956). "Notes on Bias in Estimation", *Biometrika,* 43, 353–360.

**Robins, J., Breslow, N. E., and Greenland, S.** (1986). "Estimation of the Mantel-Haenszel Variance Consistent in Both Sparse-Data and Large-Strata Limiting Models", *Biometrics,* 42, 311–324.

**Robins, J., Greenland, S., and Breslow, N. E.** (1986). "A General Estimator for the Variance of the Mantel-Haenszel Odds Ratio", *Am. J. Epidemiol.,* 124, 719–723.

**Rothman, K. J.** (1982). "Spermicide Use and Down's Syndrome", *Am. J. Publ. Health,* 72, 399–401.

**Rothman, K. J.** (1986). *Modern Epidemiology.* Little, Brown, Boston.

**Rothman, K. J. and Boice, J. D.** (1982). *Epidemiologic Analysis with a Programmable Calculator, New Edition.* Epidemiology Resources, Chestnut Hill, MA (first edition published by the U.S. Government Printing Office, Washington, D.C., NIH Publ. No. 79–1649, 1979).

**Santner, T. J. and Duffy, D. E.** (1989). *The Statistical Analysis of Discrete Data.* Springer-Verlag, New York.

**Sato, T.** (1990) "Confidence Limits for the Common Odds Ratio Based on the Asymptotic Distribution of the Mantel-Haenszel Estimator", *Biometrics,* 46, 71–80.

**Schlesselman, J. J.** (1982). *Case-Control Studies.* Oxford University Press, New York.

**StatXact,** (1995). A Statistical Package for Exact Nonparametric Inference, Version 3. Cytel Software Corporation, Cambridge, MA.

**Tarone, R. E.** (1981). "On Summary Estimators of Relative Risk", *J. Chronic Dis.,* 34, 463–468.

**Tarone, R. E.** (1985). "On Heterogeneity Tests Based on Efficient Scores", *Biometrika,* 72, 91–95.

**Tarone, R. E., Gart, J. J., and Hauck, W. W.** (1983). "On the Asymptotic Inefficiency of Certain Noniterative Estimators of a Common Relative Risk or Odds Ratio", *Biometrika,* 70, 519–522.

**Thomas, D. G.** (1975). "Exact and Asymptotic Methods for the Combination of 2 × 2 Tables", *Comput. Biomed. Res.,* 8, 423–446.

**Thomas, D. G. and Gart, J. J.** (1992). "Improved and Extended Exact and Asymptotic Methods for the Combination of 2 × 2 Tables, Version 2", *Comput. Biomed. Res.,* 25, 75–84.

**Vollset, S. E., Hirji, K. F., and Elashoff, R. M.** (1991). "Fast Computation of Exact Confidence Limits for the Common Odds Ratio in a Series of 2 × 2 Tables", *J. Am. Stat. Assoc.,* 86, 404–409.

**Walter, S. D.** (1985). "Small Sample Estimation of Log Odds Ratios from Logistic Regression and Fourfold Tables", *Stat. Med.,* 4, 437–444.

**Wolfram, S.** (1991). *Mathematica: A System for Doing Mathematics by Computers,* 2nd ed. Addison-Wesley, Reading, MA.

**Woolf, B.** (1955). "On Estimating the Relation between Blood Group and Disease", *Ann. Human Gen.,* 19, 251–253.

**Yusuf, S., Peto, R., Lewis, J., Collins, R., and Sleight, P.** (1985). "Beta Blockade During and After Myocardial Infarction: An Overview of the Randomized Trials", *Prog. Cardiovasc. Dis.,* 27, 335–371.

**Zelen, M.** (1971). "The Analysis of Several 2 × 2 Contingency Tables", *Biometrika,* 58, 129–137.

**Zelterman, D. and Le, C. T.** (1991). "Tests of Homogeneity for the Relative Risk in Multiply-Matched Case-Control Studies", *Biometrics,* 47, 751–755.

# 7 Matching

Matching refers to the process of selecting subjects so that a study group and a comparison group — cases and controls in a retrospective study and exposed and unexposed individuals in a cohort study — are similar or nearly similar with respect to extraneous variables that may act as confounders. A number of variables such as age, sex, occupation, and so forth, can be employed as a basis for matching. Matching can be individual matching, in which study and comparison subjects are paired on the basis of matching variables, or frequency matching, in which frequency distribution of matched variables is similar in study and comparison groups. (For a complete discussion of the principles of matching and its advantages and disadvantages see one of the books on epidemiologic methods, e.g., Kleinbaum et al., 1982; Schlesselman, 1982; Kelsey et al., 1986; Rothman, 1986; and Kahn and Sempos, 1989.) It should be noted that matched analysis is essentially a stratified analysis.

## 7.1 MATCHED-PAIR ANALYSIS

Another method of removing confounding effects is by matching each case with one or more randomly chosen controls, accounting for confounding variable(s). Consider the data of the Israeli Ischemic Heart Disease Study, described in Chapter 6, in which 56 cases of myocardial infarction (MI) are now matched with 56 controls of the same age as the case. Suppose that the data relating systolic blood pressure (SBP) to MI are organized as shown in Table 7.1.

Table 7.1 relates to single persons, 56 cases and 56 controls. Note that this type of representation would have been appropriate if the subjects in the case and control groups were selected independently. However, in this case they are not independent because each case-control pair is of similar age (and perhaps other characteristics as well). The correct representation of Table 7.1, relating 56 pairs of case-controls to the risk factor, is shown in Table 7.2.

In Table 7.1 persons are taken as the basic unit of analysis; one then has the sample size of 112 persons. In Table 7.2, the matched pairs are taken as the basic unit of analysis where each pair shows as to whether the case or control was exposed to the risk. Notice that now there are 56 units in the table rather than 112 as in the earlier case. Also note that in Table 7.2 there are 15 pairs for which both cases and controls were exposed to the risk, 17 pairs for which both cases and controls were unexposed, 13 pairs for which cases were exposed but

**TABLE 7.1**
**Relationship of SBP and MI: Matched-Pair Data Shown as Independent Samples**

| | SBP | | |
|---|---|---|---|
| **MI** | **≥140** | **<140** | **Total** |
| Yes | 28 | 28 | 56 |
| No | 26 | 30 | 56 |
| Total | 54 | 58 | 112 |

From Kahn, H. A. and Sempos, C. T. (1989). *Statistical Methods in Epidemiology,* Oxford University, New York, p. 109. With permission.

**TABLE 7.2**
**Relationship of SBP and MI: Matched-Pair Data Shown as Dependent Samples**

| | | Controls | | |
|---|---|---|---|---|
| | | SBP | | |
| | **SBP** | **≥140** | **<140** | **Total** |
| **Cases** | ≥140 | 15 | 13 | 28 |
| | <140 | 11 | 17 | 28 |
| | Total | 26 | 30 | 56 |

From Kahn, H. A. and Sempos, C. T. (1989). *Statistical Methods in Epidemiology,* Oxford University, New York, p. 109. With permission.

controls were unexposed, and 11 pairs for which controls were exposed but cases were unexposed. Also, we notice that for 32 pairs of persons, the cases and controls were in the same SBP category (concordant pair: a matched pair within the same category, i.e., where the outcomes are the same for each member of the pair), while for 24 pairs of persons the cases and controls are in a different SBP category (discordant pair: a matched pair within different categories, i.e., where the outcomes are different for each member of the pair).

The concordant pairs usually provide no useful information regarding differences between cases and controls, and thus are not used in the calculation of the measures of association and inferences regarding them.

### 7.1.1 Estimation of the Odds Ratio

We now consider the problem of point and interval estimation of the odds ratio (OR) in a matched-pair analysis. When a single control is matched to each case individually, then considering each pair as a separate stratum, there are only

**TABLE 7.3**
**A 2 × 2 Display of a Single Matched-Pair Stratified According to Exposure Status and Disease Outcome of Case and Control**

| | Risk factor | | | Risk factor | | | Risk factor | | | Risk factor | | |
|---|---|---|---|---|---|---|---|---|---|---|---|---|
| | + | – | Total | + | – | Total | + | – | Total | + | – | Total |
| Case | 1 | 0 | 1 | 1 | 0 | 1 | 0 | 1 | 1 | 0 | 1 | 1 |
| Control | 1 | 0 | 1 | 0 | 1 | 1 | 1 | 0 | 1 | 0 | 1 | 1 |
| Total | 2 | 0 | 2 | 1 | 1 | 2 | 1 | 1 | 2 | 0 | 2 | 2 |

**TABLE 7.4**
**A 2 × 2 Display of Sample Data in a Matched-Pair Study**

| | | Controls | | |
|---|---|---|---|---|
| | | Risk factor | | |
| | Risk factor | + | – | Total |
| Cases | + | $f$ | $g$ | $f+g$ |
| | – | $h$ | $j$ | $h+j$ |
| | Total | $f+h$ | $g+j$ | $n$ |

two subjects in each stratum. For dichotomous exposure, only four strata of exposure patterns are possible for each pair of case and control, as depicted in Table 7.3.

Note that when the exposure pattern is the same for the case and control, the marginal total for the other exposure outcome is zero in the corresponding 2 × 2 table. Thus, the first and the last of the 2 × 2 tables have a zero marginal total and consequently do not contribute in making statistical inference from the data. Combining these 2 × 2 tables from the $n$-matched pairs, the data from a matched case-control study can be exhibited as in Table 7.4, where $f$ is the number of pairs with both case and control exposed, $g$ is the number of pairs with case exposed and control unexposed, $h$ is the number of pairs with case unexposed and control exposed, and $j$ is the number of pairs with both case and control unexposed.

From Table 7.4 it can be observed that $f$ and $j$ represent the number of concordant pairs and give no useful information regarding differences between cases and controls. Thus, McNemar (1947) proposed that any inference regarding a difference in proportions, derived from matched-pair data, be made solely on the basis of discordant pairs $g$ and $h$. Cox (1958) and Kraus

(1960) proposed the same conditional form of statistical inference for the estimation of the OR.

#### 7.1.1.1 Point Estimation

We consider two estimators of the OR, the Mantel-Haenszel and the maximum likelihood estimators.

*Mantel-Haenszel Estimator*

The Mantel-Haenszel estimator can be obtained by applying Equation 6.32 for the common OR in a stratified analysis to matched pair data in which each pair is treated as a separate stratum. Note that $n_i = 2$ for all $2 \times 2$ tables in Table 7.3 and for the $i$th pair each $2 \times 2$ table of the first and last types (concordant pairs) gives

$$a_i d_i = 0 = b_i c_i,$$

and each $2 \times 2$ table of the second and third types (discordant pairs) gives

$$\text{(Second)} \quad a_i d_i = 1, \; b_i c_i = 0$$

$$\text{(Third)} \quad a_i d_i = 0, \; b_i c_i = 1$$

Therefore, on applying Equation 6.32, the Mantel-Haenszel estimator of the OR ( $\hat{\text{OR}}_{\text{MH}}$) is given by

$$\hat{\text{OR}}_{\text{MH}} = \frac{f \times 0 + g(1/2) + h \times 0 + j \times 0}{f \times 0 + g \times 0 + h \times (1/2) + j \times 0} = \frac{g}{h}. \tag{7.1}$$

*Maximum Likelihood Estimator*

One can obtain the maximum likelihood (ML) estimator of the OR conditional on the number of discordant pairs. Let $p$ be the probability that the discordant pair has an exposed case. In a matched-pair analysis the OR relating the discordant pair with exposed case to the exposed control is given by $p/(1-p)$. To determine the ML estimator of the OR, note that $g$ can be treated as a binomial random variable with a probability of success $p$ = OR/(OR + 1) and the number of trials equal to $g + h$. The ML estimator is derived by maximizing the likelihood function $f$(OR) or its logarithm:

$$f(\text{OR}) = \binom{g+h}{g} \left( \frac{\text{OR}}{\text{OR}+1} \right)^g \left( \frac{1}{\text{OR}+1} \right)^h$$

and

$$\log_e\{f(\text{OR})\} = \log_e\left\{\binom{g+h}{g}\right\} + g\log_e\left\{\frac{\text{OR}}{\text{OR}+1}\right\} + h\log_e\left\{\frac{1}{\text{OR}+1}\right\}.$$

Taking the first derivative of $\log_e\{f(\text{OR})\}$ and equating it to zero gives

$$\frac{d\log_e\{f(\text{OR})\}}{d(\text{OR})} = g - (\text{OR})h = 0. \tag{7.2}$$

Solving Equation 7.2 for the OR, one obtains

$$\hat{\text{OR}}_{\text{ML}} = g/h, \tag{7.3}$$

which yields the conditional ML estimator because

$$\frac{d^2\log_e\{f(\text{OR})\}}{d(\text{OR})^2} = -h < 0.$$

The Mantel-Haenszel formula for calculating the OR in a stratified analysis, applied to the matched-pair data in which each pair is treated as a separate stratum, also results in the ratio $g/h$ as the estimate of the OR. Thus, the Mantel-Haenszel and the maximum likelihood estimates for the OR of the matched-pair data are equivalent. The result was first pointed out by Cornfield and Haenszel (1960). The estimator (7.1) was originally given by Kraus (1958) and Mantel and Haenszel (1959) developed it via a method of stratified analysis. Miettinen (1970) obtained it using the conditional likelihood approach. Cox (1970) and Gart (1971) considered it in the framework of a linear logistic model. Ejigou and McHugh (1977) presented a derivation based on maximization of an unconditional likelihood function.

#### 7.1.1.2 McNemar and Mantel-Haenszel Chi-Square Tests

A test of the hypothesis that the OR is 1 can be carried out by treating $g$ as a binomial random variable with sample size $g + h$. An exact conditional test can be determined using binomial probability calculation. A large sample test can be carried out by treating

$$Z = \frac{g - 0.5(g+h)}{0.5\sqrt{g+h}} \tag{7.4}$$

as a standardized normal deviate.

A continuity correction may be applied by reducing the absolute value of $g - 0.5\,(g + h)$ in Equation 7.4 by 0.5. Thus, an alternate expression of Equation 7.4, with continuity correction included, is

$$Z^2 = \frac{\left(|g-h|-1\right)^2}{g+h},$$

where $Z^2$ may be treated as a chi-square variate with one degree of freedom. This test is known as McNemar's chi-square test.

It can further be shown that for matched pairs, the Mantel-Haenszel chi-square statistic (Equation 6.12) simplifies to

$$\chi^2_{\text{MH}} = \frac{(g-h)^2}{(g+h)}. \tag{7.5}$$

Thus, the statistic $Z^2$ (without continuity correction) is equivalent to the Mantel-Haenszel chi-square.

#### 7.1.1.3 Confidence Intervals

This section develops formulas for confidence intervals (CIs) of the OR using methods based on binomial proportion, maximum likelihood estimate, and the test-based approach.

*An Exact Binomial Method*

An exact CI for the OR, in a matched-pair analysis, can be obtained using a method based on a CI for the binomial proportion. Thus, let $p$ be the proportion of the binomial random variable $g$ with sample size $g + h$. A pair of $100(1 - \alpha)\%$ exact confidence limits for $p$ ($p_{\text{L}}$ and $p_{\text{U}}$) are the solutions to the equations (see, e.g., Sahai and Khurshid, 1996)

$$\sum_{k=g}^{g+h} \binom{g+h}{k} p_{\text{L}}^k \left(1-p_{\text{L}}\right)^{g+h-k} = \alpha/2 \tag{7.6}$$

and

$$\sum_{k=0}^{g} \binom{g+h}{k} p_{\text{U}}^k \left(1-p_{\text{U}}\right)^{g+h-k} = \alpha/2. \tag{7.7}$$

Equivalently, $100(1 - \alpha)\%$ exact confidence limits for the OR ($\text{OR}_{\text{L}}$ and $\text{OR}_{\text{U}}$) can be obtained by noting that $p = \text{OR}/(1 + \text{OR})$. Thus, Equations 7.6 and 7.7 can be written as

$$\sum_{k=g}^{g+h}\binom{g+h}{k}\left(\frac{\mathrm{OR_L}}{1+\mathrm{OR_L}}\right)^k\left(\frac{1}{1+\mathrm{OR_L}}\right)^{g+h-k}=\alpha/2 \tag{7.8}$$

and

$$\sum_{k=0}^{g}\binom{g+h}{k}\left(\frac{\mathrm{OR_U}}{1+\mathrm{OR_U}}\right)^k\left(\frac{1}{1+\mathrm{OR_U}}\right)^{g+h-k}=\alpha/2. \tag{7.9}$$

Equations 7.6 and 7.7, or equivalently, Equations 7.8 and 7.9, are somewhat cumbersome to solve. The detailed procedure for solving these equations is discussed in Sahai and Khurshid (1996). Alternatively, Equations 7.6 and 7.7 can be solved by using the relationship (see, e.g., Evans et al., 1993)

$$\sum_{k=0}^{x}\binom{n}{k}p^k(1-p)^{n-k}=\boldsymbol{P}\left\{\boldsymbol{F}_{\nu_1,\nu_2}>\frac{p}{1-p}\,\frac{n-x}{x+1}\right\}, \tag{7.10}$$

where $\boldsymbol{F}_{\nu_1,\nu_2}$ is a random variable having a variance ratio $\boldsymbol{F}$-distribution with $\nu_1 = 2(x + 1)$ and $\nu_2 = 2(n - x)$ degrees of freedom.

Using relationship 7.10 in Equations 7.6 and 7.7, the solutions to Equations 7.6 and 7.7 are more conveniently expressed in terms of the percentiles of the $\boldsymbol{F}$-distribution (see e.g., Sahai and Khurshid, 1996), i.e.,

$$p_\mathrm{L}=\frac{g}{g+(h+1)\boldsymbol{F}_{\alpha/2,2(h+1),2g}} \tag{7.11}$$

and

$$p_\mathrm{U}=\frac{(g+1)\boldsymbol{F}_{\alpha/2,2(g+1),2h}}{h+(g+1)\boldsymbol{F}_{\alpha/2,2(g+1),2h}}, \tag{7.12}$$

where $\boldsymbol{F}_{\gamma,m_1,m_2}$ is defined by the relationship

$$\boldsymbol{P}\left\{\boldsymbol{F}_{m_1,m_2}>\boldsymbol{F}_{\gamma,m_1,m_2}\right\}=\gamma. \tag{7.13}$$

Similarly, the solutions to Equations 7.8 and 7.9 can be written as

$$\mathrm{OR_L}=g\Big/\left[(h+1)\boldsymbol{F}_{\alpha/2,2(h+1),2g}\right] \tag{7.14}$$

and

$$\mathrm{OR}_{\mathrm{U}} = \left[(g+1)/h\right] \boldsymbol{F}_{\alpha/2,2(g+1),2h}. \tag{7.15}$$

### *An Approximate Binomial Method*

An approximate CI for the OR in a matched-pair analysis can be obtained using the large sample approximation of the binomial distribution. Thus, one can determine the large sample confidence limits for the probability that a discordant pair has an exposed case and then convert these confidence limits to the corresponding limits for the OR.

The large sample $100(1 - \alpha)\%$ approximate confidence limits for the binomial parameter $p$ with the number of Bernoulli trials $n$ are determined by

$$\hat{p} \pm Z_{\alpha/2}\sqrt{\frac{\hat{p}(1-\hat{p})}{n}}, \tag{7.16}$$

where $Z_{\alpha/2}$ is the upper $100(\alpha/2)$th percentile of the standard normal distribution. For matched case-control pairs, $n = g + h$ and $\hat{p} = g/(g + h)$ lead to the confidence limits for $p$ as

$$\frac{g}{(g+h)} \pm Z_{\alpha/2}\sqrt{\frac{gh}{(g+h)^2}}. \tag{7.17}$$

The corresponding $100(1 - \alpha)\%$ approximate confidence limits for the OR ($\mathrm{OR}_{\mathrm{L}}$ and $\mathrm{OR}_{\mathrm{U}}$) are then obtained as

$$\mathrm{OR}_{\mathrm{L}} = \frac{\dfrac{g}{(g+h)} - Z_{\alpha/2}\sqrt{\dfrac{gh}{(g+h)^3}}}{1 - \dfrac{g}{(g+h)} + Z_{\alpha 2}\sqrt{\dfrac{gh}{(g+h)^3}}} \tag{7.18}$$

and

$$\mathrm{OR}_{\mathrm{U}} = \frac{\dfrac{g}{(g+h)} + Z_{\alpha/2}\sqrt{\dfrac{gh}{(g+h)^3}}}{1 - \dfrac{g}{(g+h)} - Z_{\alpha 2}\sqrt{\dfrac{gh}{(g+h)^3}}}. \tag{7.19}$$

The approximate confidence limits (Equations 7.18 and 7.19) are fairly simple to calculate, but produce inaccurate results, unless the number of discordant pairs is fairly large. For OR values that are far from null, the number of discordant pairs must be very large for an adequate approximation. This is due to the fact the normal approximation to the binomial distribution is not very accurate for a small to moderate number of trials, especially if the probability of a success is close to 0 or 1. (For a discussion of other approximate methods that yield fairly accurate confidence limits see Sahai and Khurshid, 1996.)

*Maximum Likelihood Method*

The maximum likelihood estimator of the common OR in a matched-pair analysis is

$$\hat{\text{OR}}_{\text{ML}} = g/h.$$

Miettinen (1970) and Ejigou and McHugh (1977) derived the variance of the maximum likelihood estimate of the OR for the matched case-control data. Estimates of the large sample variances of the maximum likelihood estimates of the OR and the log OR are

$$\hat{\text{Var}}\left(\hat{\text{OR}}_{\text{ML}}\right) = \frac{g}{h}\left(\frac{1}{g} + \frac{1}{h}\right)$$

and

$$\hat{\text{Var}}\left\{\log_e\left(\hat{\text{OR}}_{\text{ML}}\right)\right\} = \left(\frac{1}{g} + \frac{1}{h}\right). \tag{7.20}$$

Thus, a $100(1 - \alpha)\%$ approximate CI for the logarithm of the OR is given by

$$\log_e\left(\hat{\text{OR}}_{\text{ML}}\right) \pm Z_{\alpha/2}\sqrt{\hat{\text{Var}}\left\{\log_e\left(\hat{\text{OR}}_{\text{ML}}\right)\right\}}, \tag{7.21}$$

where $Z_{\alpha/2}$ is the upper $100(\alpha/2)$th percentile of the standard normal distribution. From which a $100(1 - \alpha)\%$ CI for the OR is obtained by taking the antilogarithms or exponents of the endpoints of the confidence limits determined by Equation 7.21.

It is interesting to note that Equation 6.47 for the estimated variance of the logarithm of the Mantel-Haenszel estimator (Equation 6.32), when applied to the matched-pair case-control data, reduces to Equation 7.20. This should not be surprising because, as remarked earlier, the maximum likelihood and the Mantel-Haenszel estimators are the same for the matched case-control pairs.

*Test-Based Method*

An alternative approach to an approximate CI for the OR, from matched case-control pairs, is the test-based procedure. As discussed earlier, a $100(1 - \alpha)\%$ CI for $\log_e(\text{OR})$ using this method is given by

$$\log_e\left(\hat{OR}_{MH}\right) \pm Z_{\alpha/2}\sqrt{\frac{\left\{\log_e\left(\hat{OR}_{MH}\right)\right\}^2}{\chi^2_{MH}}}, \tag{7.22}$$

where $\chi^2_{MH}$ is the Mantel-Haenszel chi-square statistic given in Equation 7.5 without the continuity correction. From which a 100(1 – α)% confidence interval for the OR can be written in terms of the standard normal statistic $\chi$ as $(\hat{OR}_{MH})^{1 \pm Z_{\alpha/2}/\chi}$.

Equation 7.21 for the CI, obtained by the maximum likelihood method, provides a rather straightforward and theoretically optimum solution to constructing approximate confidence limits and should be generally preferred over other approximate procedures.

*Example 7.1*

Consider the Israeli Ischemic Heart Disease Study, described in Chapter 6, in which one control per case was selected by picking an individual of the same age as the MI case, but without any history of MI. The data on 56 pairs of matched cases and controls are shown in Table 7.2.

The following are constructions of CIs for the OR using an exact and an approximate procedure based on binomial proportion, and procedures based on the maximum likelihood estimator and the test-based approach.

**Exact binomial method** — An *exact* CI for the OR can be obtained by solving Equations 7.8 and 7.9 by trial and error for $OR_L$ and $OR_U$, or more readily by substituting the appropriate values of percentiles of $F$-distribution in Equations 7.14 and 7.15. For the data here, shown in Table 7.2 with $g = 13$ and $h = 11$, exact 95% confidence limits are given by

$$OR_L = \frac{13}{(11+1)\,F_{0.025,2(11+1),2(13)}} = \frac{13}{12(2.217)} = 0.489$$

and

$$OR_U = \frac{(13+1)}{11} F_{0.025,2(13+1),2(11)} = \frac{14(2.289)}{11} = 2.913.$$

**Approximate binomial method** — An approximate CI for the OR can be obtained by using Equations 7.18 and 7.19 as

$$OR_L = \frac{\dfrac{13}{13+11} - 1.96\sqrt{\dfrac{13\times 11}{(13+11)^3}}}{1 - \dfrac{13}{13+11} + 1.96\sqrt{\dfrac{13\times 11}{(13+11)^3}}}$$

$$= 0.521$$

and

$$\text{OR}_\text{U} = \frac{\dfrac{13}{13+11} + 1.96\sqrt{\dfrac{13\times 11}{(13+11)^3}}}{1 - \dfrac{13}{13+11} - 1.96\sqrt{\dfrac{13\times 11}{(13+11)^3}}}$$

$$= 2.861.$$

As may be noted, these limits provide a fairly good approximation to the exact limits.

**Maximum likelihood method** — To determine an approximate CI by the maximum likelihood method, we have

$$\hat{\text{OR}}_{\text{ML}} = \frac{13}{11} = 1.182$$

and

$$\hat{\text{Var}}\left[\log_e\left(\hat{\text{OR}}_{\text{ML}}\right)\right] = \frac{1}{13} + \frac{1}{11} = 0.168.$$

Thus, a 95% CI for $\log_e$(OR) is obtained as

$$\log_e(1.182) \pm 1.96\sqrt{(0.168)} = (-0.636, 0.970),$$

which yields a 95% CI for the OR of (0.529, 2.638).

Note that these limits are reasonably close to the limits determined via exact method.

**Test-based method** — To determine an approximate CI by the test-based method, using Equations 7.1 and 7.5, we have

$$\hat{\text{OR}}_{\text{MH}} = \frac{13}{11} = 1.182$$

and

$$\chi^2_{\text{MH}} = \frac{(13-11)^2}{13+11} = 0.167.$$

Thus, a 95% CI for $\log_e$(OR) is obtained as

**TABLE 7.5**
**A 2 × 2 Display of the *i*th Matched Set (*M* Controls per Case) According to Exposure Status and Disease Outcome of Case and Control**

| | Risk Factor | | |
|---|---|---|---|
| | + | – | Total |
| Case | $a_i$ | $b_i$ | 1 |
| Control | $c_i$ | $d_i$ | $M$ |
| Total | $a_i + c_i$ | $b_i + d_i$ | $1 + M$ |

$$\log_e(1.182) \pm 1.96\sqrt{\frac{\{\log_e(1.182)\}^2}{0.167}} = (-0.635, 0.969),$$

which yields a 95% CI for the OR of (0.530, 2.634).

Note that the test-based limits also provide a fairly close approximation to exact limits. Note also that the Mantel-Haenszel chi-square statistic used here does not involve correction for continuity.

## 7.2 MATCHED-SET ANALYSIS INVOLVING MULTIPLE CONTROLS PER CASE

When controls are readily and economically available, one may decide to use $M$ controls ($M \geq 2$) for each case. The procedure is also sometimes employed when the investigator may want to obtain maximum possible information from a case-control study when only a small number of cases are available. If we cross-classify each set consisting of a case and its $M$ controls, the data set gives rise to a set of $2 \times 2$ tables such as Table 7.5 for each of the $n$ case-control sets. Note that $a_i + c_i = 0, 1, 2,..., M + 1$ and $b_i + d_i = 0, 1, 2,..., M + 1$, depending upon the number of exposed cases and controls for each matched set.

### 7.2.1 Distribution Theory for Multiple Controls

The number of exposed cases $(a_i)$ in Table 7.5 may vary from 0 to 1 and the number of controls in a matched set that are exposed $(c_i)$ may vary from 0 to $M$ (i.e., $c_i = 0,1,2,...,M$). Thus, the number of possible exposure patterns is $2(M + 1)$, as shown in Table 7.6, in which entries in each cell represent the frequency of matched sets for each exposure pattern. For each possible exposure pattern, one can construct a $2 \times 2$ table, resulting in $2(M + 1)$ elementary tables, as shown in Table 7.7.

**TABLE 7.6**
**A Display of Frequency of Matched Sets for Each Possible Exposure Pattern**

| | No. of Exposed Controls | | | | |
|---|---|---|---|---|---|
| **Cases** | **0** | **1** | **2** | **. . .** | **M** |
| Exposed (1) | $n_{1,0}$ | $n_{1,1}$ | $n_{1,2}$ | . . . | $n_{1,M}$ |
| Unexposed (0) | $n_{0,0}$ | $n_{0,1}$ | $n_{0,2}$ | . . . | $n_{0,M}$ |

*Note:* 1 = Exposed; 0 = unexposed.

**TABLE 7.7**
**A 2 × 2 Display of a Single Matched Set (*M* Controls per Case) Stratified According to Exposure Status and Disease Outcome of Case and Control**

| | Risk factor | | | Risk factor | | | Risk factor | | | | Risk factor | | |
|---|---|---|---|---|---|---|---|---|---|---|---|---|---|
| **Disease** | + | – | **Total** | + | – | **Total** | + | – | **Total** | | + | – | **Total** |
| Case | 0 | 1 | 1 | 0 | 1 | 1 | 0 | 1 | 1 | | 0 | 1 | 1 |
| Controls | 0 | $M$ | $M$ | 1 | $M-1$ | $M$ | 2 | $M-2$ | $M$ | . . . | $M$ | 0 | $M$ |
| Total | 0 | $M+1$ | $M+1$ | 1 | $M$ | $M+1$ | 2 | $M-1$ | $M+1$ | | $M$ | 1 | $M+1$ |
| | **Risk factor** | | | **Risk factor** | | | **Risk factor** | | | | **Risk factor** | | |
| **Disease** | + | – | **Total** | + | – | **Total** | + | – | **Total** | | + | – | **Total** |
| Case | 1 | 0 | 1 | 1 | 0 | 1 | 1 | 0 | 1 | | 1 | 0 | 1 |
| Controls | 0 | $M$ | $M$ | 1 | $M-1$ | $M$ | 2 | $M-2$ | $M$ | . . . | $M$ | 0 | $M$ |
| Total | 1 | $M$ | $M+1$ | 2 | $M-1$ | $M+1$ | 3 | $M-2$ | $M+1$ | | $M+1$ | 0 | $M+1$ |

Note that for the first exposure pattern, none of the subjects, either case or control, are exposed. Similarly, for the last exposure pattern, none of the subjects are unexposed. Thus, these two elementary tables contain a zero marginal total and do not contribute toward any statistical inference from the data.

Let $m$ be the total number of subjects exposed in a matched set, where $m$ may vary from 0 to $M + 1$. For a given value of $m$, two patterns of exposure for the matched set are possible: the case unexposed and $m$ controls exposed, or the case exposed and $m - 1$ controls exposed. Using the notation of Table 7.6, let $n_{1,m-1}$ and $n_{0,m}$ be the number of matched sets when the case is exposed and unexposed, respectively. The results can be summarized in the 2 × 2 table

**TABLE 7.8**
**A 2 × 2 Display of a Typical Table from a Single Matched Set (*M* Controls per Case) Stratified According to Exposure Status and Disease Outcome of Case and Control**

| | Risk factor | | |
|---|---|---|---|
| | + | – | Total |
| Case | $x$ | $1-x$ | 1 |
| Control | $m-x$ | $M-m+x$ | $M$ |
| Total | $m$ | $M+1-m$ | $M+1$ |

(Table 7.8) where $x = 0$ or 1 depending on whether the case is unexposed or exposed, respectively.

From the noncentral hypergeometric distribution it follows that

$$P(X = x \mid m) = \frac{\binom{1}{x}\binom{M}{m-x}(\text{OR})^x}{\sum_{k=0}^{1}\binom{1}{k}\binom{M}{m-k}(\text{OR})^k}, \quad x = 0, 1 \tag{7.23}$$

In particular, the probabilities that the case is exposed or unexposed are obtained by letting $x = 1$ or 0 in Equation 7.23 and are given by OR/(OR + $C_m$) and $C_m$/(OR + $C_m$), respectively, where $C_m = (M + 1 - m)/m$. For a given value of $m$, the probability of obtaining exactly $n_{1,m-1}$ and $n_{0,m}$ matched sets when a case is exposed and unexposed, respectively, given a total of $n_{1,m-1} + n_{0,m}$ matched sets, follows a binomial distribution and is given by

$$P = \frac{(n_{1,m-1} + n_{0,m})!}{(n_{1,m-1})!(n_{0,m})!}\left(\frac{\text{OR}}{\text{OR} + C_m}\right)^{n_{1,m-1}}\left(\frac{C_m}{\text{OR} + C_m}\right)^{n_{0,m}}. \tag{7.24}$$

### 7.2.2 Estimation of the Odds Ratio

We now consider the problem of point and interval estimation of the OR for the matched set analysis involving multiple controls.

#### 7.2.2.1 Point Estimation

We consider two procedures of point estimation, the so-called Mantel-Haenszel and the maximum likelihood estimators as point estimates of the OR.

*Mantel-Haenszel Estimator*

The Mantel-Haenszel (MH) estimator for the common OR can be obtained by applying Equation 6.32 to matched set data in which each set is treated as a separate stratum. Using the notations of Tables 7.6 and 7.7, for a given value of $m$, let $n_{x,m-x}$ be the frequency of the matched set corresponding to $x$ exposed cases, where $x = 1$ or 0. From the entries of Tables 7.7 and 7.8,

$$\frac{a_i d_i}{n_i} = \frac{x(M-m+x)}{M+1}, \quad \begin{matrix} i = 1, 2, \ldots, n \\ x = 0, 1; m = 1, \ldots, M \end{matrix}$$

and

$$\frac{b_i c_i}{n_i} = \frac{(1-x)(m-x)}{M+1}, \quad \begin{matrix} i = 1, 2, \ldots, n \\ x = 0, 1; m = 1, \ldots, M \end{matrix}$$

Hence, the Mantel-Haenszel estimator (Equation 6.32) is given by

$$\begin{aligned} \hat{\text{OR}}_{\text{MH}} &= \frac{\sum_{i=1}^{n} \left( \frac{a_i d_i}{n_i} \right)}{\sum_{i=1}^{n} \left( \frac{b_i c_i}{n_i} \right)} = \frac{\sum_{m=1}^{M} \sum_{x=0}^{1} \frac{x(M-m+x)}{M+1} n_{x,m-x}}{\sum_{m=1}^{M} \sum_{x=0}^{1} \frac{(1-x)(m-x)}{M+1} n_{x,m-x}} \\ &= \frac{\sum_{m=1}^{M} (M-m+1) n_{1,m-1}}{\sum_{m=1}^{M} m\, n_{0,m}}. \end{aligned} \tag{7.25}$$

*Maximum Likelihood Estimator*

The likelihood function (L) of the data can be obtained as the product of binomial probabilities (Equation 7.24) for each value of $m$, from 1 to $M$, i.e.,

$$L = \prod_{m=1}^{M} \left( \frac{\left(n_{1,m-1} + n_{0,m}\right)!}{\left(n_{1,m-1}\right)!\left(n_{0,m}\right)!} \right) \left( \frac{\text{OR}}{\text{OR} + C_m} \right)^{n_{1,m-1}} \left( \frac{C_m}{\text{OR} + C_m} \right)^{n_{0,m}}.$$

The logarithm of the likelihood function is

$$\log_e(L) = \sum_{m=1}^{M} \left[ \log_e \left( \frac{(n_{1,m-1} + n_{0,m})!}{(n_{1,m-1})!(n_{0,m})!} \right) + n_{1,m-1} \log_e \left( \frac{\text{OR}}{\text{OR} + C_m} \right) \right.$$
$$\left. + n_{0,m} \log_e \left( \frac{C_m}{\text{OR} + C_m} \right) \right].$$

Taking the first derivative of $\log_e(L)$ with respect to OR and equating it to zero yields the equation (Miettinen, 1970)

$$\frac{1}{\text{OR}} \sum_{m=1}^{M} n_{1,m-1} - \sum_{m=1}^{M} \left( \frac{(n_{1,m-1} + n_{0,m})}{\text{OR} + C_m} \right) = 0. \tag{7.26}$$

For $M = 1$, Equation 7.26 is equivalent to Equation 7.2, with the solution $\hat{\text{OR}}_{\text{ML}} = n_{10}/n_{01} = g/h$. For $M = 2$, it can be written as

$$\frac{(n_{1,0} + n_{1,1})}{\text{OR}} - \frac{(n_{1,0} + n_{0,1})}{\text{OR} + 2} - \frac{(n_{1,1} + n_{0,2})}{\text{OR} + (1/2)} = 0. \tag{7.27}$$

Equation 7.27 can be solved explicitly for the OR (Miettinen, 1970):

$$\begin{aligned} \hat{\text{OR}}_{\text{ML}} &= \frac{4n_{1,0} - n_{0,1} + n_{1,1} - 4n_{0,2}}{4(n_{0,1} + n_{0,2})} \\ &\quad + \left[ \left( \frac{4n_{1,0} - n_{0,1} + n_{1,1} - 4n_{0,2}}{4(n_{0,1} + n_{0,2})} \right)^2 + \frac{n_{1,0} + n_{1,1}}{n_{0,1} + n_{0,2}} \right]^{0.5} \\ &= \frac{5\nu - S_1 - 4S_2}{4(S_1 + S_2 - \nu)} + \left[ \left( \frac{5\nu - S_1 - 4S_2}{4(S_1 + S_2 - \nu)} \right)^2 + \frac{\nu}{S_1 + S_2 - \nu} \right]^{0.5}, \end{aligned} \tag{7.28}$$

where $\nu = n_{1,0} + n_{1,1}$, $S_1 = n_{1,0} + n_{0,1}$, and $S_2 = n_{1,1} + n_{0,2}$. Note that the result of Equation 7.28 is more complicated than its analog for the case $M = 1$; i.e., one-to-one matching.

For comparison purposes, note that the Mantel-Haenszel estimator (Equation 7.25) in this case is

$$\hat{\text{OR}}_{\text{MH}} = \frac{2n_{1,0} + n_{1,1}}{n_{0,1} + 2n_{0,2}}. \tag{7.29}$$

The estimator (Equation 7.29) is not equivalent to the maximum likelihood estimator (Equation 7.28), as it was in the case of one-to-one matching. It is, however, a consistent estimator of the OR.

For $M \geq 3$, only iterative solutions to Equation 7.26 are possible. This entails a graphing of the function of OR, on the left side of Equation 7.26, to determine a reasonable starting value $\hat{\text{OR}}_0$ for its zero point. The subsequent application of the Newton-Raphson algorithm (see, e.g., Atkinson, 1989; Ralston and Wilf, 1967) generally leads to the desired solution after a finite number of iterations. It is readily seen that starting from the trial value of $\hat{\text{OR}}_0$, the result from the first cycle of iteration is (Miettinen, 1970):

$$\hat{\text{OR}}_1 = \hat{\text{OR}}_0 + \frac{\dfrac{1}{\hat{\text{OR}}_0}\displaystyle\sum_{m=1}^{M} n_{1,m-1} - \sum_{m=1}^{M}\left(\frac{\left(n_{1,m-1} + n_{0,m}\right)}{\hat{\text{OR}}_0 + C_m}\right)}{\dfrac{1}{\hat{\text{OR}}_0^2}\displaystyle\sum_{m=1}^{M} n_{1,m-1} - \sum_{m=1}^{M}\left(\frac{\left(n_{1,m-1} + n_{0,m}\right)}{\left(\hat{\text{OR}}_0 + C_m\right)^2}\right)}. \tag{7.30}$$

The subsequent iterations can be carried out with $\hat{\text{OR}}_1$ in place of $\hat{\text{OR}}_0$, $\hat{\text{OR}}_2$ in place of $\hat{\text{OR}}_1$, etc., until the solution converges.

*Other Estimators*

In recent statistical literature, there are several other estimators which have been proposed. The interested reader is referred to the papers by Ejigou and McHugh (1981), Jewel (1984) and Schuster (1986). For some small sample properties with regard to bias and mean squared error, see Lubin (1981) and Ejigou (1990).

#### 7.2.2.2 Confidence Intervals

We consider three approximate methods for determining CIs for the OR, the Mantel-Haenszel, maximum likelihood, and test-based methods, as well as an exact method, which generally requires the use of a computer program. For a discussion of some other methods of confidence intervals see Ejigou (1990).

*Mantel-Haenszel Method*

An approximate CI for the common OR can be obtained by using an estimate of the variance for the Mantel-Haenszel estimator (Equation 7.25). To obtain an estimate of the variance, one can use one of the formulas (Equations 6.45, 6.46, or 6.47) for the general stratified analysis and apply it to the matched-set data. For example, the components of Equation 6.47, when applied to the matched-set data, are

$$
\begin{aligned}
&\sum_{i=1}^{k} P_i R_i = \sum_{m=1}^{M} n_{1,m-1} \frac{(M+2-m)(M+1-m)}{(M+1)^2}, \\
&\sum_{i=1}^{k} Q_i R_i = \sum_{m=1}^{M} n_{1,m-1} \frac{(m-1)(M+1-m)}{(M+1)^2}, \\
&\sum_{i=1}^{k} P_i S_i = \sum_{m=1}^{M} n_{0,m} \frac{m(M-m)}{(M+1)^2}, \quad \sum_{i=1}^{k} Q_i S_i = \sum_{m=1}^{M} n_{0,m} \frac{m(m+1)}{(M+1)^2}, \\
&\sum_{i=1}^{k} R_i = \sum_{m=1}^{M} n_{1,m-1} \frac{(M+1-m)}{(M+1)}, \quad \sum_{i=1}^{k} S_i = \sum_{m=1}^{M} n_{0,m} \frac{m}{(M+1)}.
\end{aligned}
\tag{7.31}
$$

The required confidence limits can then be calculated in the usual way.

*Test-Based Method*

An approximate CI for the common OR can be obtained using the test-based procedure. The Mantel-Haenszel chi-square statistic in this case may be expressed as (Miettinen, 1969; Pike and Morrow, 1970; Rothman, 1986)

$$
\chi^2_{\mathrm{MH}} = \frac{\left\{ \sum_{m=1}^{M} \left[ n_{1,m-1} - \frac{m}{M+1} \left( n_{1,m-1} + n_{0,m} \right) \right] \right\}^2}{\sum_{m=1}^{M} \left[ \left( n_{1,m-1} + n_{0,m} \right) \frac{m(M+1-m)}{(M+1)^2} \right]}, \tag{7.32}
$$

which is obtained from the general formula (Equation 6.12) for the stratified analysis, applied to the 1-to-$M$ controls matched set, in which each set is treated as a separate stratum. The statistic (7.32) was proposed independently by Miettinen (1969) and Pike and Morrow (1970), and is commonly referred to as the *Miettinen statistic.* Notice that for $M = 1$, statistic (7.32) reduces to the McNemar's chi-square statistic (without continuity correction) as defined by Equation 7.5.*

The required confidence limits can be calculated in the usual way.

*Maximum Likelihood Method*

An approximate CI for the common OR can be obtained by calculating the variance of the maximum likelihood estimator for the case of 1-to-$M$ matching.

* The efficiency *(E)* of the test based on statistic (7.32) relative to McNemar's test, with one control matched per case, is $E = 2M/(M + 1)$ (Ury, 1975). Thus, the unit increase in efficiency per unit increase in $M$ decreases rather rapidly for $M \geq 5$. As $M$ becomes infinitely large, $E$ approaches a maximum value of 2.

The estimate of the variance that represents a simple extension of Equation 7.20 is given by (Miettinen, 1970)

$$\hat{\text{Var}}\left\{\log_e\left(\hat{\text{OR}}_{\text{ML}}\right)\right\} = \frac{1}{\hat{\text{OR}}_{\text{ML}} \sum_{m=1}^{M} \frac{\left(n_{1,m-1} + n_{0,m}\right)C_m}{\left(\hat{\text{OR}}_{\text{ML}} + C_m\right)^2}}, \tag{7.33}$$

where $C_m = (M + 1 - m)/m$ and $\hat{\text{OR}}_{\text{ML}}$ is the conditional maximum likelihood estimate obtained as the iterative solution to Equation 7.26.

The required confidence limits can be calculated in the usual way.

*An Exact Method*

An exact CI for the common OR can be obtained by using the result of the binomial probability expression, Equation 7.24 (Miettinen, 1970). Thus, the joint probability function for all the observations can be written as the product of $M$ binomial probabilities and is given by

$$\boldsymbol{P} = \prod_{m=1}^{M} \left( \frac{\left(n_{1,m-1} + n_{0,m}\right)!}{\left(n_{1,m-1}\right)!\left(n_{0,m}\right)!} \left(\frac{\text{OR}}{\text{OR} + C_m}\right)^{n_{1,m-1}} \left(\frac{C_m}{\text{OR} + C_m}\right)^{n_{0,m}} \right). \tag{7.34}$$

The probability expression (7.34) can be rewritten as

$$\boldsymbol{P} = \prod_{m=1}^{M} \mathrm{C}_{k_m}^{s_m} \left(\frac{\text{OR}}{\text{OR} + C_m}\right)^{k_m} \left(\frac{C_m}{\text{OR} + C_m}\right)^{s_m - k_m}, \tag{7.35}$$

where, for a given value of $m$, $s_m = n_{1,m-1} + n_{0,m}$ is the total number of matched sets and $k_m = n_{1,m-1}$ is the number of matched sets when the case is exposed.

Exact confidence limits can be determined iteratively by solving the probability expression (7.35) for every possible outcome of the data that deviates equally or more extreme from the null value, beginning with the observed data. The sum is calculated for all permissible values of the OR until the tail area equals the specified value. Thus, the lower confidence limit of a $100(1 - \alpha)\%$ CI is the the OR value, $\text{OR}_{\text{L}}$, determined in such a way that it yields an upper tail probability of $\alpha/2$:

$$\sum_{k=a}^{b} \prod_{m=1}^{M} \mathrm{C}_{k_m}^{s_m} \left(\frac{\text{OR}_{\text{L}}}{\text{OR}_{\text{L}} + C_m}\right)^{k_m} \left(\frac{C_m}{\text{OR}_{\text{L}} + C_m}\right)^{s_m - k_m} = \alpha/2, \tag{7.36}$$

where $a$ is the total number of exposed cases in matched sets with at least one control unexposed ($a = \sum_{m=1}^{M} n_{1,m-1}$), $b$ is the total number of matched sets that are not completely concordant ($b = \sum_{m=1}^{M} s_m$), and $k = \sum_{m=1}^{M} k_m$. Similarly, the upper confidence limit is the value of the OR, $\mathrm{OR_U}$, determined so that it yields a lower tail probability of $\alpha/2$:

$$\sum_{k=0}^{a}\prod_{m=1}^{M} C_{k_m}^{s_m}\left(\frac{\mathrm{OR_U}}{\mathrm{OR_U}+C_m}\right)^{k_m}\left(\frac{C_m}{\mathrm{OR_U}+C_m}\right)^{s_m-k_m}=\alpha/2. \qquad (7.37)$$

As indicated earlier, the determination of exact limits by solving Equations 7.36 and 7.37 through trial and error in most situations is extremely tedious. Computer programs and approximations are generally needed to reach solutions (see Thomas and Gart, 1992).

*Example 7.2*

Consider the matched case-control study described by Miettinen (1969, 1970), who examined the data from an unpublished study evaluating the hypothesis that induced abortions increase the risk of tubal implantation in subsequent pregnancies. The data were described and analyzed further by Rothman (1986). The study entailed cases with ectopic pregnancy and the controls were women without ectopic pregnancy selected from the same source population and then matched individually to the cases for the number of pregnancies, age, and husband's educational level. All women reported at least one previous pregnancy, and a positive history shows that the woman had at least one induced abortion. There were 18 cases and 4 controls matched to each case. The results on exposure for each case and the corresponding controls are summarized in Table 7.9. The distribution of exposed patterns for cases and controls is displayed in Table 7.10.

First, we compute the Mantel-Haenszel and the maximum likelihood estimates of the odds ratio.

**Mantel-Haenszel estimate** — Equation 7.25, applied to the data in Table 7.10, yields

$$\hat{\mathrm{OR}}_{\mathrm{MH}}=\frac{4(3)+3(5)+2(3)+1(0)}{1(1)+2(0)+3(0)+4(0)}=33.$$

**Maximum likelihood estimate** — Note that for $M = 4$, the likelihood equation (7.26) can be written as

$$\frac{1}{\mathrm{OR}}\sum_{m=1}^{4} n_{1,m-1}-\sum_{m=1}^{4}\left(\frac{\left(n_{1,m-1}+n_{0,m}\right)}{\mathrm{OR}+(5-m)/m}\right). \qquad (7.38)$$

**TABLE 7.9**
**Previous History of Induced Abortions Among Women with Tubal Pregnancy and Matched Controls**

| Case | History of induced abortion (control no.) 1 | 2 | 3 | 4 |
|---|---|---|---|---|
| – | – | – | – | – |
| + | – | + | – | – |
| + | – | – | – | – |
| – | – | – | – | – |
| – | + | – | – | – |
| + | – | – | – | – |
| + | – | – | – | – |
| – | – | – | – | – |
| + | + | – | – | + |
| + | – | + | – | – |
| + | – | + | + | – |
| – | – | – | – | – |
| + | + | + | + | + |
| + | – | – | + | – |
| + | – | – | + | – |
| + | + | – | – | – |
| – | – | – | – | – |
| + | + | – | – | + |

*Note:* +: previous induced abortion; – : no previous induced abortion.

From Miettinen, O. S. (1969). *Biometrics,* 25, 339–355. With permission. Original data from Trichopoulos, D. et al. (1969). Unpublished.

**TABLE 7.10**
**Patterns of Exposure for the 18 Matched Sets in Table 7.9**

| | No. of exposed controls 0 | 1 | 2 | 3 | 4 |
|---|---|---|---|---|---|
| Exposed cases | 3 | 5 | 3 | 0 | 1 |
| Unexposed cases | 5 | 1 | 0 | 0 | 0 |

From Table 7.10, $n_{1,0} = 3$, $n_{1,1} = 5$, $n_{1,2} = 3$, $n_{1,3} = 0$, $n_{0,1} = 1$, $n_{0,2} = n_{0,3} = n_{0,4} = 0$. Substituting these values in Equation 7.38, the likelihood equation becomes

$$\frac{11}{\text{OR}} - \frac{4}{\text{OR}+4} - \frac{5}{\text{OR}+(3/2)} - \frac{3}{\text{OR}+(2/3)} = 0. \tag{7.39}$$

To solve the above equation for the OR, it is seen by trial and error that the solution to the equation lies somewhere in the vicinity of 20. Starting from the initial trial value of $\hat{OR}_0 = 20$, the left side of Equation 7.39 is equal to 0.005614. Substituting $\hat{OR}_0 = 20$ in Equation 7.30, the result from the first cycle of iteration is $\hat{OR}_1 = 22.07$. Substituting OR = 22.07 in Equation 7.39 makes the left side equal to 0.0009015. Again, substituting $\hat{OR}_1 = 22.07$ in place of $\hat{OR}_0$ in Equation 7.30, the result from the second iteration yields $\hat{OR}_2 = 22.55$. Repeating the process, the result from the third cycle of iteration gives $\hat{OR}_3 = 22.57$, which may be taken as the maximum likelihood estimate of the OR. The conditional maximum likelihood estimate using a computer program (Thomas and Gart, 1992) is 22.566, which is exactly the same value as obtained above. Note also that the conditional maximum likelihood estimate of 22.57 is appreciably different from the Mantel-Haenszel estimate of 33. Although the Mantel-Haenszel estimator is consistent and nearly as efficient as the maximum likelihood estimator for the OR near unity (Breslow, 1981), the present example typifies a strong positive association with sparse data.

We now compute CIs for the OR using the Mantel-Haenszel, maximum likelihood, and test-based methods as well as an exact method described earlier.

**Mantel-Haenszel method** — For the data of Table 7.10, the Mantel-Haenszel estimate of the OR was found to be $\hat{OR}_{MH} = 33.0$. An estimate of the variance of the logarithm of the estimator can be calculated by the use of Equation 6.47, whose components are determined by applying the data of Table 7.10 to the expressions in Equation 7.31. The resulting variance estimate is calculated as 1.518. A 95% CI for $\log_e$(OR) is

$$\log_e(33.0) \pm 1.96\sqrt{1.518} = (1.082, 5.912),$$

which yields a 95% CI for the OR of (2.951, 369.444).

**Maximum likelihood method** — For the data of Table 7.10, the maximum likelihood estimate of the OR was determined as $\hat{OR}_{ML} = 22.57$. An estimate of the variance of the logarithm of the OR can be calculated by Equation 7.33. The resulting variance estimate is

$$\hat{Var}\left\{\log_e\left(\hat{OR}_{ML}\right)\right\} = \frac{1}{22.57\left[\dfrac{4(4)}{(22.57+4)^2} + \dfrac{5(3/2)}{(22.57+3/2)^2} + \dfrac{3(2/3)}{(22.57+2/3)^2}\right]}$$

$$= 1.127.$$

Note that the estimated variance of the logarithm of the Mantel-Haenszel estimate was calculated to be 1.518, which is larger than 1.127. This is to be expected because the OR value departs considerably from the null value of unity. It is only in the neighborhood of unity that the maximum likelihood and the Mantel-Haenszel estimators are equally efficient. A 95% CI for $\log_e$(OR) is

$$\log_e(22.57) \pm 1.96\sqrt{1.127} = (1.036, 5.197),$$

which yields a 95% CI for the OR of (2.818, 180.729).

**Test-based method** — For the data of Table 7.10, the value of the Mantel-Haenszel chi-square statistic using Equation 7.32 is calculated as 16.000. A 95% CI of $\log_e$(OR) using this method is

$$= \log_e(33.0) \pm 1.96\sqrt{\{\log_e(33.0)\}^2 / 16.000} = (1.784, 5.210),$$

which yields a 95% CI for the OR of (5.954, 183.094). It is clear that these limits are too narrow and do not provide an adequate approximation to the corresponding exact limits. The reader should recall from an earlier discussion that the test-based limits are usually satisfactory in the vicinity of the null value of the OR, but if the data depart too strongly from the null value, the test-based limits yield a rather poor approximation.

**Exact method** — In order to obtain exact confidence limits, one would require the tail summation of the probabilities in Equations 7.36 and 7.37 until the solution is reached. The computational details are somewhat involved and cannot be carried out manually. Using a computer program (Thomas and Gart, 1992), for a 95% CI, the solutions are $OR_L = 3.066$ and $OR_U = 1005.696$.

## 7.3 MATCHED-SET ANALYSIS INVOLVING A VARYING NUMBER OF CONTROLS PER CASE

With a varying number of controls matched to each case, the frequency of matched sets for each possible exposure pattern can be summarized by a set of displays such as the one in Table 7.6, each for a different value of *M*.

### 7.3.1 Estimation of Odds Ratio

We consider the problem of point and interval estimation of the OR for the matched-set analysis involving varying number of controls per case.

#### 7.3.1.1 Point Estimation

We describe two procedures of point estimation, the Mantel-Haenszel and the maximum likelihood estimators. (For a further discussion of maximum likelihood estimation, tests of hypothesis, and other related problems, see Walter, 1980.)

*Mantel-Haenszel Estimator*

The formula for the Mantel-Haenszel estimator of the OR is a simple extension of Equation 7.25, and can be written as

$$\hat{\text{OR}}_{\text{MH}} = \frac{\sum_{l=1}^{R}\sum_{m=1}^{M_l}\left(\frac{(M_l+1-m)n_{1,m-1}}{M_l+1}\right)}{\sum_{l=1}^{R}\sum_{m=1}^{M_l}\frac{mn_{0,m}}{M_l+1}}, \tag{7.40}$$

where $R$ is the number of distinct sets of matched controls and $M_l$ ($l = 1,2,...,R$) represents the number of matched controls in the $l$th set. Note that in Equation 7.40, the summation would be performed $R$ times: first for the matched sets with $M_1$ controls, second with $M_2$ controls, and so on; and finally for the matched sets with $M_R$ controls.

*Maximum Likelihood Estimator*

The likelihood function for the varying number of controls to each case is a simple generalization of the likelihood function for the equal number of controls to each case, and the equation that yields the maximum likelihood estimate of the OR is a simple extension of Equation 7.26:

$$\sum_{l=1}^{R}\left(\frac{1}{\text{OR}}\sum_{m=1}^{M_l}n_{1,m-1} - \sum_{m=1}^{M_l}\frac{(n_{1,m-1}+n_{0,m})}{\text{OR}+C_m}\right) = 0, \tag{7.41}$$

where the notations follow as before.

#### 7.3.1.2 Confidence Intervals

Three approximate methods of determining CIs for the OR are briefly outlined: the Mantel-Haenszel, maximum likelihood, and test-based methods, as well as an exact method, which generally requires the use of a computer program.

*Mantel-Haenszel Method*

An approximate interval for the common odds ratio can be obtained by using an estimate of the variance for the Mantel-Haenszel estimator. An estimate of the variance can be obtained by extending result of (Equation 7.31) for the case of varying number of controls. The components of formula (Equation 6.47), when applied to the case of varying number of controls, are

$$
\begin{aligned}
\sum_{i=1}^{k} P_i R_i &= \sum_{l=1}^{R} \sum_{m=1}^{M_l} n_{1,m-1} \frac{(M_l + 2 - m)(M_l + 1 - m)}{(M_l + 1)^2}, \\
\sum_{i=1}^{k} Q_i R_i &= \sum_{l=1}^{R} \sum_{m=1}^{M_l} n_{1,m-1} \frac{(m-1)(M_l + 1 - m)}{(M_l + 1)^2}, \\
\sum_{i=1}^{k} P_i S_i &= \sum_{l=1}^{R} \sum_{m=1}^{M_l} n_{0,m} \frac{m(M_l - m)}{(M_l + 1)^2}, \\
\sum_{i=1}^{k} Q_i S_i &= \sum_{l=1}^{R} \sum_{m=1}^{M_l} n_{0,m} \frac{m(m+1)}{(M_l + 1)^2}, \\
\sum_{i=1}^{k} R_i &= \sum_{l=1}^{R} \sum_{m=1}^{M_l} n_{1,m-1} \frac{(M_l + 1 - m)}{(M_l + 1)}, \\
\sum_{i=1}^{k} S_i &= \sum_{l=1}^{R} \sum_{m=1}^{M_l} n_{0,m} \frac{m}{(M_l + 1)}.
\end{aligned}
\tag{7.42}
$$

*Maximum Likelihood Method*

An approximate CI for the common OR can be obtained through the result of the variance of the maximum likelihood estimator. The formula that extends the result of Equation 7.33, for the varying number of matched controls, is (Miettinen, 1970)

$$
\hat{\text{Var}}\left\{\log_e\left(\hat{\text{OR}}_{\text{ML}}\right)\right\} = \frac{1}{\hat{\text{OR}}_{\text{ML}} \sum_{l=1}^{R} \sum_{m=1}^{M_l} \frac{\left(n_{1,m-1} + n_{0,m}\right) C_m}{\left(\hat{\text{OR}}_{\text{ML}} + C_m\right)^2}}, \tag{7.43}
$$

where the notations follow as before.

*Test-Based Method*

An approximate CI for the common OR can be obtained using the test-based method. However, the accuracy of the procedure is affected depending on how much the data deviate from the null case. The Mantel-Haenszel chi-square statistic used for this purpose, which is a simple extension of Equation 7.32, is (Miettinen, 1975; Rothman, 1986)

**TABLE 7.11**
**Distribution of Cases of MI and Matched Controls According to Amount of Coffee Consumption**

| | No. of controls consuming 6+ cups/d | | | | |
|---|---|---|---|---|---|
| | Matched Pairs | | Matched triplets | | |
| | (M = 1) | | (M = 2) | | |
| **Cases** | **0** | **1** | **0** | **1** | **2** |
| 6+ cups/d | 8 | 8 | 16 | 23 | 4 |
| 0 cups/d | 8 | 3 | 20 | 22 | 3 |

From Jick, H. et al. (1973). *N. Engl. J. Med.*, 289, 63–77. With permission.

$$\chi^2_{\text{MH}} = \frac{\left\{\sum_{l=1}^{R}\sum_{m=1}^{M_l}\left[n_{1,m-1} - \frac{m}{M_l+1}\left(n_{1,m-1}+n_{0,m}\right)\right]\right\}^2}{\sum_{l=1}^{R}\sum_{m=1}^{M_l}\left[\left(n_{1,m-1}+n_{0,m}\right)\frac{m\left(M_l+1-m\right)}{\left(M_l+1\right)^2}\right]}. \tag{7.44}$$

Note that statistic (7.44) is essentially the sum of each component of the chi-square statistic as determined for different values of $M$ using Equation 7.32.

*An Exact Method*

With a varying number of controls, the probability function for the observations, as a function of the OR, is a simple extension of Equation 7.35, and is obtained by taking the product of the probabilities over each distinct set of $M$ values, and can be written as

$$\prod_{l=1}^{R}\prod_{m=1}^{M_l} C_{k_m}^{s_m}\left(\frac{\text{OR}}{\text{OR}+C_m}\right)^{k_m}\left(\frac{C_m}{\text{OR}+C_m}\right)^{s_m-k_m}. \tag{7.45}$$

The equations entailing the tail probabilities for the calculation of exact confidence limits can be written analogous to Equations 7.36 and 7.37.

*Example 7.3*

The following data were obtained from a case-control study of myocardial infarction (MI) and the history of coffee consumption as reported by Jick et al. (1973) and further discussed by Rothman (1986). Two controls were matched to each case, but for 27 cases only one matched control was used. The resulting data consist of 27 matched pairs and 88 matched triplets, and are summarized in Table 7.11 according to the number of cups of coffee consumed per day. Subjects consuming one to five cups of coffee per day were excluded from the study.

The Mantel-Haenszel estimate can be obtained by applying Equation 7.40 to the data in Table 7.11:

$$\hat{OR}_{MH} = \frac{8/2 + [2(16) + 23]/3}{3/2 + [22 + 2(3)]/3} = 2.062.$$

The maximum likelihood estimate is obtained by solving the likelihood equation (7.41) as applied to the data in Table 7.11. The resulting equation is

$$\left(\frac{8}{OR} - \frac{11}{OR+1}\right) + \left(\frac{16+23}{OR} - \frac{16+22}{OR+2} + \frac{23+3}{OR+1/2}\right) = 0.$$

A trial and error solution to the above equation yields $\hat{OR}_{ML}$ = 2.000. The conditional maximum likelihood estimate using a computer program (Thomas and Gart, 1992) is 1.984. The solution to the asymptotic maximum likelihood using the same program is 2.002. Thus, the Mantel-Haenszel and the maximum likelihood estimates yield fairly similar results.

We now compute CIs for the OR using the approximate procedures of the Mantel-Haenszel, maximum likelihood, and test-based methods, as well as the exact method.

**Mantel-Haenszel method** — For the data of Table 7.11, the Mantel-Haenszel estimate of the OR was $\hat{OR}_{MH}$ = 2.062. An estimate of the variance of the logarithm of the estimate can be calculated by the use of Equation 6.47, whose components are determined by applying the data of Table 7.11 to the expressions in Equation 7.42. The resulting variance calculated in this way is 0.066. A 95% CI for $\log_e$(OR) is

$$\log_e(2.062) \pm 1.96\sqrt{0.066} = (0.220, 1.227),$$

which yields a 95% CI for the OR of (1.246, 3.411).

**Maximum likelihood method** — For the data of Table 7.11, the maximum likelihood estimate of the OR was determined as $\hat{OR}_{ML}$ = 2.000, and an estimate of the variance of the logarithm of the $\hat{OR}_{ML}$ can be calculated using Equation 7.43:

$$\hat{Var}\left\{\log_e\left(\hat{OR}_{ML}\right)\right\} = \frac{1}{2.000\left[\frac{11}{(2.000+1)^2} + \frac{38(2)}{(2.000+2)^2} + \frac{26(1/2)}{(2.000+1/2)^2}\right]}$$

$$= 0.063.$$

As expected, this variance is slightly smaller than the Mantel-Haenszel variance of 0.066. A 95% CI for $\log_e$(OR) is

$$\log_e(2.000) \pm 1.96\sqrt{0.063} = (0.201, 1.185),$$

which yields a 95% CI for the OR of (1.223, 3.271).

**Test-based method** — For the data of Table 7.11, the value of the Mantel-Haenszel chi-square statistic, using Equation 7.44, is calculated as 7.784. A 95% CI for $\log_e$(OR), using this method, is

$$\log_e(2.062) \pm 1.96\sqrt{\{\log_e(2.062)\}^2 / 7.784} = (0.215, 1.232),$$

which yields a 95% CI for the OR of (1.240, 3.428). These limits seem rather close to the limits obtained by the Mantel-Haenszel and the maximum likelihood methods. This should not be surprising because in this example the data depart only moderately from the null value, and thus one would expect better performance for the test-based procedure.

**Exact method** — In order to obtain exact confidence limits, one would require the tail summation of the probabilities in Equation 7.45 iteratively until the solution is reached. The computational details are somewhat involved and cannot be carried out manually. The required 95% confidence limits, using a computer program (Thomas and Gart, 1992), are calculated as $OR_L = 1.189$ and $OR_U = 3.360$.

## 7.4 EFFICACY OF MATCHING

The efficacy of matching methods in controlling confounding can be assessed by evaluating the correlation of exposure within matched sets. For a matched pair design, the correlation coefficient *(r)* is determined by (Miettinen, 1975)

$$r = \frac{fj - gh}{\sqrt{(f+g)(h+j)(f+h)(g+j)}},$$

where the notations are as shown in Table 7.4. For matching with $M$ controls per case, one can calculate the correlation coefficient by assuming that each case has been paired repeatedly with each control, and thereby counting each case $M$ times rather than only once. This scheme avoids overestimates of the correlation which may result from the greater precision in the exposure rate among controls when multiple controls are matched to each case. The resulting value of the correlation can be interpreted as the value of the correlation, which would have been obtained had a matched-pair design been employed. Miettinen (1975) describes a procedure for testing the departure of the correlation of exposures from the null value. The resulting test is equivalent to a test of the linear trend in the proportion of sets in which the case is exposed according to the number of controls being exposed.

**TABLE 7.12**
**A 2 × 2 Display of Sample Data in Matched-Pair Follow-Up Study**

| | | Exposed | | |
|---|---|---|---|---|
| | | **Case** | **Noncase** | **Total** |
| **Unexposed** | Case | $f$ | $g$ | $f+g$ |
| | Noncase | $h$ | $j$ | $h+j$ |
| | Total | $f+h$ | $g+j$ | $n$ |

## 7.5 MATCHED FOLLOW-UP STUDIES

Matched follow-up studies are relatively free of bias with respect to matching factors because of the lack of correlation between the exposure and the matching factors among the subjects at the commencement of the study. However, such studies are not very common and only a brief, limited discussion of the topic is provided.

Consider a matched follow-up study with $n$ matched pairs of exposed and unexposed subjects. The results of the disease outcomes from the exposed and unexposed groups after the follow-up period are summarized in Table 7.12.

The risk difference (RD) and risk ratio (RR) can be estimated by

$$\hat{\text{RD}} = \frac{f+h}{n} - \frac{f+g}{n} = \frac{h-g}{n} \tag{7.46}$$

and

$$\hat{\text{RR}} = \frac{(f+h)/n}{(f+g)/n} = \frac{(f+h)}{(f+g)}. \tag{7.47}$$

The variance estimates for $\hat{\text{RD}}$ and $\log_e(\hat{\text{RR}})$ are (Fleiss, 1981; Rothman, 1986):

$$\hat{\text{Var}}\left(\hat{\text{RD}}\right) = \frac{n(g+h)-(g-h)^2}{n^3} \tag{7.48}$$

and

$$\hat{\text{Var}}\left\{\log_e\left(\hat{\text{RR}}\right)\right\} \approx \frac{g+h}{(f+g)(f+h)}. \tag{7.49}$$

The approximate CIs for the RD and the RR can be obtained using the variance Equations 7.48 and 7.49 or the test-based procedures with Mantel-Haenszel chi-square statistic given by Equation 7.5. The analysis of matched follow-up studies with several unexposed subjects matched to each exposed subject is analogous to the analysis of matched-pair data.

# References


**Atkinson, K. E.** (1989). *An Introduction to Numerical Analysis,* 2nd ed. John Wiley & Sons, New York.

**Breslow, N. E.** (1981). "Odds Ratio Estimators when the Data are Sparse", *Biometrika,* 68, 73–84.

**Cornfield, J. and Haenszel, W.** (1960). "Some Aspects of Retrospective Studies", *J. Chronic Dis.,* 11, 523–534.

**Cox, D. R.** (1958). "Two Further Applications of a Model for Binary Regression", *Biometrika,* 45, 562–565.

**Cox, D. R.** (1966). "A Simple Example of a Comparison Involving Quantal Data", *Biometrika,* 53, 215–220.

**Cox, D. R.** (1970). *Analysis of Binary Data.* Methuen, London.

**Ejigou, A.** (1990). "Small Sample Properties of Odds Ratio Estimators Under Multiple Matching in Case-Control Studies", *Biometrics,* 46, 61–69.

**Ejigou, A. and McHugh, R.** (1977). "Estimation of Relative Risk from Matched Pairs in Epidemiologic Research", *Biometrics,* 33, 552–556.

**Ejigou, A. and McHugh, R.** (1981). "Relative Risk Estimation Under Multiple Matching", *Biometrika,* 68, 85–92.

**Evans, M., Hastings, N. A. J., and Peacock, J. B.** (1993). *Statistical Distributions,* 2nd ed. John Wiley & Sons, New York.

**Fleiss, J. L.** (1981). *Statistical Methods for Rates and Proportions,* 2nd ed. John Wiley & Sons, New York.

**Gart, J. J.** (1971). "The Comparison of Proportions: A Review of Significance Tests, Confidence Intervals, and Adjustments for Stratification", *Rev. Int. Stat. Inst.,* 39, 148–169 (Errata, ibid., 1972, 40, 221).

**Jewell, N. P.** (1984). "Small-Sample Bias of Point Estimators of the Odds Ratio from Matched Sets", *Biometrics*, 40, 421–435.

**Jick, H., Miettinen, O. S., Neff, R. K., Shapiro, S., Heinonen, O. P., and Slone, D.** (1973). "Coffee and Myocardial Infarction", *N. Engl. J. Med.,* 289, 63–77.

**Kahn, H. A. and Sempos, C. T.** (1989). *Statistical Methods in Epidemiology.* Oxford University Press, New York.

**Kelsey, J. L., Thompson, W. D., and Evans, A. S.** (1986). *Methods in Observational Epidemiology.* Oxford University Press, New York.

**Kleinbaum, D. G., Kupper, L. L., and Morgenstern, H.** (1982). *Epidemiologic Research: Principles and Quantitative Methods.* Lifetime Learning Publications, Belmont, CA.

**Kraus, A. S.** (1958). "The Use of Family Members as Controls in the Study of the Possible Etiologic Factors of a Disease", Sc.D. Thesis, University of Pittsburgh, Pennsylvania.

**Kraus, A. S.** (1960). "Comparison of a Group with a Disease and a Control Group from the Same Families in the Search for Possible Etiologic Factors", *Am. J. Publ. Health,* 50, 303–311.

**Lubin, J. H.** (1981). "An Empirical Evaluation of the Use of Conditional and Unconditional Likelihoods for Case-Control Data", *Biometrika*, 68, 567–571.

**Mantel, N. and Haenszel, W. M.** (1959). "Statistical Aspects of the Analysis of Data from Retrospective Studies of Disease", *J. Nat. Cancer Inst.,* 22, 719–748.

**McNemar, Q.** (1947). "Note on the Sampling Error of the Difference Between Correlated Proportions or Percentages", *Psychometrika,* 12, 153–157.

**Miettinen, O. S.** (1969). "Individual Matching with Multiple Controls in the Case of All-or-None Responses", *Biometrics,* 25, 339–355.

**Miettinen, O. S.** (1970). "Estimation of Relative Risks from Individually Matched Series", *Biometrics,* 26, 75–86.

**Miettinen, O. S.** (1975). Principles of Epidemiologic Research, unpublished course text, Department of Epidemiology and Biostatistics, School of Public Health, Harvard University, Cambridge, MA.

**Pike, M. C. and Morrow, R. H.** (1970). "Statistical Analysis of Patient-Control Studies in Epidemiology: Factor Under Investigation on All-or-None Variable", *Br. J. Prevent. Social Med.,* 24, 42–44.

**Ralston, A. and Wilf, H.** (1967). *Mathematical Methods for Digital Computers.* John Wiley & Sons, New York.

**Rothman, K. J.** (1986). *Modern Epidemiology.* Little, Brown, Boston.

**Sahai, H. and Khurshid, A.** (1996). "Confidence Intervals for the Probability of Success in the Binomial Distribution: A Review", *Metron*, LIV, 153–180.

**Schesselman, J. J.** (1982). *Case-Control Studies.* Oxford University Press, New York.

**Schuster, J. J.** (1986). "The Cross-Product Estimator in Matched Case-Control Studies", *Biometrika,* 73, 212–216.

**Thomas, D. G. and Gart, J. J.** (1992). "Improved and Extended Exact and Asymptotic Methods for the Combination of 2 ¥ 2 Tables, Version 2", *Comput. Biomed. Res.,* 25, 75–84.

**Ury, H. K.** (1975). "Efficiency of Case-Control Studies with Multiple Controls Per Case: Continuous or Discontinuous Data", *Biometrics,* 31, 643–649.

**Walter, S. D.** (1980). "Matched Case-Control Studies with a Variable Number of Controls Per Case", *Appl. Stat.,* 29, 172–179.

# 8 Multivariate Models

Multivariate models refer to statistical techniques involving several variables which permit the adjustment for confounding and evaluation of an effect modifier in an epidemiologic study involving various potentially confounding factors with great computational and statistical efficiency. Statistical analysis involving multivariate models for adjusting confounding is an extremely useful analytic approach when the use of stratified analysis and matching becomes impractical. For example, in stratified analysis involving numerous strata, the data will be dispersed too thinly over various subcategories and the analysis will be inefficient, resulting in imprecise estimates of an effect measure. Multivariate analysis provides an efficient way of obtaining precise estimates, while controlling for potentially confounding factors, with the aid of mathematical models which allow simultaneous estimation of many effects. Moreover, the use of modern high-speed computing devices permits the realization of these analytic goals with relative ease, unencumbered by computational and mathematical chores.

## 8.1 LINEAR MODELS

Let $Y$ denote a response variate and $X_1, X_2, ..., X_k$ be a set of $k$ explanatory variables. A mathematical model relating $Y$ to $X_1, X_2, ..., X_k$, for specified values of $X_1 = x_1, X_2 = x_2, ..., X_k = x_k$, is

$$Y = \beta_0 + \beta_1 x_1 + \beta_2 x_2 + \ldots + \beta_k x_k + e$$

$$E(Y) = \beta_0 + \sum_{i=1}^{k} \beta_i x_i, \tag{8.1}$$

where $E(Y)$ can represent the risk, rate or odds of disease in persons with characteristics $X_1$, $X_2, ..., X_k$, and $e$ is a random error term. In statistical jargon, the variable $Y$ is called the *dependent variable,* the variables $X_1, X_2, ..., X_k$ are known as *independent variables, e* is an *error term,* and the mathematical equation (8.1) is called a *linear model.*

Classical linear models of the type depicted in Equation 8.1 stipulate the assumption which underlies this analysis; that is, for specified values of $X_1 = x_1, X_2 = x_2, ..., X_k = x_k$, the distribution of $Y$ is normal with mean $\beta_0 + \sum_{i=1}^{k} \beta_i x_i$.

. Thus, the model (8.1) can give values for *E(Y)* that are larger than 1.0 or smaller than zero. Hence, the model (8.1) is rarely used directly in medical and epidemiologic studies because the risk, rate, or odds of disease cannot be less than zero and the disease risk cannot be greater than one. Therefore, generally, a logarithmic transformation is used which yields a function that has a theoretical range of $-\infty$ to $\infty$. A family of models exists which involves logarithmic transformation and we consider a special case of this family, the logistic model, which is particularly suited to the estimation of effect measures of risk ratio (RR) and odds ratio (OR).

The importance of multivariate analysis by using mathematical models such as Equation 8.1 lies in the fact that the inferences based on the coefficient for any independent variable in the model is conditional on the remaining independent variables in the model. This means that in an epidemiologic study involving many confounding variates and effect modifiers, all the confounding factors can be controlled simultaneously in a single model, and the effect of each factor adjusted for the other factors in the model can be estimated. Multivariate analysis is a specialized topic and a full discussion of its application is not possible here. An excellent reference on the use of multivariate models for epidemiologic data is Kleinbaum et al. (1988).

## 8.2 BINARY LOGISTIC REGRESSION

One reason that linear regression is not used frequently in epidemiologic and medical research is that the outcome variable cannot be assumed to have a normal distribution. A common type of response or outcome variable in medical research is a binary variable. This type of response variable takes one of the two values such as developing an outcome or not, among others.

Because the dependent variable $Y$ can assume only two possible values, it would be unrealistic to describe a linear regression model such as

$$
\begin{aligned}
Y &= \beta_0 + \beta_1 x_1 + \beta_2 x_2 + \ldots + \beta_k x_k + e \\
E(Y) &= \beta_0 + \sum_{i=1}^{k} \beta_i x_i .
\end{aligned}
\tag{8.2}
$$

Note that theoretically, $-\infty < E(Y) < \infty$, because in a linear regression model $E(Y)$ is assumed to be the expected value (mean) of a normal distribution. In a logistic regression, however, the dependent variable $Y$ can take only two values, for example, 0 and 1. Thus,

$$
\begin{aligned}
E(Y) &= 0 \times P(Y = 0) + 1 \times P(Y = 1) \\
&= P(Y = 1) = p.
\end{aligned}
$$

Note that

$$0 < p < 1,$$

$$0 < \frac{p}{1-p} < \infty,$$

$$-\infty < \log_e\left(\frac{p}{1-p}\right) < \infty.$$

Therefore, a reasonable regression model is

$$\log_e\left(\frac{p}{1-p}\right) = \beta_0 + \sum_{i=1}^{k} \beta_i x_i$$

$$\frac{p}{1-p} = \exp\left(\beta_0 + \sum_{i=1}^{k} \beta_i x_i\right) \tag{8.3}$$

$$p = \frac{\exp\left(\beta_0 + \sum_{i=1}^{k} \beta_i x_i\right)}{1 + \exp\left(\beta_0 + \sum_{i=1}^{k} \beta_i x_i\right)}.$$

Logistic regression model (8.3) can be used to describe the relationship between a dichotomous response variable and a set of explanatory variables (e.g., age, treatment, sex). Such analysis is of interest for the evaluation of treatment effects as well as interaction effects of treatment with other explanatory variables. The details of calculations in estimating a logistic regression model are somewhat involved, requiring complex numerical algorithms, and are not presented here. A general method of estimation, called the maximum likelihood, for estimating parameters of a logistic regression model is described in Appendix L. The results using the maximum likelihood estimates for the logistic regression model can be calculated with the aid of the SAS procedures CATMOD or LOGIST (SAS Institute, 1992); the BMDP procedure LR, documented in Dixon (1992); or the LOGISTIC procedure, documented in SPSS-Advanced Statistics (SPSS, Inc., 1994). Some general purpose and epidemiologic software for microcomputers also implement this procedure (see EGRET, 1994; STATA, 1994; SYSTAT, 1994; TRUE EPISTAT, 1994). Most logistic regression software currently available provide results on $p$-values and confidence intervals (CIs) based on asymptotic or large sample approximation. The LogXact (1992) developed by CYTEL Software Corporation supports both exact and asymptotic inferences.

As in a linear regression analysis, if $\beta_i$ is zero, then the factor represented by $X_i$ is not associated with the outcome variable $Y$. A suitable statistic for testing the hypothesis that the regression coefficient $\beta_i$ equals zero is

$$Z = \frac{\hat{\beta}_i}{\hat{SE}(\hat{\beta}_i)}, \tag{8.4}$$

where for a large sample size $Z$ can be treated as a standard normal variate under the null hypothesis that the $i$th independent variable has no association with the dependent variable after controlling for the other variables. Thus, the null hypothesis will be rejected for either large positive or large negative values of the test statistic $Z$ as defined in (8.4).

The test given above is commonly known as the Wald test, and is obtained by dividing the maximum likelihood estimate of the parameter to an estimate of its standard error. The method of estimating standard error of an estimated coefficient follows from the theory of maximum likelihood estimation (see Rao, 1973). Most computer programs on logistic regression produce the estimates of standard errors of the estimated parameters as an essential part of their output. (For a discussion of the adequacy of inference of the Wald test in a logistic regression analysis, see Hauck and Donner, 1977 and Jennings, 1986.) In addition to Wald test, two other tests are applied to hypotheses in logistic regression. These are the likelihood ratio test and the score test. (For a detailed discussion of these tests, see Cox and Hinkley, 1974 and Dobson, 1983.)

### 8.2.1 Estimation of Odds Ratio

In a logistic regression analysis, in addition to assessing statistical significance, an OR also can be calculated to measure the strength of the association between each independent variable and the dependent variable after controlling for the other variables in the model. The procedure is described below for both dichotomous and continuous independent random variables.

#### 8.2.1.1 Dichotomous Independent Variable

Consider a dichotomous independent variable ($X_i$), which is coded as 1 if present and 0 if absent. For the multiple logistic regression model (Equation 8.3), the OR relating this independent variable to the dependent variable is estimated by

$$\hat{OR} = \exp\left(\hat{\beta}_i\right). \tag{8.5}$$

The relationship (Equation 8.5) expresses the ratio of the odds in favor of the outcome when $x_i = 1$ to the odds in favor of the outcome when $x_i = 0$, after controlling for all other variables in the logistic regression model.

An approximate CI for the OR can be obtained from the corresponding interval for $\beta_i$. Thus, a two-sided 100(1 – α)% CI for the true OR is given by

$$\left[\exp\left\{\hat{\beta}_i - Z_{\alpha/2}\,\hat{\mathrm{SE}}\left(\hat{\beta}_i\right)\right\}, \exp\left\{\hat{\beta}_i + Z_{\alpha/2}\,\hat{\mathrm{SE}}\left(\hat{\beta}_i\right)\right\}\right], \tag{8.6}$$

where $Z_{\alpha/2}$ is the upper 100(α/2)th percentile of the standard normal distribution.

### 8.2.1.2 Continuous Independent Variable

We are also interested in expressing the magnitude of association between a continuous or nondichotomous independent variable and the dependent variable after controlling for the other independent variables in the model. Let $X_i$ be a continuous independent variable of interest. Suppose we wish to express the risk of certain condition at level $x_i'$ compared to that at level $x_i''$ for the independent variable $x_i$, adjusting for other variables considered in the model. It is readily seen that the OR relating the exposure level $x_i''$ to $x_i'$ is estimated by

$$\hat{\mathrm{OR}} = \exp\left\{\hat{\beta}_i\left(x_i'' - x_i'\right)\right\}. \tag{8.7}$$

The relationship (Equation 8.7) expresses the ratio of the odds in favor of the outcome when $x_i = x_i''$ to the odds in favor of the outcome when $x_i = x_i'$, after controlling for all other variables in the logistic regression model.

An approximate CI for the OR can be obtained from the corresponding interval for $\beta_i$. Thus, a two-sided 100(1 – α)% CI for the true OR is given by

$$\left[\exp\left\{\left(\hat{\beta}_i - Z_{\alpha/2}\,\hat{\mathrm{SE}}\left(\hat{\beta}_i\right)\right)\left(x_i'' - x_i'\right)\right\}, \exp\left\{\left(\hat{\beta}_i + Z_{\alpha/2}\,\hat{\mathrm{SE}}\left(\hat{\beta}_i\right)\right)\left(x_i'' - x_i'\right)\right\}\right]. \tag{8.8}$$

*Example 8.1*

Melo-Villalobos and Weber (1992) analyzed data from a case-control study for Hodgkin's disease (HD). The study was performed to test the hypothesis that HD is associated with prior exposure to an infectious agent, which in turn is associated with low economic conditions. The study population was confined to children under 16 years of age from low socioeconomic groups. A sample of 91 cases was obtained from those registered at the Instituto Nacional de Cancerologia (INC) in Santafé de Bogota, Colombia, and diagnosed with HD. Another sample of 182 controls was taken from those registered at the INC during the same period as the cases but diagnosed with a cancer other than HD. From the clinical history of each case and control, the data were obtained on age, sex, and a number of other sociodemographic and family history variables, including prior exposure to an infectious agent. The age was treated as a

**TABLE 8.1**
**Multiple Logistic Regression Analysis Relating Prevalence of Hodgkin's Disease to Sex, Age, and Exposure to an Infectious Agent**

| Risk factor | Regression coefficient $[(\hat{\beta}_i)]$ | Standard error $[\hat{SE}(\hat{\beta}_i)]$ | Z $[(\hat{\beta}_i)/\hat{SE}(\hat{\beta}_i)]$ | *p*-Value |
|---|---|---|---|---|
| Constant | 0.527 | 0.239 | 2.205 | 0.028 |
| Sex | 0.718 | 0.155 | 4.632 | <0.001 |
| Age 1 | –0.487 | 0.186 | –2.618 | 0.009 |
| Age 2 | 0.494 | 0.167 | 2.958 | 0.006 |
| Infectious agent | 0.516 | 0.192 | 2.688 | 0.007 |

From Melo-Villalobos, B. and Weber, S. (1992). *Rev. Col. Estad.*, No. 25–26, 13–32. With permission.

categorical variable with the following three categories: 1 to 4 (years), 5 to 9, and 10 to 15 (number of years completed). Several logistic regression models were fitted using the CATMOD procedure from SAS. In addition to the variables on age and sex, the full analysis included all socioeconomic and family history variables, which were not statistically significant. The results of a logistic regression analysis relating HD to the risk factors of age, sex, and prior exposure to an infectious agent, including estimates of parameters, standard errors, and test statistics, are shown in Table 8.1.

To assess the significance of each one of the risk factors, we first examine the values of the test statistic *Z*, or equivalently the *p*-value, as shown in Table 8.1. For a two-sided test with an $\alpha$ level of 0.05, we compare $|Z|$ to $Z_{0.025} = 1.96$ for each one of the risk factors. Because all factors satisfy the criterion, they are all significant at the 5% level of significance.

We can also determine an OR to measure the strength of the association for each one of the risk factors. For example, the odds in favor of HD for male children after controlling for other variables can be estimated by*

$$\hat{OR} = \exp(2 \times 0.718) = 4.204.$$

Thus, the odds in favor of HD for male children is nearly four times as large as that for female children after controlling for other variables. An approximate 95% CI for the OR is calculated using Equation 8.6:

* Because the CATMOD uses the marginal method of coding, assigning the value of –1 to the lower code and 1 to the upper code, the coefficients must be multiplied by 2 before exponentiating for the determination of the OR and CI.

**TABLE 8.2**
**Estimated ORs and CIs for Logistic Regression Analysis in Table 8.1**

| Variable | $\hat{OR}$ | $\hat{OR}_L$ | $\hat{OR}_U$ |
|---|---|---|---|
| Sex | 4.204 | 2.290 | 7.718 |
| Age 1 | 0.378 | 0.182 | 0.783 |
| Age 2 | 2.686 | 1.396 | 5.169 |
| Infectious agent | 2.807 | 1.322 | 5.957 |

$$\left[\exp\{2(0.718 - 1.96 \times 0.155)\}, \exp\{2(0.718 + 1.96 \times 0.155)\}\right]$$

$$= [2.290, 7.718].$$

The OR relating the odds of HD to other variables and corresponding CIs can be determined similarly and are summarized in Table 8.2.

Thus, the OR for HD relating exposure to an infectious agent is 2.807, which means that the risk of acquiring HD is nearly three times as large as the risk of getting any other type of cancer or disease. The OR for age 1 is 0.378, which is interpreted as the estimated relative risk of HD for children <5 years old as compared to children between 5 and 15 years of age. The relative risk for those between 5 and 15 years of age as compared to children <5 years old is approximately equal to 1/0.378 = 2.646. Comparing the latter value to the estimated relative risk of 2.686 for age 2 (i.e., children between 5 and 9 years to other age groups), one may conclude that the relative risk for the age group 5 to 9 years does not seem to be of any real importance.

### 8.2.2 Estimation of Relative Risk in Cohort and Case-Control Studies

We now indicate the estimation of relative risk using logistic regression models under two well-known epidemiologic designs, prospective cohort studies and retrospective case-control studies.

#### 8.2.2.1 Cohort Studies

Several variations of the cohort design are in common use. The simplest cohort design entails a random sample of subjects who are followed through for a certain period of time and the response outcome, including the covariates, is measured. A simple modification of this design is the clinical trial, in which a simple random sample of subjects is selected, the members of which are then allocated independently into two treatment groups. The subjects are then followed and the response outcome and the covariates are recorded. Another modification of this design may involve the stratification of subjects by location, clinic, or year of recruitment to account for stratum-specific response.

In some cohort studies the response variate of interest is the time to the occurrence of some event or endpoint. In these studies the time to the occurrence is generally modeled using the proportional hazards regression described in Section 8.3. Another method of analysis for such data which is sometimes used is to ignore the time of occurrence and to analyze the occurrence or nonoccurrence of the event using a logistic regression model. (For a discussion of the use of logistic regression with survival data, see Green and Symmons, 1983; Abbot, 1985; Bren and Arnesen, 1985; Hauck 1985; and Efron, 1988.)

In all cohort studies relative risk is estimated as RR and can be estimated directly from the logistic model (8.3) by assuming mean values for all other independent variables.

#### 8.2.2.2 Case-Control Studies

In case-control studies involving a rare disease, relative risk is estimated by the OR. Note that in a case-control study the sampling is performed on the condition of the outcome variable, in which samples of fixed sizes are chosen from the two groups defined by the outcome variable. Thus, the dependent variables in the study are one or more exposure variables or risk factors. However, the OR is invariant under study design, cohort, or case-control (Cornfield, 1951; Farewell, 1979; Prentice and Pyke, 1979). A derivation of the result is given in Appendix M. Thus, the dependent variable in a logistic regression model, for a case-control design, can be taken as the outcome variable of interest to the investigator, and the regression analysis can be carried out in the same way as in cohort studies (Breslow and Powers, 1978). Let the outcome variable $Y$ represent the disease state; in other words, $Y = 1$ corresponds to the case and $Y = 0$ corresponds to noncase. Let $X_i$ be a risk factor of interest. The OR relating the risk factor $X_i$ to the disease state $Y$ can be estimated using Equations 8.5 or 8.7, according to whether $X_i$ is a dichotomous or continuous variate.

The OR from logistic regression models can also be estimated for matched case-control studies involving 1–1 or 1–$M$ matched designs. The logistic regression model for a matched design makes use of the conditional likelihood analysis to obtain the maximum likelihood estimator of the slope coefficients. (For a discussion of the logistic regression analysis for the matched case-control design, see Breslow et al., 1978; Holford et al., 1978; Breslow and Day, 1980; Thomas, 1981; Kleinbaum et al., 1982; Schlesselman, 1982; Moolgavakar et al., 1985; Hosmer and Lemeshow, 1989; and Collett, 1991.) The 1–1 matched design can be analyzed using a standard logistic regression software. For a 1–$M$ design ($M > 1$), the requisite software is given in EGRET (1994). The LogXact (1992) performs both exact and asymptotic logistic analyses for the general $m{:}n$ matched design. In addition, Breslow and Day (1980) list programs that will perform the necessary computations.

**TABLE 8.3**
**A 2 × 2 Table Relating the Outcome and Risk Variable**

| | | Risk Variable ($X$) | |
|---|---|---|---|
| | | x = 1 (+) | x = 0 (–) |
| Outcome Variable ($Y$) | | | |
| | $y = 1$ (+) | $a$ | $b$ |
| | $y = 0$ (–) | $c$ | $d$ |

### 8.2.3 Logistic Regression in a 2 × 2 Table

Consider a 2 × 2 table relating the outcome variable $Y$ to the risk variable $X$, as shown in Table 8.3. The mathematical model for a binary logistic regression is

$$P(Y = 1 \mid X = x) = \frac{\exp(\beta_0 + \beta_1 x)}{1 + \exp(\beta_0 + \beta_1 x)}.$$

Note that the OR relating the risk variable $X$ to the outcome variable $Y$ is given by

$$\begin{aligned}
\text{OR} &= \frac{P(y=1 \mid x=1) \div P(y=0 \mid x=1)}{P(y=1 \mid x=0) \div P(y=0 \mid x=0)} \\
&= \frac{\left[\dfrac{\exp(\beta_0+\beta_1)}{1+\exp(\beta_0+\beta_1)}\right] \div \left[1 - \dfrac{\exp(\beta_0+\beta_1)}{1+\exp(\beta_0+\beta_1)}\right]}{\left[\dfrac{\exp(\beta_0)}{1+\exp(\beta_0)}\right] \div \left[1 - \dfrac{\exp(\beta_0)}{1+\exp(\beta_0)}\right]} \\
&= \exp(\beta_1).
\end{aligned}$$

Hence, for the logistic regression involving a dichotomous independent variable, OR = $\exp(\beta_1)$ and $\log_e(\text{OR}) = \beta_1$.

Thus, the antilogarithm of the coefficient for a binary independent variable in a logistic regression is equal to the OR. This interpretation of the coefficients in a logistic regression model has made the logistic regression analysis a very useful analytic approach for analyzing epidemiologic data. We previously discussed the use of stratification to test for no association in a 2 × 2 table, adjusting for possible confounding variable(s) in the study population. In general, logistic regression models are designed to make such adjustments more efficiently, but the stratification approach can be shown to be a special case of a logistic regression model. (For further details and references concerning logistic regression analysis, see Breslow and Day, 1980; Schesselman, 1982; Kleinbaum et al., 1982; Koch et al., 1982, 1985; Cox and Snell, 1989; Hosmer and Lemeshow, 1989; Neter et al., 1989; Glantz and Slinker, 1990; Darlington, 1991; and Kleinbaum, 1994.)

## 8.3 PROPORTIONAL HAZARDS REGRESSION

The logistic regression model is useful for identifying risk factors related to the presence or absence of a disease or condition. However, in many medical and epidemiologic studies, interest is focused not on the particular outcome of a disease or condition, but the time of its occurrence. For example, in many studies of chronic diseases, perhaps the most common endpoint of interest is survival time. The proportional hazards regression is one of the most frequently used regression models to relate survival time to a host of risk factors. This model relates events to the individuals at risk at the time of the event and uses a mathematical model to adjust for covariates.

Survival function, denoted by $S(t)$, is defined as the probability that an individual survives at least up to time $t$:

$$S(t) = P(T > t),$$

where $T$ is a random variable denoting survival time. Hazard function, denoted by $h(t)$, is defined as the conditional probability of failure (not surviving) during a very small time interval, assuming that the individual has survived to the beginning of the interval. It is the conditional instantaneous probability of having an event at time $t$ and can be obtained as the limit of the probability that the individual fails in a very short interval, $(t, t + \Delta t)$, given that the individual has survived to time $t$:

$$h(t) = \lim_{\Delta t \to 0} \frac{S(t) - S(t + \Delta t)}{\Delta t} \Big/ S(t).$$

Let $h_j(t)$ be the hazard function for a specific individual at time $t$ and $h_0(t)$ be the hazard to the general population, or more specifically, the baseline hazard at time $t$. Under the proportional hazards regression, the ratio $h_j(t)/h_0(t)$ is considered constant and is modeled as the exponential of the characteristics of the individual:

$$\frac{h_j(t)}{h_0(t)} = \exp\left(\beta_1 x_{1j} + \beta_2 x_{2j} + \ldots + \beta_k x_{kj}\right), \quad j = 1, 2, \ldots, n, \qquad (8.9)$$

where $x_{1j}, x_{2j}, \ldots, x_{kj}$ are the observed values of the characteristics of the $j$th individual, also known as explanatory variables, covariates, or independent variables, and $\beta_1,\beta_2,\ldots,\beta_k$ are the corresponding coefficients. Note that the baseline hazard $h_0(t)$ represents the hazard at time $t$ for an individual whose covariates are all zero (i.e., $x_{1j} = 0$, $x_{2j} = 0,\ldots,x_{kj} = 0$). It is not necessary that an individual having all values of the covariates equal to zero be realistic, but rather $h_0(t)$ is simply a reference point and serves the same role as the intercept in a general regression model. The only difference is that whereas the intercept is a single numerical constant, $h_0(t)$ changes as $t$ varies. Note also that the hazard ratio $h_j(t)/h_0(t)$ is the relative risk of an individual as compared to the individual with baseline characteristics or the general population. Equation (8.9) can also be written as

$$\log_e\left\{\frac{h_j(t)}{h_0(t)}\right\} = \beta_1 x_{1j} + \beta_2 x_{2j} + \ldots + \beta_k x_{kj}. \tag{8.10}$$

The left side of Equation 8.10 is a function of the hazard for the $j$th individual, and the right side is a linear combination of the explanatory variables. If we let $y_j = \log_e[h_j(t)/h_0(t)]$, then Equation 8.10 is simply written

$$y_j = \beta_1 x_{1j} + \beta_2 x_{2j} + \ldots + \beta_k x_{kj},$$

which represents the standard multiple regression model.

The methods of estimation of the coefficients $\beta_1,\beta_2,\ldots,\beta_k$, from the observed data on survival and the covariates, are analogous to those used for the standard multiple regression and are not presented here. Maximum likelihood equations for estimating the $\beta_i$ and their variance–covariance matrix are given in Lawless (1982). The results using the maximum likelihood estimates for the proportional hazards regression can be calculated with the aid of SAS procedures PHREG (SAS Institute, 1992) and PHGLM (Proportional Hazards General Linear Model), documented in Harrell (1986). Some general purpose and epidemiologic software for microcomputers also implement this procedure (see, e.g., EGRET, 1994; STATA, 1994; SYSTAT, 1994; TRUE EPISTAT, 1994).

As in a linear regression analysis, if $\beta_i$ is zero, then the covariate $x_i$ is not associated with the hazard. A suitable statistic for testing the hypothesis $H_0$ : $\beta_i = 0$ vs. $\beta_i \neq 0$ is

$$Z = \frac{\hat{\beta}_i}{\hat{\mathrm{SE}}\left(\hat{\beta}_i\right)}, \tag{8.11}$$

where for a large sample size $Z$ can be treated as a standard normal variate under the null hypothesis that the $i$th covariate has no association with the hazard function after controlling for the other covariates. Thus, the null hypothesis will be rejected for either large positive or large negative values of the test statistic $Z$, as defined in Equation 8.11.

### 8.3.1 Estimation of Relative Risk of Hazards

Equation 8.9 is similar to the logistic regression model (Equation 8.3), and the coefficients of a proportional hazards model can be interpreted in a manner similar to that of a logistic regression model. Thus, $\hat{\beta}_i$ represents the estimated change in log hazard ratio for each unit change in $x_i$ after adjusting for the effects of other covariates included in the model. In addition, the results of the model can be used to calculate the ratio of hazards for two individuals with different characteristics. For example, let $x_1', x_2', \ldots, x_k'$ be the values of the characteristics or covariates of an individual or group, and let $x_1'', x_2'', \ldots, x_k''$ be the corresponding values of another individual or group. Then the relative risk (RR) of hazards of two individuals or two groups is given by

$$\hat{\text{RR}} = \exp\left\{\hat{\beta}_1\left(x_1'' - x_1'\right) + \hat{\beta}_2\left(x_2'' - x_2'\right) + \ldots + \hat{\beta}_k\left(x_k'' - x_k'\right)\right\}.$$

The results are summarized below for dichotomous and continuous independent variables.

#### 8.3.1.1 Dichotomous Independent Variable

Consider a dichotomous independent variable $(x_i)$ which is coded as 1 if present and 0 if absent. For the proportional hazards model (Equation 8.9), the ratio of hazards for two individuals, one with the risk factor present and the other with the risk factor absent, given that the individuals have the same values for other covariates, is estimated by

$$\hat{\text{RR}} = \exp\left\{\hat{\beta}_i\right\}. \tag{8.12}$$

The relationship in Equation 8.12 represents the ratio of the instantaneous hazard of an event per unit of time for an individual with the risk factor present as compared to an individual with the risk factor absent, given that both individuals have survived until time $t$.

An approximate CI for the hazards ratio can be obtained from the corresponding interval for $\beta_i$. Thus, a two-sided $100(1 - \alpha)\%$ CI for the true hazards ratio is given by

$$\left[\exp\left\{\hat{\beta}_i - Z_{\alpha/2}\,\hat{\text{SE}}\left(\hat{\beta}_i\right)\right\}, \exp\left\{\hat{\beta}_i + Z_{\alpha/2}\,\hat{\text{SE}}\left(\hat{\beta}_i\right)\right\}\right], \tag{8.13}$$

where $Z_{\alpha/2}$ is the upper $100(\alpha/2)$th percentile of the standard normal distribution.

#### 8.3.1.2 Continuous Independent Variable

Consider a continuous independent variable $(x_i)$ of interest. For the proportional hazards model (Equation 8.9), the ratio of hazards for two individuals, one with the value of the risk factor $x_i'$ and the other with the value of $x_i''$, given that the two individuals have the same values for other covariates, is estimated by

$$\hat{RR} = \exp\left\{\hat{\beta}_i\left(x_i'' - x_i'\right)\right\}. \tag{8.14}$$

The relationship in Equation 8.14 represents the ratio of the instantaneous hazard of an event per unit of time for an individual with the value of the risk factor $x_i'$ as compared to an individual with the risk factor value $x_i''$, given that both individuals have survived until time $t$.

An approximate CI for the true hazards ratio can be obtained from the corresponding interval for $\beta_i$. Thus, a two-sided $100(1 - \alpha)\%$ CI for the hazards ratio is given by

$$\left[\exp\left\{\left(\hat{\beta}_i - Z_{\alpha/2}\,\hat{SE}\left(\hat{\beta}_i\right)\right)\left(x_i'' - x_i'\right)\right\}, \exp\left\{\left(\hat{\beta}_i + Z_{\alpha/2}\,\hat{SE}\left(\hat{\beta}_i\right)\right)\left(x_i'' - x_i'\right)\right\}\right]. \tag{8.15}$$

The proportional hazards regression was developed by Cox (1972) and is frequently referred to as *Cox's regression.* It is now widely used to report the results of longitudinal studies on survival data in the epidemiologic literature. This regression also has become the standard method for analyses of these types of data in many other fields. Numerous other models are introduced for these types of data to relate survival to a set of other risk factors or covariates. An enormous literature deals with the subject, including a number of textbooks (e.g., Kalbfleisch and Prentice, 1980; Miller, 1981; Lawless, 1982; Cox and Oakes, 1984; Harris and Albert, 1991; Lee, 1992; Collett, 1994; and Marubini and Valsecchi, 1995).

*Example 8.2*

Feigel and Zelen (1965) reported and analyzed data to investigate the relationship among survival of acute myclogenous leukemia patients, white blood cell (WBC) counts, and a white cell morphologic characteristic. The morphologic characteristic is the presence or absence of Auer rods, called AG positive and AG negative. The data on survival times in weeks and the WBC count for AG positive and AG negative patients are summarized in Table 8.4. Feigel and Zelen analyzed the data, assuming an exponential model for survivorship. These data also have been referred, reported, and analyzed by Lawless (1982), Harris and Albert (1991), and Selvin (1991).

Selvin (1991) analyzed the data using a proportional hazards regression in order to describe the influence of AG status on survival while accounting for the influence of WBC level. The full model relating WBC count and AG status to survival time (including interaction term) is

**TABLE 8.4**
**Survival Times and White Blood Cell (WBC) Counts**

| | AG positive | | | AG negative | |
|---|---|---|---|---|---|
| | Weeks | WBC | | Weeks | WBC |
| 1 | 65 | 2,300 | 1 | 65 | 3,000 |
| 2 | 156 | 750 | 2 | 17 | 4,000 |
| 3 | 100 | 4,300 | 3 | 7 | 1,500 |
| 4 | 134 | 2,600 | 4 | 16 | 9,000 |
| 5 | 16 | 6,000 | 5 | 22 | 5,300 |
| 6 | 108 | 10,500 | 6 | 3 | 10,000 |
| 7 | 121 | 10,000 | 7 | 4 | 19,000 |
| 8 | 4 | 17,000 | 8 | 2 | 27,000 |
| 9 | 39 | 5,400 | 9 | 3 | 28,000 |
| 10 | 143 | 7,000 | 10 | 8 | 31,000 |
| 11 | 56 | 9,400 | 11 | 4 | 26,000 |
| 12 | 26 | 32,000 | 12 | 3 | 21,000 |
| 13 | 22 | 35,000 | 13 | 30 | 79,000 |
| 14 | 1 | 100,000 | 14 | 4 | 100,000 |
| 15 | 1 | 100,000 | 15 | 43 | 100,000 |
| 16 | 5 | 52,000 | 16 | 56 | 4,400 |
| 17 | 65 | 100,000 | | | |

From Selvin, S. (1991). *Statistical Analysis of Epidemiologic Data.* Oxford University Press, New York, p. 333. (Original data from Feigel and Zelen, 1965). With permission.

$$\frac{h_j(t)}{h_0(t)} = \exp\left(\beta_1 x_{1j} + \beta_2 x_{2j} + \beta_3 x_{1j} x_{2j}\right), \quad j = 1, 2, \ldots, 33$$

where $x_{1j}$ is an indicator of AG status and $x_{2j}$ is the WBC count. The results of the analysis, including estimates of parameters, standard errors, and test statistics are given in Table 8.5.

To assess the significance of each one of the risk factors, AG status, WBC, and the interaction term, we examine the values of the test statistic *Z*, or equivalently the *p*-value, as shown in Table 8.5. The results show that AG status significantly affects survival while adjusting for the effect of WBC. The test of interaction coefficient is also significant, indicating that the relationship between survival patterns is not the same for two types of AG status. The presence of interaction limits the interpretation of findings and additional analyses are needed.

The effect of AG status can be quantified in terms of relative risk of hazards. For example, given an AG positive individual or group and the other AG negative, the instantaneous relative risk of death of one being AG positive, compared to the other being AG negative, is given by

**TABLE 8.5**
**Proportional Hazards Regression Analysis Relating Survival to AG Status and WBC**

| Risk factor | Regression coefficient $[(\hat{\beta}_i)]$ | Standard error $[\widehat{SE}(\hat{\beta}_i)]$ | $Z$ $[(\hat{\beta}_i)/\widehat{SE}(\hat{\beta}_i)]$ | $p$-Value |
|---|---|---|---|---|
| AG status | 1.816 | 0.583 | 3.115 | 0.002 |
| WBC | 0.0000415 | 0.000017 | 2.441 | 0.015 |
| AG status × WBC | −0.0000209 | 0.0000105 | −1.991 | 0.047 |

From Selvin, S. (1991). *Statistical Analysis of Epidemiologic Data,* Oxford University Press, New York, p. 334. With permission.

$$\hat{RR} = \exp(1.816) = 6.147.$$

Thus, given that the two individuals survived up to time $t$, the AG positive person is nearly six times as likely to die over a short period of time than the AG negative person. A 95% CI for the true relative risk of hazards (death) can be calculated using Equation 8.13, and is given by

$$\left[\exp\{1.816 - 1.96(0.583)\}, \exp\{1.816 + 1.96(0.583)\}\right]$$

$$= (1.961, 19.273).$$

(For further discussion of this problem, including some additional analyses, see Selvin, 1991.)

*Example 8.3*

Krall et al. (1975) reported and analyzed the data on the survivorship experience of 65 patients who were diagnosed with the presence of multiple myeloma. The original study included 16 covariates, but after screening for their statistical significance, the following three covariates measured at diagnosis were retained:

1. $X_1$: Logarithm of blood urea nitrogen (mg/100 ml)
2. $X_2$: Hemoglobin (%)
3. $X_3$: Serum calcium (mg/100 ml)

Table 8.6 shows the data for these variables and for $X_4$ (sex) and $X_5$ (age at diagnosis). These data also have been referred, reported, and analyzed by Lawless (1982) and Harris and Albert (1991). The data contain a number of tied survival times for both censored and noncensored cases. (For a discussion of various methods proposed to adjust for tied values, see Lawless, 1982, and Harris and Albert, 1991.)

**TABLE 8.6**
**Survival Times and Covariates for 65 Multiple Myeloma Patients**

| *t* (month) | $X_1$ | $X_2$ | $X_3$ | $X_4$ | $X_5$ | *t* (month) | $X_1$ | $X_2$ | $X_3$ | $X_4$ | $X_5$ |
|---|---|---|---|---|---|---|---|---|---|---|---|
| 1 | 2.218 | 9.4 | 10 | 0 | 67 | 26 | 1.230 | 11.2 | 11 | 1 | 49 |
| 1 | 1.940 | 12.0 | 18 | 0 | 38 | 32 | 1.322 | 10.6 | 9 | 0 | 46 |
| 2 | 1.519 | 9.8 | 15 | 0 | 81 | 35 | 1.114 | 7.0 | 10 | 0 | 48 |
| 2 | 1.748 | 11.3 | 12 | 0 | 75 | 37 | 1.602 | 11.0 | 9 | 0 | 63 |
| 2 | 1.301 | 5.1 | 9 | 0 | 57 | 41 | 1.000 | 10.2 | 10 | 0 | 69 |
| 3 | 1.544 | 6.7 | 10 | 1 | 46 | 42 | 1.146 | 5.0 | 9 | 1 | 70 |
| 5 | 2.236 | 10.1 | 9 | 1 | 50 | 51 | 1.568 | 7.7 | 13 | 0 | 74 |
| 5 | 1.681 | 6.5 | 9 | 0 | 74 | 52 | 1.000 | 10.1 | 10 | 1 | 60 |
| 6 | 1.362 | 9.0 | 8 | 0 | 77 | 54 | 1.255 | 9.0 | 10 | 0 | 49 |
| 6 | 2.114 | 10.2 | 8 | 1 | 70 | 58 | 1.204 | 12.1 | 10 | 1 | 42 |
| 6 | 1.114 | 9.7 | 10 | 0 | 60 | 66 | 1.447 | 6.6 | 9 | 0 | 59 |
| 6 | 1.415 | 10.4 | 8 | 1 | 67 | 67 | 1.322 | 12.8 | 10 | 0 | 52 |
| 7 | 1.978 | 9.5 | 10 | 0 | 48 | 88 | 1.176 | 10.6 | 9 | 1 | 47 |
| 7 | 1.041 | 5.1 | 10 | 1 | 61 | 89 | 1.322 | 14.0 | 9 | 0 | 63 |
| 7 | 1.176 | 11.4 | 13 | 1 | 53 | 92 | 1.431 | 11.0 | 11 | 1 | 58 |
| 9 | 1.724 | 8.2 | 12 | 0 | 55 | 4* | 1.945 | 10.2 | 10 | 0 | 59 |
| 11 | 1.114 | 14.0 | 10 | 0 | 61 | 4* | 1.924 | 10.0 | 13 | 1 | 49 |
| 11 | 1.230 | 12.0 | 9 | 0 | 43 | 7* | 1.114 | 12.4 | 10 | 1 | 48 |
| 11 | 1.301 | 13.2 | 10 | 0 | 65 | 7* | 1.532 | 10.2 | 11 | 0 | 81 |
| 11 | 1.508 | 7.5 | 12 | 0 | 70 | 8* | 1.079 | 9.9 | 8 | 1 | 57 |
| 11 | 1.079 | 9.6 | 9 | 1 | 51 | 11* | 1.613 | 14.0 | 9 | 0 | 60 |
| 13 | 0.778 | 5.5 | 10 | 1 | 60 | 12* | 1.146 | 11.6 | 7 | 1 | 46 |
| 14 | 1.398 | 14.6 | 10 | 0 | 66 | 12* | 1.398 | 8.8 | 9 | 1 | 66 |
| 15 | 1.602 | 10.6 | 11 | 0 | 70 | 13* | 1.663 | 4.9 | 9 | 1 | 71 |
| 16 | 1.342 | 9.0 | 10 | 0 | 48 | 16* | 1.146 | 13.0 | 9 | 0 | 55 |
| 16 | 1.322 | 8.8 | 10 | 1 | 62 | 19* | 1.322 | 13.0 | 10 | 1 | 59 |
| 17 | 1.230 | 10.0 | 9 | 0 | 53 | 19* | 1.322 | 10.8 | 10 | 1 | 69 |
| 17 | 1.591 | 11.2 | 10 | 0 | 68 | 28* | 1.230 | 7.3 | 9 | 1 | 82 |
| 18 | 1.447 | 7.5 | 8 | 1 | 65 | 41* | 1.756 | 12.8 | 9 | 0 | 72 |
| 19 | 1.079 | 14.4 | 15 | 0 | 51 | 53* | 1.114 | 12.0 | 11 | 0 | 66 |
| 19 | 1.255 | 7.5 | 9 | 1 | 60 | 57* | 1.255 | 12.5 | 11 | 0 | 66 |
| 24 | 1.301 | 14.6 | 9 | 1 | 56 | 77* | 1.079 | 14.0 | 12 | 0 | 60 |
| 25 | 1.000 | 12.4 | 10 | 0 | 67 | | | | | | |

* Censored survival time.

From Harris, E. K. and Albert, A. (1991). *Survivalship Analysis for Clinical Studies.* Marcel Dekker, New York, pp. 97–98. (Original data from Krall et al., 1975). With permission.

The proportional hazards model relating all five covariates is

$$\frac{h_j(t)}{h_0(t)} = \exp\left(\beta_1 x_{1j} + \beta_2 x_{2j} + \beta_3 x_{3j} + \beta_4 x_{4j} + \beta_5 x_{5j}\right), \quad j = 1, 2, \ldots, 65$$

**TABLE 8.7**
**Proportional Hazards Regression Analysis Relating Survival to Covariates**

| Covariates | Regression coefficient $[(\hat{\beta}_i)]$ | Standard error $[\widehat{SE}(\hat{\beta}_i)]$ | $Z$ $[(\hat{\beta}_i)/\widehat{SE}(\hat{\beta}_i)]$ | $p$-Value |
|---|---|---|---|---|
| Logarithm of blood urea nitrogen | 1.770 | 0.645 | 2.744 | 0.006 |
| Hemoglobin | –0.149 | 0.062 | –2.403 | 0.016 |
| Serum calcium | –0.022 | 0.016 | 1.375 | 0.169 |
| Sex | –0.185 | 0.324 | –0.571 | 0.568 |
| Age | 0.150 | 0.104 | 1.442 | 0.149 |

From Harris, E. K. and Albert, A. (1991). *Survivalship Analysis for Clinical Studies*, Marcel Dekker, New York, p. 100. With permission.

where $X_{ij}(i = 1,...,5)$ represent the covariates, as defined above. The results of the analysis, when ties are broken randomly, including estimates of parameters, standard errors, and test statistics, are given in Table 8.7.

To assess the significance of each one of the covariates, we examine the values of the test statistic $Z$, or equivalently the $p$-value, as shown in Table 8.7. Note that the covariates sex and age are not statistically significant. The covariate, serum calcium, is not significant at either the 5 or 10% levels. The effect of covariates can be quantified in terms of relative risk of hazards. For example, given an individual with hemoglobin of 5.0 mg/100 ml and another with 10.0 mg/100 ml, the instantaneous relative risk of death of the latter as compared to the former is given by

$$\widehat{RR} = \exp\{-0.149(10.0 - 5.0)\} = 0.475.$$

Thus, given that the two individuals have survived up to time $t$, the one with 5.0 mg/100 ml higher hemoglobin has a nearly 52% less risk of dying over a short period of time. The instantaneous relative risk of the former compared to the latter individual is approximately 1/0.475 = 2.105, that is nearly 110% more. A 95% CI for the true relative risk of hazards (death) can be calculated using Equation 8.15:

$$\begin{aligned} &\big[\exp\{(-0.149 - 1.96(0.062))(10.0 - 5.0), \\ &\qquad (-0.149 + 1.96(0.062))(10.0 - 5.0)\}\big] \\ &= (0.259, 0.872). \end{aligned}$$

## 8.4 POISSON REGRESSION

The Poisson regression assumes that the underlying distribution of the dependent or response variable *(Y)* is Poisson. In many epidemiologic and health studies $Y$ denotes the observed number of cases from certain rare conditions and is adequately described by Poisson distribution. For example, the Poisson distribution is often used to describe the number of new cases of lung cancer developing in some population over a certain period of time, the number of automobile accidents occurring at a certain location per year, and other similar phenomena.

In Poisson regression analysis the mean of the dependent variable, $E(Y)$, is modeled as the exponential of the characteristics of the individuals. Let $Y_j$ denote the Poisson random variable designating the count of health failures in the $j$th category formed by a set of predictors or explanatory variables $X_1, X_2, \ldots, X_k$, with $x_{1j}, x_{2j}, \ldots, x_{kj}$ as the set of values of the predictors specific to the $j$th category. Then the Poisson regression model is defined by

$$E(Y_j) = \lambda_j = \lambda_0 \exp(\beta_1 x_{1j} + \beta_2 x_{2j} + \ldots + \beta_k x_{kj}), \tag{8.16}$$

where $\beta_1, \beta_2, \ldots, \beta_k$ are the coefficients corresponding to the predictor variates $X_1, X_2, \ldots, X_k$ and $\lambda_0$ is the baseline hazard rate when all the characteristics are zero, i.e., $x_{1j} = 0$, $x_{2j} = 0, \ldots, x_{kj} = 0$.

Equation (8.16) can also be written as

$$\log_e\left(\frac{\lambda_j}{\lambda_0}\right) = \beta_1 x_{1j} + \beta_2 x_{2j} + \ldots + \beta_k x_{kj}. \tag{8.17}$$

Note that the quantity $\log_e(\lambda_j/\lambda_0)$, on the left side of Equation 8.17, represents the log rate ratio* of an individual pertaining to the $j$th category as compared to the individual with baseline characteristics, and the right side is a linear combination of the explanatory variables. If we let $U_j = \log_e(\lambda_j/\lambda_0)$, Equation 8.17 can be written simply as

$$U_j = \beta_1 x_{1j} + \beta_2 x_{2j} + \ldots + \beta_k x_{kj},$$

which represents the standard multiple regression model.

The method of estimation of the regression coefficients is generally based on the maximum likelihood principle. For example, the likelihood function *(L)* for the Poisson regression model (Equation 8.17), under the assumption of the Poisson probability function, can be written as

* The quantity $\lambda_j/\lambda_0$ is commonly referred to as *rate ratio* (RR). Other terms used are *incidence density ratio* and *hazard ratio.*

$$L=\prod_{j=1}^{n}P\left(Y_j=y_j\right)=\prod_{j=1}^{n}\frac{\exp\left(-\lambda_j\right)\left(\lambda_j\right)^{y_j}}{y_j!}$$

$$=\prod_{j=1}^{n}\frac{\exp\left\{-\lambda_0\, e^{\sum\limits_{i=1}^{k}\beta_i x_{ij}}\right\}\left\{\lambda_0\, e^{\sum\limits_{i=1}^{k}\beta_i x_{ij}}\right\}^{y_j}}{y_j!} \tag{8.18}$$

$$=\frac{\exp\left\{-\lambda_0\, e^{\sum\limits_{i=1}^{k}\sum\limits_{j=1}^{n}\beta_i x_{ij}}\right\}\prod\limits_{j=1}^{n}\left\{\lambda_0\, e^{\sum\limits_{i=1}^{k}\beta_i x_{ij}}\right\}^{y_j}}{\prod\limits_{j=1}^{n}y_j!}.$$

The maximum likelihood estimates of the parameters $\beta_1,\beta_2,\ldots,\beta_k$ are obtained as the solution to the likelihood equations

$$\frac{\partial}{\partial\beta_i}\left[\log_e(L)\right]=0,\quad i=1,2,\ldots,k. \tag{8.19}$$

The solution to the likelihood equations given by Equation 8.19 must generally be obtained via the use of a computer algorithm. Some computational algorithms were discussed by Frome (1983). Certain statistical packages such as GLIM (Aitkin et al., 1989; Baker and Nelder, 1991), SAS MACRO CATMAX (Stokes and Koch, 1983), SAS PROC GENMOD (SAS Institute, 1992), BMDP-P45 (Brown, 1988), PREG (Frome, 1983), and EGRET (1994) also can be utilized to find the maximum likelihood estimates of the regression coefficients. Frome et al. (1973) discussed various other methods of estimating the parameters $\beta_1,\beta_2,\ldots,\beta_k$ and the extent to which the maximum likelihood, minimum chi-square, and weighted least-squares procedures yield equivalent results. They also provide several illustrative examples from the biological and physical sciences. Similarly, Charnes et al. (1976) list conditions under which iterative least squares and maximum likelihood estimates give equivalent results.

The Poisson regression model as a special case of the generalized linear models is presented in the books by McCullagh and Nelder (1983, 1989), Dobson (1990) and Hinkly et al. (1991). In addition, there are several recently published papers which illustrate applications of Poisson regression methodology in epidemiologic and medical research. For example, Breslow et al. (1983)

and Rosenbaum and Rubin (1984) used Poisson regression in the analysis of standard mortality ratio. Frome (1983) presented the analysis of rates using Poisson regression models. Frome and Checkoway (1985) used Poisson regression models in estimating incidence rates and ratios. Frome and Morris (1989) discussed the evaluation of goodness of fit of Poisson regression models in cohort studies. Gallagher et al. (1989) used Poisson regression to study the effect of calcitriol on patients with postmenopausal osteoporosis involving a therapeutic trial. Parker (1989) presented the results of a Poisson regression analysis of surveillance data on the number of abortion-related deaths. Vonesh (1989) employed Poisson regression to investigate potential risk factors associated with the number of bacterial infections of the peritoneum for patients on continuous ambulatory peritoneal dialysis. Campbell et al. (1991) modeled the Poisson regression on factors influencing the number of involuntary expulsions of a vaginal ring used as a contraceptive device. Rochon et al. (1992) performed Poisson regression to examine the number of "rejection episodes" experienced by renal transplant patients during the first 3 months of transplantations. Similarly, Neugebauer et al. (1994) used Poisson regression to study the impact of various stressful life events on the seizure frequency in patients with epilepsy. An historically relevant application of Poisson regression for the analysis of Poisson distributed data was given by Cochran (1940). For a concise review of the basic methodology of Poisson regression analysis and its application to clinical research, including issues of model diagnostics and sample size determination, see Kianifard and Gallo (1995). The problem of sample size determination in Poisson regression is also discussed by Signorini (1991). For some further discussion and numerical examples, the reader is referred to the books by Kleinbaum et al. (1988) and Myers (1990).

Finally, note that the only real conceptual difference between the Poisson regression and standard multiple regression is that the former entails the assumption of the Poisson distribution in place of the normal distribution. The analytic goal in both cases is the same: to fit a regression equation with mean as a function of a set of independent variables. The Poisson regression analysis uses the Poisson model formulation to derive a likelihood function that can be maximized to enable the determination of the maximum likelihood estimates of the parameters, estimated standard errors, and other relevant information. With widespread availability of computer software to carry out such analysis, the reader may need to specify only the model to be fitted; the program will then produce all the relevant statistics of interest.

# References

**Abbot, R. D.** (1985). "Logistic Regression in Survival Analysis", *Am. J. Epidemiol.*, 121, 465–471.

**Aitkin, M., Anderson, D., Francis, B., and Hinde, J.** (1985). *Statistical Modelling in GLIM*. Oxford University Press, Oxford.

**Baker, R. J. and Nelder, J. A.** (1991). *Generalized Linear Interactive Modelling (GLIM)*. Release 3.77. Numerical Algorithms Group, Oxford, U.K.

**Bren T. and Arnesen, E.** (1985). "Selecting Risk Factors: A Comparison of Discriminant Analysis, Logistic Regression and Cox's Regression Model Using Data from the Tromsø Heart Study", *Stat. Med.*, 4, 413–423.

**Breslow, N. E. and Day, N. E.** (1980). *Statistical Methods in Cancer Research, Vol. 1: The Analysis of Case-Control Studies*. International Agency for Research on Cancer, Lyons, France.

**Breslow, N. E., Day, N. E., Halvorsen, K. T., Prentice, R. L., and Sabai, C.** (1978). "Estimation of Multiple Relative Risk Functions in Matched Case-Control Studies", *Am. J. Epidemiol.*, 108, 299–307.

**Breslow, N. E., Lubin, J. H., Marek, P., and Langholz, B.** (1983). "Multiplicative Models and Cohort Analyses", *J. Am. Stat. Assoc.*, 78, 1–12.

**Breslow, N. E. and Powers, W.** (1978). "Are There Two Logistic Regressions for Retrospective Studies?", *Biometrics*, 34, 100–105.

**Brown, M. B.** (1988). "P45: Poisson Regression", In: *BMDP Statistical Software* (Chapter 11) (Eds. W. J. Dixon et al.). University of California Press, Los Angeles.

**Campbell, M. J., Machin, D., and D'Arcangues, C.** (1991). "Coping with Extra Poisson Variability in the Analysis of Factors Influencing Vaginal Ring Expulsions", *Stat. Med.*, 10, 241–254.

**Charnes, A., Frome, E. L., and Yu, P. L.** (1976). "The Equivalence of Generalized Least Squares and Maximum Likelihood Estimates in the Exponential Family", *J. Am. Stat. Assoc.*, 71, 169–171.

**Cochran, W. G.** (1940). "The Analysis of Variance When Experimental Errors Follow Poisson and Binomial Laws", *Ann. Math. Stat.*, 11, 335–347.

**Collett, D.** (1991). *Modeling Binary Data*. Chapman & Hall, London.

**Collett, D.** (1994). *Modelling Survival Data in Medical Research*. Chapman & Hall, London.

**Cornfield, J.** (1951). "A Method of Estimating Comparative Rates from Clinical Data: Applications to Cancer of the Lung, Breast and Cervix", *J. Nat. Cancer Inst.*, 11, 1269–1275.

**Cox, D. R.** (1972). "Regression Models and Life Tables", *J. R. Stat. Soc.*, B, 34, 187–220.

**Cox, D. R. and Hinkley, D. V.** (1974). *Theoretical Statistics*. Chapman & Hall, London.

**Cox, D. R. and Oakes, D.** (1984). *Analysis of Survival Data*. Chapman & Hall, London.

**Cox, D. R. and Snell, E. J.** (1989). *The Analysis of Binary Data,* 2nd ed. Chapman & Hall, London.

**Darlington, R. B.** (1991). *Regression and Linear Models.* McGraw-Hill, New York.

**Dixon, W. J.** (1992). "LR: Stepwise Logistic Regression", In: *BMDP Statistical Software,* Vol. 2. pp. 1105–1114. University of California Press, Los Angeles.

**Dobson, A. J.** (1983). *An Introduction to Statistical Modelling.* Chapman & Hall, London.

**Dobson, A. J.** (1990) *An Introduction to Generalized Linear Models.* Chapman & Hall, London.

**EGRET** (1994). *EGRET: State of the Art Epidemiologic Computing.* Statistics and Epidemiology Research Corporation, Seattle, WA.

**Efron, B.** (1988). "Logistic Regression, Survival Analysis and the Kaplan-Meir Curve", *J. Am. Stat. Assoc.,* 83, 414–425.

**Farewell, V. T.** (1979). "Some Results on the Estimation of Logistic Models Based on Retrospective Data", *Biometrika,* 66, 27–32.

**Feigel, P. and Zelen, M.** (1965). "Estimation of Exponential Survival Probabilities with Concomitant Information", *Biometrics,* 21, 826–838.

**Frome, E. L.** (1983). "The Analysis of Rates Using Poisson Regression Models", *Biometrics,* 39, 665–674.

**Frome, E. L. and Checkoway, H.** (1985). "Use of Poisson Regression Models in Estimating Incidence Rates and Ratios", *Am. J. Epidemiol.,* 121, 309–323.

**Frome, E. L., Kutner, M. H., and Beauchamp, J. J.** (1973). "Regression Analysis of Poisson Distributed Data", *J. Am. Stat. Assoc.,* 68, 935–940.

**Frome, E. L. and Morris, M. D.** (1989). "Evaluating Goodness of Fit of Poisson Regression Models in Cohort Studies", *Am. Statist.,* 43, 144–147.

**Gallagher, J. C., Riggs, B. L., Recker, R. R., and Goldgar, D.** (1989). "The Effect of Calcitrol on Patients with Postmenopausal Osteoporosis with Special Reference to Fracture Frequency", *Proc. Soc. Exp. Biol. Med.,* 191, 287–292.

**Glantz, S. A. and Slinker, B. K.** (1990). *Primer of Applied Regression and Analysis of Variance.* McGraw-Hill, New York.

**Green, M. S. and Symmons, M. J.** (1983). "A Comparison of the Logistic Risk Function and Proportional Hazards Model in Prospective Epidemiologic Studies", *J. Chronic Dis.,* 36, 715–724.

**Harrell, F. E.** (1986). *The PHLGM Procedure, SUGI Supplementary User's Guide,* Version 5 Edition, pp. 437–466. SAS Institute, Inc., Cary, NC.

**Harris, E. K. and Albert, A.** (1991). *Survivorship Analysis for Clinical Studies.* Marcel Dekker, New York.

**Hauck, W. W.** (1985). "A Comparison of the Logistic Risk Function and the Proportional Hazards Model in Prospective Epidemiologic Studies", *J. Chronic Dis.,* 38, 125–126.

**Hauck, W. W. and Donner, A.** (1977). "Wald's Test as Applied to Hypothesis in Logit Analysis", *J. Am. Stat. Assoc.,* 72, 851–853 (correction, *ibid.,* 75, 482).

**Hinkley, D. V., Reid, N., and Snell, E. J. (Eds.)** (1991). *Statistical Theory and Modelling,* Chapman & Hall, London.

**Holford, T. R., White, C., and Kelsey, J. L.** (1978). "Multivariate Analysis for Matched Case-Control Studies", *Am. J. Epidemiol.,* 107, 245–256.

**Hosmer, D. W. and Lemeshow, S.** (1989). *Applied Logistic Regression.* John Wiley & Sons, New York.

**Jennings, D. E.** (1986). "Judging Inferences Adequacy in Logistic Regression", *J. Am. Stat. Assoc.,* 81, 471–476.

**Kalbfleisch, J. D. and Prentice, R. L.** (1980). *The Statistical Analysis of Failure Time Data.* John Wiley & Sons, New York.

**Kianifard, F. and Gallo, P. P.** (1995). "Poisson Regression Analysis in Clinical Research", *J. Biopharmaceut. Stat.,* 5, 115–129.

**Kleinbaum, D. G.** (1994). *Logistic Regression.* Springer-Verlag, New York.

**Kleinbaum, D. G., Kupper, L. L., and Morgenstern, H.** (1982). *Epidemiologic Research: Principles and Quantitative Methods.* Lifetime Learning Publications, Belmont, CA.

**Kleinbaum, D. G., Kupper, L. L., and Muller, K. E.** (1988). *Applied Regression Analysis and Other Multivariate Methods.* PWS-Kent Publishing Company, Boston.

**Koch, G. G., Amara, I. A., Davis, G. W., and Gillings, D. B.** (1982). "A Review of Some Statistical Methods for Covariance Analysis of Categorical Data", *Biometrics,* 38, 563–595.

**Koch, G. G., Imery, P. B., Singer, J. M., Atkinson, S. S., and Stokes, M. E.** (1985). *Analysis of Categorical Data.* Les Presses de l'Université de Montréal, Montréal, Canada.

**Krall, J. M., Uthoff, V. A., and Harley, J. B.** (1975). "A Step-Up Procedure for Selecting Variables Associated With Survival", *Biometrics,* 31, 49–57.

**Lawless, J. F.** (1982). *Statistical Models and Methods for Life-Time Data.* John Wiley & Sons, New York.

**Lee, E. T.** (1992). *Statistical Methods for Survival Data Analysis,* 2nd ed. John Wiley & Sons, New York.

**LogXact,** (1992). *A Statistical Package for Exact Logistic Regression.* Cytel Software Corporation, Cambridge, MA.

**Marubini, E. and Valsecchi, M. G.** (1995). *Analyzing Survival Data from Clinical Trials and Observational Studies.* John Wiley & Sons, Chichester, U.K.

**McCullagh, P. and Nelder, J. A.** (1983, 1989). *Generalized Linear Models,* 1st and 2nd eds. Chapman & Hall, New York.

**Melo-Villalobos, B. and Weber, S.** (1992). "Regressión Logística en Estudios Epidemiologicos de Casos y Controles", *Rev. Col. Estad.,* No. 25–26, 13–32.

**Miller, R. G., Jr.** (1981). *Survival Analysis.* John Wiley & Sons, New York.

**Moolgavakar, S. S., Lustbader, E. D., and Venzan, D. J.** (1985). "Assessing the Adequacy of the Logistic Regression Model for Matched Case-Control Studies", *Stat. Med.,* 4, 425–435.

**Myers, R. H.** (1990). *Classical and Modern Regression with Applications,* 2nd ed. PWS-Kent, Boston.

**Neter, J., Wasserman, W., and Kutner, M. H.** (1989). *Applied Linear Regression Models,* 2nd ed. Richard D. Irwin, Homewood, IL.

**Neugebauer, R., Paik, M., Hauser, W. A., Nadel, E., Leppik, I., and Susser, M.** (1994). "Stressful Life Events and Seizure Frequency in Patients with Epilepsy", *Epilepsia,* 35, 336–343.

**Parker, R. A.** (1989). "Analysis of Surveillance Data with Posson Regression: A Case Study", *Stat. Med.,* 8, 285–294.

**Prentice, R. L. and Pyke, R.** (1979). "Logistic Disease Incidence Models and Case-Control Studies", *Biometrika,* 66, 404–411.

**Rao, C. R.** (1973). *Linear Statistical Inference and Its Applications,* 2nd ed. John Wiley & Sons, New York.

**Rochon, J., Aprile, M. A., and Cardella, C. J.** (1992). "Analyzing the Number of Rejection Episodes in Renal Transplant Studies", *Transplantation*, 53, 1236–1242.

**Rosenbaum, P. R. and Rubin, D. B.** (1984). "Difficulties with Regression Analyses of Age-Adjusted Rates", *Biometrics,* 40, 437–443.

**SAS Institute** (1992). *SAS User's Guide: Statistics,* Version 6 Edition. SAS Institute, Inc., Cary, NC.

**Signorini, D. F.** (1991). "Sample Size for Poisson Regression", *Biometrika,* 78, 446–450.

**SPSS, Inc**. (1994). *SPSS-Advanced Statistics.* SPSS, Inc., Chicago.

**STATA** (1994). STATA, Version 3.1. Stata Corporation, College Station, Texas.

**SYSTAT** (1994). *SYSTAT: The System for Statistics,* Version 3. Systat, Inc., Evanston, IL.

**Schesselman, J. J.** (1982). *Case-Control Studies.* Oxford University Press, New York

**Selvin, S.** (1991). *Statistical Analysis of Epidemiologic Data.* Oxford University Press, New York.

**Stokes, M. E. and Koch, G. G.** (1983). "A Macro for Maximum Likelihood Fitting of Log-Linear Models to Poisson and Multinomial Counts with Contrast Matrix Capability for Hypothesis Testing", In: *Proc. 8th Annu.* SAS *Users Group Int. Conf.* pp. 795–800.

**Thomas, D. C.** (1981). "General Relative-Risk Models for Survival Time and Matched Case-Control Studies", *Stat. Med.,* 4, 425–435.

**TRUE EPISTAT** (1994). *TRUE EPISTAT: The Stat/Graphics Package for Physicians.* Epistat Services, Richardson, TX.

**Vonesh, E. F.** (1989). "Modelling Peritonitis Rates and Associated Risk Factors for Individuals on Continuous Ambulatory Peritoneal Dialysis", *Stat. Med.,* 9, 263–271.

# 9 Prospective (Cohort) Studies with Person-Time Data

The measures of association presented in the preceding chapters assume that the entire cohort under risk at the beginning of the study period has been followed through for the specified time interval for the development of the outcome under investigation. Often, however, participants will enter into a study over a period of one or several years. Furthermore, even if all the subjects enter the study at the same time, some may be lost during the follow-up, so that the same information will not be available on all the subjects at the completion of the study. The major distinguishing feature in such a study is that the follow-up period is not uniform for all the participants. To account for these varying time intervals for different subjects, it is essential to specify for each individual the time period at risk or the period each person remained under observation and free from disease.

Thus, in prospective studies with varying length of follow-up periods, a different form of $2 \times 2$ table is used for data presentation because the number of person-time units for each individual are recorded rather than the number of persons in each exposed and unexposed group. Suppose that each subject is classified as exposed or unexposed according to certain risk factors, and is followed through, with the resulting data comparing the total number of cases and person-time units for both exposed and unexposed categories as shown in Table 9.1.

Note that in Table 9.1 the second row margins now indicate the total number of person-time units (e.g., person-years) of follow-up among all exposed and unexposed subjects, referred to as $PT_1$ and $PT_2$, respectively. Thus, $PT_1$ and $PT_2$ represent length of observation on each individual summed over all subjects in the exposed and unexposed groups, respectively. Moreover, because of the use of person-time units rather than the number of persons in the margins, it is not possible to derive the values of cell counts for the number of noncases in the exposed and unexposed categories.

**TABLE 9.1**
**A 2 × 2 Display of Person-Time Data in a Prospective Study**

| | Exposed | Unexposed | Total |
|---|---|---|---|
| Cases | *a* | *b* | *m* |
| Person-time | $PT_1$ | $PT_2$ | PT |

## 9.1 MEASURES OF RISK

In the fixed cohort studies discussed in Chapter 3, the concept of *risk* was introduced. Risk is the probability of developing a condition or dying from a particular disease during a specified time period. In prospective cohort studies with person-time data, a precise estimate of the effect of exposure in a population using such data is called *incidence rate, incidence density, force of morbidity,* or *hazard function,* and is defined as the number of new cases of disease during a given time period divided by the total person-time of observation. (For a more mathematical explanation of the difference between risk and rate, refer to Elandt-Johnson, 1975.)* This section considers the problem of estimating the difference and the ratio measures of effect involving the *difference or ratio* of the observed values of incidence rates.

### 9.1.1 Incidence Rate Difference

We now consider methods of point and interval estimation of incidence rate difference.

#### 9.1.1.1 Point Estimation

A point estimate of the incidence rate difference (IRD) is given by

$$\widehat{\text{IRD}} = \frac{a}{\text{PT}_1} - \frac{b}{\text{PT}_2}. \tag{9.1}$$

Thus, for cohort studies with person-time data, the IRD is calculated as the ratio of difference of incidence rates or densities in those exposed to that among those unexposed. An IRD of zero indicates that the incidence rates of disease in the exposed and unexposed groups are similar, and thus no association exists between the exposure and the disease. A value greater than zero indicates a positive association or increased risk and a value less than zero indicates a negative association or decreased risk among those exposed.

* The risk or probability $(p)$ of developing the disease during a given observation period is related to the incidence rate by the equation $p = 1 - \exp(-\lambda t)$, where $\lambda$ is the per person incidence rate (i.e., the rate expressed in terms of individual person at risk rather than in terms of 1000, 10,000, 100,000, etc.) and $t$ is the length of the observation period.

### 9.1.1.2 Confidence Intervals

An approximate method using the Poisson model and the test-based method for determining confidence intervals (CIs) for the IRD are described. An exact method of determining the CI does not exist because the total number of cases is not independent of the rate difference.

*An Approximate Poisson Method*

By assuming a Poisson model for the incidence of disease in the exposed and unexposed categories, we have

$$\mathrm{Var}\left(\hat{\mathrm{IRD}}\right) = \frac{\lambda_1}{\left(\mathrm{PT}_1\right)^2} + \frac{\lambda_2}{\left(\mathrm{PT}_2\right)^2}, \tag{9.2}$$

where $\lambda_1$ and $\lambda_2$ denote the mean incidence of disease in the population for the two groups. A good sample estimate of the variance (Equation 9.2) is given by

$$\hat{\mathrm{Var}}\left(\hat{\mathrm{IRD}}\right) = \frac{a}{\left(\mathrm{PT}_1\right)^2} + \frac{b}{\left(\mathrm{PT}_2\right)^2}. \tag{9.3}$$

Thus, an approximate $100(1 - \alpha)\%$ CI for the IRD is

$$\left(\frac{a}{\mathrm{PT}_1} - \frac{b}{\mathrm{PT}_2}\right) \pm Z_{\alpha/2}\sqrt{\frac{a}{\left(\mathrm{PT}_1\right)^2} + \frac{b}{\left(\mathrm{PT}_2\right)^2}}, \tag{9.4}$$

where $Z_{\alpha/2}$ denotes the upper $100(\alpha/2)$th percentile of the standard normal distribution.

*Test-Based Method*

Another approach is to determine the test-based limits, similar to Equation 3.6, given by

$$\hat{\mathrm{IRD}} \pm Z_{\alpha/2}\sqrt{\left(\hat{\mathrm{IRD}}\right)^2 / \chi^2_{\mathrm{MH}}}, \tag{9.5}$$

where $Z_{\alpha/2}$ denotes the $100(\alpha/2)$th upper percentile of the standard normal distribution and $\chi^2_{\mathrm{MH}}$ is defined by the formula (Oleinick and Mantel, 1970; Rothman, 1986):

$$\chi^2_{\mathrm{MH}} = \frac{\left[a - \dfrac{(m)\left(\mathrm{PT}_1\right)}{\mathrm{PT}}\right]^2}{\dfrac{(m)\left(\mathrm{PT}_1\right)\left(\mathrm{PT}_2\right)}{(\mathrm{PT})^2}}. \tag{9.6}$$

**TABLE 9.2**
**Person-Time Data from a Postmenopausal Hormone and Coronary Heart Disease Cohort Study**

| | Postmenopausal hormone use | | |
|---|---|---|---|
| | **Yes** | **No** | **Total** |
| CHD | 30 | 60 | 90 |
| Person-years | 54308.7 | 51477.5 | 105786.2 |

From Stampfer, M. J. et al. (1985). *N. Engl. J. Med.*, 313, 1044–1049. With permission.

The chi-square statistic (Equation 9.6) is based on the normal approximation to the binomial distribution, using the number of exposed cases as the binomial random variable, with null mean and variance given by $(m)(\mathrm{PT}_1)/\mathrm{PT}$ and $(m)(\mathrm{PT}_1)(\mathrm{PT}_2)/(\mathrm{PT})^2$, respectively.

Again, in terms of the standard normal statistic $\chi$, Equation 9.5 can be expressed more simply as

$$\widehat{\mathrm{IRD}}\left(1 \pm Z_{\alpha/2}/\chi\right),$$

where $\chi$ represents the square root of the chi-square statistic (Equation 9.6).

*Example 9.1*

Consider the data from a cohort study of postmenopausal hormone (MPH) and the coronary heart disease (CHD) among female nurses, as reported by Stampfer et al. (1985). The relevant results are summarized in Table 9.2.

We first calculate an estimate of the IRD. From Table 9.2, we obtain

$$\widehat{\mathrm{IR}}_1 = 30/54308.7 = 0.0006$$

and

$$\widehat{\mathrm{IR}}_2 = 60/51477.5 = 0.0012.$$

Thus, an estimate of the IRD is given by

$$\widehat{\mathrm{IRD}} = \widehat{\mathrm{IR}}_1 - \widehat{\mathrm{IR}}_2 = -0.0006.$$

We obtain 95% approximate CIs of the IRD using the Poisson model and test-based procedures.

**Poisson model method** — A 95% CI for the IRD using this method is

$$-0.0006 \pm 1.96\sqrt{\frac{30}{(54308.7)^2}+\frac{60}{(51477.5)^2}} = (-0.001, -0.0002).$$

**Test-based method** — To obtain a CI for the IRD using the test-based method, note that

$$\chi^2_{\text{MH}} = \frac{\left[30 - \frac{90(54308.7)}{105786.2}\right]^2}{\frac{90(54308.7)(51477.5)}{(105786.2)^2}}$$

$$= 11.6786.$$

Therefore, a 95% CI for the IRD using this method is given by

$$-0.0006 \pm 1.96\sqrt{(-0.0006)^2/11.6786} = (-0.001, -0.0002).$$

These limits are the same as those obtained using the Poisson model approach. However, in general, the two methods may yield different results.

### 9.1.2 Incidence Rate Ratio

We now consider various methods of point and interval estimation of incidence rate ratio.

#### 9.1.2.1 Point Estimation

A point estimate of the incidence rate ratio (IRR) is given by

$$\hat{\text{IRR}} = \frac{a/\text{PT}_1}{b/\text{PT}_2}. \tag{9.7}$$

Thus, for cohort studies with person-time data, the IRR is calculated as the ratio of incidence rates or densities in those exposed to that among those unexposed. An IRR of 1 indicates that the incidence rates of disease in the exposed and unexposed groups are similar, and thus no association exists between the exposure and the disease. A value >1 indicates a positive association or increased risk, and a value <1 indicates a negative association or decreased risk among those exposed.

#### 9.1.2.2 Confidence Intervals

An approximate method and an exact method using the Poisson model and test-based limits for determining CIs for the IRR are described.

*An Approximate Poisson Method*

By assuming a Poisson model and considering the logarithm of the IRR, we have (see Appendix B)

$$\mathrm{Var}\left\{\log_e\left(\hat{\mathrm{IRR}}\right)\right\} \simeq \frac{1}{\lambda_1} + \frac{1}{\lambda_2}, \tag{9.8}$$

where, as before, $\lambda_1$ and $\lambda_2$ denote the mean incidence of disease in the population for the two groups. A good sample estimate of the variance (Equation 9.8) is given by

$$\hat{\mathrm{Var}}\left\{\log_e\left(\hat{\mathrm{IRR}}\right)\right\} \simeq \frac{1}{a} + \frac{1}{b}. \tag{9.9}$$

Thus, an approximate 100(1 – α)% CI for $\log_e$(IRR) is given by

$$\log_e\left(\frac{a/\mathrm{PT}_1}{b/\mathrm{PT}_2}\right) \pm Z_{\alpha/2}\sqrt{\frac{1}{a} + \frac{1}{b}}, \tag{9.10}$$

from which a 100(1 – α)% CI for the IRR is obtained by taking the antilogarithms of the corresponding endpoints of the interval (9.10).

*Test-Based Method*

An alternative approach is to use the test-based limits. Thus, an approximate 100(1 – α)% CI for $\log_e$(IRR) is given by

$$\left\{\log_e\left(\hat{\mathrm{IRR}}\right)\right\} \pm Z_{\alpha/2}\sqrt{\left\{\log_e\left(\hat{\mathrm{IRR}}\right)\right\}^2 / \chi^2_{\mathrm{MH}}}, \tag{9.11}$$

where $\chi^2_{\mathrm{MH}}$ is defined as in Equation 9.6.

Again, in terms of the standard normal statistic $\chi$, Equation 9.11 can be expressed more simply as

$$\log_e\left(\hat{\mathrm{IRR}}\right)\left(1 \pm Z_{\alpha/2}/\chi\right),$$

from which a 100(1 – α)% CI for the IRR can be written as

$$\left(\hat{\mathrm{IRR}}\right)^{\left(1 \pm Z_{\alpha/2}/\chi\right)}.$$

*An Exact Poisson Method*

An exact CI for the IRR with person-time data can be obtained using a double Poisson model. Thus, if it is assumed that the random variables *A* and *B* have independent Poisson distributions with parameters $\lambda_1$ and $\lambda_2$, respectively, then the IRR, using the person-time data, is defined by

$$\text{IRR} = \left(\frac{\text{PT}_2}{\text{PT}_1}\right)\left(\frac{\lambda_1}{\lambda_2}\right).$$

If $a$ and $b$ are the observed number of cases in the exposed and unexposed categories, respectively, then, given $a + b = m$, $A$ has a binomial distribution with parameters: the number of trials equal to $m = a + b$ and the probability of success equal to $p = \lambda_1/(\lambda_1 + \lambda_2)$ (see, e.g., Sahai and Misra, 1992).

An exact CI for the IRR can be obtained by first determining an exact CI for $p = \lambda_1/(\lambda_1 + \lambda_2)$. Thus, if $p_\text{L}$ and $p_\text{U}$ are the lower and upper confidence limits of $p$ and $\text{IRR}_\text{L}$ and $\text{IRR}_\text{U}$ are the lower and upper confidence limits of IRR, it readily follows that

$$\text{IRR}_\text{L} = \left(\frac{\text{PT}_2}{\text{PT}_1}\right)\left(\frac{p_\text{L}}{1 - p_\text{L}}\right)$$

and (9.12)

$$\text{IRR}_\text{U} = \left(\frac{\text{PT}_2}{\text{PT}_1}\right)\left(\frac{p_\text{U}}{1 - p_\text{U}}\right).$$

By using an argument tied to hypothesis testing, it can be shown that a pair of $100(1 - \alpha)\%$ confidence limits, $p_\text{L}$ and $p_\text{U}$, are the solutions to the equations (see, e.g., Sahai and Khurshid, 1996):

$$\sum_{k=a}^{a+b} \binom{a+b}{k} p_\text{L}^k (1 - p_\text{L})^{a+b-k} = \alpha/2 \tag{9.13}$$

and

$$\sum_{k=0}^{a} \binom{a+b}{k} p_\text{U}^k (1 - p_\text{U})^{a+b-k} = \alpha/2. \tag{9.14}$$

Equations 9.13 and 9.14 are somewhat cumbersome to solve manually, but are more readily resolved using a computer program. Alternatively, Equations 9.13 and 9.14 can be solved by using the relationship (see, e.g., Evans et al., 1993)

$$\sum_{k=0}^{x} \binom{n}{k} p^k (1 - p)^{n-k} = P\left\{F_{\nu_1,\nu_2} > \frac{p}{1-p}\,\frac{n-x}{x+1}\right\}, \tag{9.15}$$

where $F_{\nu_1,\nu_2}$ is a random variable having a variance ratio $F$ distribution with $\nu_1 = 2(x + 1)$ and $\nu_2 = 2(n - x)$ degrees of freedom.

Using relationship (9.15) in Equations 9.13 and 9.14, the solutions to Equations 9.13 and 9.14 are more conveniently expressed in terms of percentiles of the $F$-distribution (see, e.g., Sahai and Khurshid, 1996):

$$p_L = \left( \frac{a}{a + (b+1)F_{\alpha/2,2(b+1),2a}} \right) \tag{9.16}$$

and

$$p_U = \left( \frac{(a+1)F_{\alpha/2,2(a+1),2b}}{b + (a+1)F_{\alpha/2,2(a+1),2b}} \right), \tag{9.17}$$

where $F_{\gamma,m_1,m_2}$ is defined by the relationship

$$P\left\{F_{m_1,m_2} > F_{\gamma,m_1,m_2}\right\} = \gamma.$$

From Equation 9.12 it follows that

$$\text{IRR}_L = \left( \frac{\text{PT}_2}{\text{PT}_1} \right) \left( \frac{a}{b+1} \right) \frac{1}{F_{\alpha/2,2(b+1),2a}} \tag{9.18}$$

and

$$\text{IRR}_U = \left( \frac{\text{PT}_2}{\text{PT}_1} \right) \left( \frac{a+1}{b} \right) F_{\alpha/2,2(a+1),2b}. \tag{9.19}$$

*Example 9.2*

Consider the person-time data from the cohort study of PMH use described in Example 9.1. An estimate of the IRR is

$$\hat{\text{IRR}} = \frac{30/54308.7}{60/51477.5} = 0.474.$$

Illustrated below is the computation of CIs for the IRR using the approximate and exact Poisson methods as well as the test-based method.

**Approximate Poisson method** — An approximate 95% CI for $\log_e$(IRR) using this method is given by

$$\log_e(0.474) \pm 1.96\sqrt{\frac{1}{30}+\frac{1}{60}} = (-1.185, -0.309),$$

from which a 95% CI for the IRR is given by (0.306, 0.734).

**Test-based method** — To obtain a CI for the IRR using the test-based method, note that from Example 9.1, $\chi^2_{MH} = 11.6786$. Therefore, a 95% CI for $\log_e$(IRR) using this method is

$$\log_e(0.474) \pm 1.96\sqrt{\{\log_e(0.474)\}^2/11.6786} = (-1.175, -0.319),$$

from which a 95% CI for the IRR is given by (0.309, 0.727).

**Exact Poisson method** — To obtain a 95% CI for the IRR using the exact Poisson method, note that

$$a = 30, \quad PT_1 = 54308.7$$

$$b = 60, \quad PT_2 = 51477.5$$

$$F_{\alpha/2,2(b+1),2a} = F_{0.025,122,60} = 1.5795$$

$$F_{\alpha/2,2(a+1),2b} = F_{0.025,62,120} = 1.5241$$

Using Equations 9.18 and 9.19, the lower and upper confidence limits, $IRR_L$ and $IRR_U$, are given by

$$IRR_L = \left(\frac{51477.5}{54308.7}\right)\left(\frac{30}{61}\right)\frac{1}{1.5795} = 0.295$$

and

$$IRR_U = \left(\frac{51477.5}{54308.7}\right)\left(\frac{31}{60}\right)1.5241 = 0.746.$$

Thus, the approximate limits obtained via Poisson model and test-based methods agree well with the exact limits given above.

# References

**Elandt-Johnson, R. C.** (1975). "Definitions of Rates: Some Remarks on Their Use and Misuse", *Am. J. Epidemiol.*, 102, 267–271.

**Evans, M., Hastings, N. A. J., and Peacock, J. B.** (1993). *Statistical Distributions,* 2nd ed. John Wiley & Sons, New York.

**Oleinick, A. and Mantel, N.** (1970). "Family Studies in Systemic Lupus Erythmatous, II: Mortality Among Siblings and Offspring of Index Cases with a Statistical Appendix Concerning Life Table Analysis", *J. Chronic Dis.*, 22, 617–623.

**Rothman, K. J.** (1986). *Modern Epidemiology.* Little, Brown, Boston.

**Sahai, H. and Khurshid, A.** (1996). "Confidence Intervals for the Probability of Success in the Binomial Distribution: A Review", *Metron*, LIV, 153–180.

**Sahai, H. and Misra, S. C.** (1992). "Comparing Means of Two Poisson Distributions", *Math. Sci.,* 17, 60–67.

**Stampfer, M. J., Willett, W. C., Colitz, G. A., Rosner, B., Speizer, F. E., and Hennekens, C. H.** (1985). "A Prospective Study of Post Menopausal Hormones and Coronary Heart Disease", *N. Engl. J. Med.,* 313, 1044–1049.

# 10 Stratified Analysis with Person-Time Data

This chapter describes the methods of stratified analysis to estimate an overall summary risk difference and risk ratio based on person-time data after adjusting for confounding variables. The methods discussed are similar to those described in Chapter 6 for count data.

Consider the person-time data stratified into $k$ strata, with the results in the stratum $i$ ($i = 1,2,...,k$), as shown in Table 10.1.

## 10.1 MEASURES OF RISK

In this section we develop methods of point and interval estimation of incidence rate difference and incidence rate ratio using stratified analysis.

### 10.1.1 Incidence Rate Difference

We now consider methods of point and interval estimation for incidence rate difference.

#### 10.1.1.1 Point Estimation

Two methods of point estimation for the common incidence rate difference (IRD) are described: pooling with inverse variances and the maximum likelihood procedure. The specific procedure used for a given problem will depend on the type of data and the study being analyzed.

*Pooled Estimator*

An estimate of the IRD and its variance estimate from a single stratum are given by

$$\hat{\text{IRD}}_i = \frac{a_i}{\text{PT}_{1i}} - \frac{b_i}{\text{PT}_{2i}} \tag{10.1}$$

and

$$\hat{\text{Var}}\left(\hat{\text{IRD}}_i\right) = \frac{a_i}{\left(\text{PT}_{1i}\right)^2} + \frac{b_i}{\left(\text{PT}_{2i}\right)^2}. \tag{10.2}$$

**TABLE 10.1**
**A 2 × 2 Display of Person-Time Data in a Stratified Analysis**

| | Exposed | Unexposed | Total |
|---|---|---|---|
| Cases | $a_i$ | $b_i$ | $m_i$ |
| Person-time | $\text{PT}_{1i}$ | $\text{PT}_{2i}$ | $\text{PT}_i$ |

Therefore, a pooled or weighted estimator for the IRD that is constant over strata can be obtained as

$$\widehat{\text{IRD}}_w = \frac{\sum_{i=1}^{k} W_i \widehat{\text{IRD}}_i}{\sum_{i=1}^{k} W_i}, \tag{10.3}$$

where the weight $W_i$ is inversely proportional to the stratum-specific variance estimate:

$$W_i = \frac{1}{\widehat{\text{Var}}\left(\widehat{\text{IRD}}_i\right)} = \frac{\left(\text{PT}_{1i}\right)^2 \left(\text{PT}_{2i}\right)^2}{\left(a_i\right)\left(\text{PT}_{2i}\right)^2 + \left(b_i\right)\left(\text{PT}_{1i}\right)^2}. \tag{10.4}$$

*Maximum Likelihood Estimator*

The maximum likelihood (ML) estimator of the common IRD requires the solution of the following likelihood equations (Miettinen, 1975; Rothman and Boice, 1982; Rothman, 1986):

$$\sum_{i=1}^{k}\left[\frac{a_i}{\widehat{\text{IR}}_{u_i} + \widehat{\text{IRD}}_{\text{ML}}}\right] - \sum_{i=1}^{k}\left(\text{PT}_{1i}\right) = 0 \tag{10.5}$$

and for each stratum $i$ ($i = 1,2,\ldots,k$)

$$\frac{a_i}{\widehat{\text{IR}}_{u_i} + \widehat{\text{IRD}}_{\text{ML}}} + \frac{b_i}{\widehat{\text{IR}}_{u_i}} - \text{PT}_i = 0, \tag{10.6}$$

where $\hat{\text{IRD}}_{\text{ML}}$ is the maximum likelihood estimator of the IRD and $\hat{\text{IR}}_{u_i}$ is the maximum likelihood estimator of the incidence rate among the unexposed group in the $i$th stratum. The statistics $\hat{\text{IR}}_{u_i}$ ($i = 1,2,...,k$) are the estimators of the nuisance parameters that need to be estimated in order to solve for the desired estimate of the overall IRD ($\hat{\text{IRD}}_{\text{ML}}$).

Again, note that there are $k + 1$ equations, one more than the number of strata, to be solved. Thus, in addition to solving for $\hat{\text{IRD}}_{\text{ML}}$, it is necessary to solve for $\hat{\text{IR}}_{u_i}$. Under the large sample conditions, an initial approximation to the value of $\hat{\text{IRD}}_{\text{ML}}$ in the solution to Equations 10.5 and 10.6 can be (see Miettinen, 1975):

$$\hat{\text{IRD}}_{\text{ML}} = \frac{\sum_{i=1}^{k} W_i \hat{\text{IRD}}_i}{\sum_{i=1}^{k} W_i},$$

where $\hat{\text{IRD}}_i$ is defined as in Equation 10.1 and

$$W_i = \frac{(\text{PT}_{1i})(\text{PT}_{2i})}{m_i}.$$

#### 10.1.1.2 Confidence Intervals

Two approximate methods, based on pooling with inverse variances using Poisson model and its improvement using the maximum likelihood estimates, and the test-based procedure for determining CIs for the common IRD are described. As indicated in the case of simple analysis, an exact method does not exist for determining the CI for this problem.

*Pooling Method*

An approximate $100(1 - \alpha)\%$ CI for the IRD can be obtained by determining an estimate of the variance of the pooled estimator (Equation 10.3) and using the formula

$$\hat{\text{IRD}}_w \pm Z_{\alpha/2}\sqrt{\hat{\text{Var}}(\hat{\text{IRD}}_w)}, \tag{10.7}$$

where $Z_{\alpha/2}$ denotes the upper $100(\alpha/2)$th percentile of the standard normal distribution, and an estimate of the variance of the $\hat{\text{IRD}}_w$ can be obtained as

$$\hat{\mathrm{Var}}\left(\hat{\mathrm{IRD}}_w\right) = \hat{\mathrm{Var}}\left[\frac{\sum_{i=1}^{k} W_i \hat{\mathrm{Var}}\left(\hat{\mathrm{IRD}}_i\right)}{\sum_{i=1}^{k} W_i}\right]$$

$$= \frac{1}{\left(\sum_{i=1}^{k} W_i\right)^2}\left[\sum_{i=1}^{k} W_i^2 \frac{1}{W_i}\right] \tag{10.8}$$

$$= \frac{1}{\sum_{i=1}^{k} W_i},$$

with $W_i$ being given as in Equation 10.4.

*Maximum Likelihood Method*

The maximum likelihood estimator of the IRD requires the simultaneous maximum likelihood estimation of the nuisance parameters $\mathrm{IR}_{ui}$ for each stratum. The estimates of $\mathrm{IR}_{ui}$ can be used, in conjunction with the maximum likelihood estimate $\hat{\mathrm{IRD}}_{\mathrm{ML}}$, to obtain an improved estimate of the variance for the IRD in each stratum by substituting $\hat{\mathrm{IR}}_{u_i}$ for $b_i/\mathrm{PT}_{2i}$ and $\hat{\mathrm{IR}}_{u_i} + \hat{\mathrm{IRD}}_{\mathrm{ML}}$ for $a_i/\mathrm{PT}_{1i}$ in Equation 10.2. Thus, the the resulting weights ($W_i$) are determined by using the maximum likelihood estimates $\hat{\mathrm{IRD}}_{\mathrm{ML}}$ and $\hat{\mathrm{IR}}_{u_i}$ as delineated by Equations 10.5 and 10.6. The modified weights are then obtained by taking the inverses of improved estimates of Var( $\hat{\mathrm{IRD}}_i$) given by

$$\hat{\mathrm{Var}}\left(\hat{\mathrm{IRD}}_i\right) = \frac{\hat{\mathrm{IR}}_{u_i} + \hat{\mathrm{IRD}}_{\mathrm{ML}}}{\mathrm{PT}_{1i}} + \frac{\hat{\mathrm{IR}}_{u_i}}{\mathrm{PT}_{2i}}.$$

Hence, the new weights $W_i$ to be used in Equation 10.8 to obtain an estimate of the variance of the maximum likelihood estimator are determined by

$$W_i = \frac{\mathrm{PT}_{1i}\,\mathrm{PT}_{2i}}{\mathrm{PT}_{1i}\,\hat{\mathrm{IR}}_{ui} + \mathrm{PT}_{2i}\left(\hat{\mathrm{IR}}_{ui} + \hat{\mathrm{IRD}}_{\mathrm{ML}}\right)}.$$

An approximate $100(1-\alpha)\%$ CI for the IRD, using this method, is given by

$$\hat{\mathrm{IRD}}_{\mathrm{ML}} \pm Z_{\alpha/2}\sqrt{\hat{\mathrm{Var}}\left(\hat{\mathrm{IRD}}_{\mathrm{ML}}\right)}. \tag{10.9}$$

**TABLE 10.2**
**Person-Time Data on Mortality by Sex and Age for Patients with Trigeminal Neuralgia**

| | Age <65 | | | Age ≥65 | | |
|---|---|---|---|---|---|---|
| | **Males** | **Females** | **Total** | **Males** | **Females** | **Total** |
| Deaths | 14 | 10 | 24 | 76 | 121 | 197 |
| Person-years | 1516 | 1701 | 3217 | 949 | 2245 | 3194 |

From Rothman, K. J. and Monson, R. R. (1973). *J. Chronic Dis.*, 26, 303–309. With permission.

*Test-Based Method*

A third method of obtaining the CI is to determine the test-based limits, similar to Equation 9.5, given by

$$\hat{\text{IRD}} \pm Z_{\alpha/2}\sqrt{\left(\hat{\text{IRD}}\right)^2 / \chi^2_{\text{MH}}}, \tag{10.10}$$

where $\chi^2_{\text{MH}}$ is determined by (Shore et al., 1976; Rothman, 1986)

$$\chi^2_{\text{MH}} = \frac{\left[\sum_{i=1}^{k} a_i - \sum_{i=1}^{k}\left[\frac{(m_i)(\text{PT}_{1i})}{\text{PT}_i}\right]\right]^2}{\sum_{i=1}^{k}\left[\frac{(m_i)(\text{PT}_{1i})(\text{PT}_{2i})}{(\text{PT}_i)^2}\right]}. \tag{10.11}$$

Note that Equation 10.11 is identical to Equation 9.6 for person-time data in the simple analysis, except that $m$, $\text{PT}_1$, $\text{PT}_2$, and PT are obtained by summing the stratum-specific contributions over all the strata.

Again, in terms of the standard normal statistic $\chi$, Equation 10.10 can be expressed more simply as

$$\hat{\text{IRD}}\left(1 \pm Z_{\alpha/2}/\chi\right),$$

where $\chi$ represents the square root of the chi-square statistic (Equation 10.11).

*Example 10.1*

Consider the data from a survival study of patients with trigeminal neuralgia reported by Rothman and Monson (1973) and further discussed by Rothman (1986). The results stratified by age groups are summarized in Table 10.2.

First, we obtain point estimates of the IRD using the method of pooling and the maximum likelihood procedure. From the stratified data of Table 10.2, we have

$$\widehat{\mathrm{IRD}}_1 = \frac{14}{1516} - \frac{10}{1701} = 0.0034$$

and

$$\widehat{\mathrm{IRD}}_2 = \frac{76}{949} - \frac{121}{2245} = 0.0262.$$

In order to obtain a pooled estimate of the IRD, we first find

$$W_1 = \frac{(1516)^2\,(1701)^2}{14(1701)^2 + 10(1516)^2} = 104{,}737.0922$$

and

$$W_2 = \frac{(949)^2\,(2245)^2}{76(2245)^2 + 121(949)^2} = 9{,}225.4404.$$

Using Equation 10.3, the pooled (weighted) estimate of the IRD is given by

$$\widehat{\mathrm{IRD}}_w = \frac{(104{,}737.0922)(0.0034) + (9{,}225.4404)(0.0262)}{104{,}737.0922 + 9{,}225.4404} = 0.0052.$$

In order to obtain the maximum likelihood estimate of the IRD, the likelihood equations are

$$\frac{14}{\widehat{\mathrm{IR}}_{u_1} + \widehat{\mathrm{IRD}}_{\mathrm{ML}}} + \frac{76}{\widehat{\mathrm{IR}}_{u_2} + \widehat{\mathrm{IRD}}_{\mathrm{ML}}} - (1516 + 949) = 0,$$

$$\frac{14}{\widehat{\mathrm{IR}}_{u_1} + \widehat{\mathrm{IRD}}_{\mathrm{ML}}} + \frac{10}{\widehat{\mathrm{IR}}_{u_1}} - 3217 = 0,$$

and

$$\frac{76}{\widehat{\mathrm{IR}}_{u_2} + \widehat{\mathrm{IRD}}_{\mathrm{ML}}} + \frac{121}{\widehat{\mathrm{IR}}_{u_2}} - 3194 = 0.$$

The maximum likelihood solution for $\widehat{\mathrm{IRD}}_{\mathrm{ML}}$ using a computer program (Wolfram, 1991) is 0.0056, which is in close agreement with the pooled estimate of 0.0052.

Next, we construct CIs for the IRD using methods based on pooling, the maximum likelihood, and the test-based approach.

**Pooling method** — $\hat{\text{IRD}}_w = 0.0052$, and using Equation 10.8, we have

$$\hat{\text{Var}}\left(\hat{\text{IRD}}_w\right) = \frac{1}{104737.0922 + 9225.4404} = 0.0000087748.$$

Thus, a 95% CI for the IRD using this method is given by

$$0.0052 \pm 1.96\sqrt{0.0000087748} = (-0.0006, 0.0110).$$

**Maximum likelihood method** — From the likelihood equations given above, $\hat{\text{IRD}}_{\text{ML}} = 0.0056$, $\hat{\text{IR}}_{u_1} = 0.0052$, $\hat{\text{IR}}_{u_2} = 0.0597$, and the weights based on the maximum likelihood estimates are

$$W_1 = \frac{(1516)(1701)}{1701(0.0052 + 0.0056) + 1516(0.0052)} = 9,8221.833$$

and

$$W_2 = \frac{(949)(2245)}{2245(0.0597 + 0.0056) + 949(0.0597)} = 10,481.993.$$

Using Equation 10.8, an estimate of the variance of $\hat{\text{IRD}}_{\text{ML}}$ is

$$\hat{\text{Var}}\left(\hat{\text{IRD}}_{\text{ML}}\right) = \frac{1}{98221.833 + 10481.993} = 0.000009199.$$

Thus, a 95% CI for the IRD using this method is given by

$$0.0056 \pm 1.96\sqrt{0.000009199} = (-0.0003, 0.0115).$$

**Test-based method** — To obtain a 95% CI for the IRD by the test-based method, note that

$$\chi^2_{\text{MH}} = \frac{\left[(14 + 76) - \left(\frac{(24)(1516)}{3217} + \frac{(197)(949)}{3194}\right)\right]^2}{\frac{(24)(1516)(1701)}{(3217)^2} + \frac{(197)(949)(2245)}{(3194)^2}} = 8.6229.$$

Therefore, a 95% CI for the IRD is given by

$$0.0052 \pm 1.96\sqrt{(0.0052)^2/8.6229} = (0.0017, 0.0087).$$

Note that the test-based limits are too narrow, which contradicts the nonsignificance of the results obtained using the pooling and the maximum likelihood methods.

#### 10.1.1.3 Test for Homogeneity of Incidence Rate Differences

An important assumption in the methods of estimation described earlier is the uniformity of IRDs over all strata. A test for homogeneity of effect over strata in terms of uniform IRD can be carried out by the statistic

$$\sum_{i=1}^{k}\left[\frac{\left(\hat{\text{IRD}}_i - \hat{\text{IRD}}_w\right)^2}{\hat{\text{Var}}\left(\hat{\text{IRD}}_i\right)}\right],$$

which asymptotically has a chi-square distribution with $k - 1$ degrees of freedom. Note that $\hat{\text{IRD}}_i$, $\hat{\text{Var}}(\hat{\text{IRD}}_i)$, and $\hat{\text{IRD}}_w$ are defined by Equations 10.1, 10.2, and 10.3, respectively.

The test statistic for the data in Example 10.1, is calculated as

$$\frac{(0.0034 - 0.0052)^2}{0.000009548} + \frac{(0.0262 - 0.0052)^2}{0.0001084} = 4.408,$$

and from the chi-square table

$$P\left(\chi_1^2 > 4.408\right) = 0.036.$$

Thus, the hypothesis of the homogeneity of IRDs for the two age strata is rejected and there is evidence of some heterogeneity.

### 10.1.2 Incidence Rate Ratio

We now consider various methods of point and interval estimation of incidence rate ratio.

#### 10.1.2.1 Point Estimation

Three methods of point estimation for the incidence rate ratio (IRR) are described: pooling with inverse variances, the maximum likelihood estimator, and the Mantel-Haenszel estimator.

*Pooled Estimator*

For the IRR, pooling is performed after logarithmic transformation of the stratum-specific estimates in order to stabilize the variances. The estimate of the incidence rate ratio for the *i*th stratum ($\hat{\text{IRR}}_i$) is

$$\hat{\text{IRR}}_i = \frac{a_i/\text{PT}_{1i}}{b_i/\text{PT}_{2i}}. \tag{10.12}$$

An approximate variance estimate for $\log_e(\hat{\text{IRR}}_i)$ can be obtained as (see Appendix B):

$$\hat{\text{Var}}\left[\log_e\left(\hat{\text{IRR}}_i\right)\right] \simeq \frac{1}{a_i} + \frac{1}{b_i}. \tag{10.13}$$

Thus, a pooled estimator of the logarithm of the common IRR can be obtained as the weighted average of $\log_e(\hat{\text{IRR}}_i)$, with stratum-specific weight as the inverse of the stratum variance estimate:

$$\log_e\left(\hat{\text{IRR}}_w\right) = \frac{\sum_{i=1}^{k} W_i \log_e\left(\hat{\text{IRR}}_i\right)}{\sum_{i=1}^{k} W_i} \tag{10.14}$$

and

$$\hat{\text{IRR}}_w = \exp\left[\log_e\left(\hat{\text{IRR}}_w\right)\right], \tag{10.15}$$

where

$$W_i = \frac{a_i b_i}{a_i + b_i}. \tag{10.16}$$

*Maximum Likelihood Estimator*

The maximum likelihood estimate of the IRR ($\hat{\text{IRR}}_{\text{ML}}$) is obtained as an iterative solution to a single equation (Miettinen, 1975; Rothman and Boice, 1982; Rothman, 1986; Breslow and Day, 1987):

$$\sum_{i=1}^{k} a_i - \hat{\text{IRR}}_{\text{ML}} \sum_{i=1}^{k} \left[ \frac{\left(a_i + b_i\right)}{\hat{\text{IRR}}_{\text{ML}} + \dfrac{\text{PT}_{2i}}{\text{PT}_{1i}}} \right] = 0. \tag{10.17}$$

Equation 10.17 does not involve any nuisance parameter and is relatively simple to solve. However, the iterative nature of the solution generally requires the use of a computer program. Under the large sample conditions, an initial approximation to the value of $\hat{\text{IRR}}_{\text{ML}}$ in the solution to Equation 10.17 is (Miettinen, 1975)

$$\widehat{\text{IRR}}_{\text{ML}} = \exp\left[\frac{\sum_{i=1}^{k} W_i \log_e\left(\widehat{\text{IRR}}_i\right)}{\sum_{i=1}^{k} W_i}\right],$$

where $\widehat{\text{IRR}}_i$ is defined as it was in Equation 10.12 and

$$W_i = \frac{(m_i)(\text{PT}_{1i})(\text{PT}_{2i})}{\text{PT}_i^2}.$$

Note that the likelihood equation (10.17) was developed under the Poisson model, and the usual problems with the maximum likelihood equation of the common odds ratio in a large series of small 2 × 2 tables do not apply to the present case (Breslow, 1981). Under the Poisson model, conditional and unconditional likelihood estimators are the same (Haberman, 1974).

*Mantel-Haenszel Estimator**

In an analogy with the Mantel-Haenszel (MH) estimator (Equation 6.19) of the risk ratio for the count data, an overall estimator of the IRR can be obtained (Rothman and Boice, 1982; Rothman, 1986):

$$\widehat{\text{IRR}}_{\text{MH}} = \frac{\sum_{i=1}^{k} (a_i \text{PT}_{2i})/\text{PT}_i}{\sum_{i=1}^{k} (b_i \text{PT}_{1i})/\text{PT}_i}. \tag{10.18}$$

Equation 10.18 represents a simple noniterative estimator of the common IRR and can be considered to be a weighted average of stratum-specific estimates of the IRR with weights equal to $(b_i\text{PT}_{1i})/\text{PT}_i$. The estimator is nearly as efficient as the maximum likelihood estimator (Walker, 1985). Thus, the Mantel-Haenszel estimator (Equation 10.18) provides a simple and robust alternative to the maximum likelihood estimator determined by Equation 10.17. Clayton (1982) showed that this estimate arises at the first stage of iteration of one of the computational procedures used to determine the maximum likelihood estimate.

* The term *Mantel-Haenszel (MH) estimator* is used here analogously with the MH type estimator (Equation 6.19) and in no way refers to the authors of the procedure.

#### 10.1.2.2 Confidence Intervals

The CIs for the IRR for the stratified data can be determined by an exact method as well as by various approximate procedures. We describe four approximate methods based on pooling with inverse variances, the maximum likelihood, the Mantel-Haenszel, and the test-based approach, as well as an exact method.

*Pooling Method*

An approximate 100(1 – α)% CI for $\log_e$(IRR) can be obtained by first determining an estimate of the variance of the logarithm of the pooled estimator (Equation 10.14) and then using the formula

$$\log_e\left(\hat{\text{IRR}}_w\right) \pm Z_{\alpha/2}\sqrt{\hat{\text{Var}}\left\{\log_e\left(\hat{\text{IRR}}_w\right)\right\}}, \tag{10.19}$$

from which a 100(1 – α)% CI for the IRR can be obtained by taking the antilogarithms of the corresponding endpoints of the CI for $\log_e$(IRR).

A formula for an estimate of the variance of $\log_e(\hat{\text{IRR}}_w)$ can be obtained:

$$\begin{aligned}\hat{\text{Var}}\left\{\log_e\left(\hat{\text{IRR}}_w\right)\right\} &= \hat{\text{Var}}\left[\frac{\sum_{i=1}^{k} W_i \hat{\text{Var}}\left\{\log_e\left(\hat{\text{IRR}}_i\right)\right\}}{\sum_{i=1}^{k} W_i}\right] \\ &= \frac{1}{\left(\sum_{i=1}^{k} W_i\right)^2}\left[\sum_{i=1}^{k} W_i^2 \frac{1}{W_i}\right] \\ &= \frac{1}{\sum_{i=1}^{k} W_i},\end{aligned} \tag{10.20}$$

where $W_i$ is estimated approximately as it is in Equation 10.16.

*Mantel-Haenszel Method*

An approximate 100(1 – α)% CI for $\log_e$(IRR) using this method can be obtained by first determining an estimate of the variance of the logarithm of the Mantel-Haenszel estimator (Equation 10.18) and then using the formula

$$\log_e\left(\hat{\text{IRR}}_{\text{MH}}\right) \pm Z_{\alpha/2}\sqrt{\hat{\text{Var}}\left\{\log_e\left(\hat{\text{IRR}}_{\text{MH}}\right)\right\}}. \tag{10.21}$$

A formula for an estimate of the variance can be derived by assuming each $a_i$ and $b_i$ to have independent Poisson distributions (Tarone, 1981) or each $a_i$ and $b_i$ to have independent binomial distributions conditional on $\text{PT}_{1i}$ and $\text{PT}_{2i}$, respectively (Greenland and Robins, 1985). The variance formulas using these two approaches are

$$\hat{\text{Var}}\left\{\log_e\left(\hat{\text{IRR}}_{\text{MH}}\right)\right\} = \frac{\sum_{i=1}^{k}\left[\frac{\text{PT}_{2i}}{\text{PT}_i}\right]^2 a_i + \left(\hat{\text{IRR}}_{\text{MH}}\right)^2 \sum_{i=1}^{k}\left[\frac{\text{PT}_{1i}}{\text{PT}_i}\right]^2 b_i}{\sum_{i=1}^{k}\left[\frac{\text{PT}_{1i}}{\text{PT}_i}\right]^2} \tag{10.22}$$

and

$$\hat{\text{Var}}\left\{\log_e\left(\hat{\text{IRR}}_{\text{MH}}\right)\right\} = \frac{\left[\sum_{i=1}^{k}\left(\frac{m_i \text{PT}_{1i}\text{PT}_{2i}}{\left(\text{PT}_i\right)^2}\right)\right]}{\left[\sum_{i=1}^{k}\left(\frac{\text{PT}_{2i}}{\text{PT}_i}\right)a_i\right]\left[\sum_{i=1}^{k}\left(\frac{\text{PT}_{1i}}{\text{PT}_i}\right)b_i\right]}. \tag{10.23}$$

*Maximum Likelihood Method*

An approximate $100(1 - \alpha)\%$ CI for $\log_e(\text{IRR})$ using the maximum likelihood method can be obtained by first determining the maximum likelihood estimate and an estimate of its variance, and then using the formula

$$\log_e\left(\hat{\text{IRR}}_{\text{ML}}\right) \pm Z_{\alpha/2}\sqrt{\hat{\text{Var}}\left\{\log_e\left(\hat{\text{IRR}}_{\text{ML}}\right)\right\}}. \tag{10.24}$$

The maximum likelihood estimate is determined as an iterative solution to Equation 10.17, and a large sample variance estimate is given by (Rothman, 1986)

$$\hat{\text{Var}}\left\{\log_e\left(\hat{\text{IRR}}_{\text{ML}}\right)\right\} = \frac{1}{\hat{\text{IRR}}_{\text{ML}} \sum_{i=1}^{k} \frac{m_i \text{PT}_{2i}/\text{PT}_{1i}}{\left(\hat{\text{IRR}}_{\text{ML}} + \text{PT}_{2i}/\text{PT}_{1i}\right)^2}}. \tag{10.25}$$

*Test-Based Method*

Another alternative is to use test-based limits. As previously discussed, a 100(1 – α)% approximate CI for $\log_e$(IRR), using this method, is obtained by the formula

$$\log_e\left(\hat{\text{IRR}}_{\text{MH}}\right) \pm Z_{\alpha/2}\sqrt{\left\{\log_e\left(\hat{\text{IRR}}_{\text{MH}}\right)\right\}^2 / \chi^2_{\text{MH}}}, \tag{10.26}$$

where $\hat{\text{IRR}}_{\text{MH}}$ is the Mantel-Haenszel estimator (Equation 10.18) and $\chi^2_{\text{MH}}$ is the chi-square statistic given by Equation 10.11.

Again, in terms of the standard normal statistic $\chi$, Equation 10.26 can be expressed more simply as

$$\log_e\left(\hat{\text{IRR}}_{\text{MH}}\right)\left(1 \pm Z_{\alpha/2}/\chi\right),$$

from which a 100(1 – α)% CI for the IRR can be written:

$$\hat{\text{IRR}}^{\left(1 \pm Z_{\alpha/2}/\chi\right)}.$$

*An Exact Method*

Following the assumption of the Poisson model and the uniform IRR, the common IRR, using the person-time data, is defined by

$$\text{IRR} = \frac{\text{PT}_{2i}}{\text{PT}_{1i}}\left(\frac{\lambda_{1i}}{\lambda_{2i}}\right),$$

where $\lambda_{1i}$ and $\lambda_{2i}$ are the Poisson means for the exposed and unexposed groups, respectively. For each stratum, given $a_i + b_i = m_i$, $A_i$ has a binomial distribution with parameters: the number of trials equal to $m_i = a_i + b_i$ and the probability of success equal to $p_i = \lambda_{1i}/(\lambda_{1i} + \lambda_{2i})$. If $p_{\text{L}_i}$ and $p_{\text{U}_i}$ are the lower and upper confidence limits of $p_i$ and $\text{IRR}_\text{L}$ and $\text{IRR}_\text{U}$ are the lower and upper confidence limits of the common IRR, then it follows that

$$\text{IRR}_\text{L} = \frac{\text{PT}_{2i}}{\text{PT}_{1i}}\left(\frac{p_{\text{L}_i}}{1 - p_{\text{L}_i}}\right) \tag{10.27}$$

and

$$\text{IRR}_\text{U} = \frac{\text{PT}_{2i}}{\text{PT}_{1i}}\left(\frac{p_{\text{U}_i}}{1 - p_{\text{U}_i}}\right). \tag{10.28}$$

Further, given $a_i + b_i = m_i$, the probability formula for the number of exposed cases in a single stratum can be written as

$$P(a_i) = \binom{m_i}{a_i} p_i^{a_i} (1 - p_i)^{m_i - a_i}.$$

Hence, the probability of obtaining the outcomes $\{a_1, a_2, ..., a_k\}$ in a set of $k$ 2 × 2 tables is given by

$$P\{a_1, a_2, \ldots, a_k\} = \prod_{i=1}^{k} \binom{m_i}{a_i} p_i^{a_i} (1 - p_i)^{m_i - a_i}. \tag{10.29}$$

The upper (lower) tail probability for the exact confidence limits, $p_{L_i}$ and $p_{U_i}$ can be evaluated by taking the sum of the probabilities in Equation 10.29 for all possible values of $\sum_{i=1}^{k} a_i$ equal to or greater (less) than the actual value observed, for example, $a$. Thus, given a pair of 100(1 – α)% confidence limits $p_{L_i}$ and $p_{U_i}$

$$\sum_{l=a}^{m} \prod_{i=1}^{k} \binom{m_i}{a_i} p_{L_i}^{a_i} \left(1 - p_{L_i}\right)^{m_i - a_i} = \alpha/2 \tag{10.30}$$

and

$$\sum_{l=0}^{a} \prod_{i=1}^{k} \binom{m_i}{a_i} p_{U_i}^{a_i} \left(1 - p_{U_i}\right)^{m_i - a_i} = \alpha/2, \tag{10.31}$$

where $m = \sum_{i=1}^{k} m_i$. The value of $IRR_L$ that satisfies Equations 10.27 and 10.30 corresponds to the lower confidence limit. Similarly, the value of $IRR_U$ that satisfies Equations 10.28 and 10.31 corresponds to the upper confidence limit.

It should be noticed that exact limits for the IRR have been obtained from the convolution of the $k$ binomial distributions. They are similar to the determination of exact limits for the OR discussed in Chapter 6 (Section 6.3.3.2), which were obtained from the convolution of the $k$ hypergeometric distributions. The computation of exact limits, however, is quite complicated and must be evaluated iteratively using a computer program.

*Example 10.2*

Consider the data from the survival study of patients with trigeminal neuralgia, as summarized in Table 10.2. First, we obtain point estimates using the methods of pooling, maximum likelihood, and the Mantel-Haenszel approach. From the stratified data of Table 10.2, we have

$$\hat{\text{IRR}}_1 = \frac{14/1516}{10/1701} = 1.571$$

and

$$\hat{\text{IRR}}_2 = \frac{76/949}{121/2245} = 1.486.$$

In order to obtain a pooled estimate of the common IRR, we first obtain stratum-specific weights ($W_i$) as follows:

$$W_1 = \frac{(14)(10)}{14+10} = 5.833$$

and

$$W_2 = \frac{(76)(121)}{76+121} = 46.680.$$

Using Equations 10.14 and 10.15, the pooled (weighted) estimate of the IRR is given by

$$\log_e\left(\hat{\text{IRR}}_w\right) = \frac{(5.833)\log_e(1.571) + (46.680)\log_e(1.486)}{5.833 + 46.680} = 0.402.$$

or

$$\hat{\text{IRR}}_w = 1.495.$$

In order to obtain the maximum likelihood estimate of the IRR, the likelihood equation is

$$(14+76) - \hat{\text{IRR}}_{\text{ML}}\left[\frac{(14+10)}{\hat{\text{IRR}}_{\text{ML}} + 1701/1516} + \frac{(76+121)}{\hat{\text{IRR}}_{\text{ML}} + 2245/949}\right].$$

The maximum likelihood solution for $\hat{\text{IRR}}_{\text{ML}}$ using a computer program (Wolfram, 1991) is obtained as 1.495, which is the same as the value of the pooled estimate determined above.

The Mantel-Haenszel estimate of the IRR, using Equation 10.18, is

$$\hat{\text{IRR}}_{\text{MH}} = \frac{\dfrac{14(1701)}{3217} + \dfrac{76(2245)}{3194}}{\dfrac{10(1516)}{3217} + \dfrac{121(949)}{3194}} = 1.496.$$

Next, we construct CIs for the IRR using the methods based on pooling, the maximum likelihood, the Mantel-Haenszel procedure, the test-based procedure, and the exact procedure.

**Pooling method** — As obtained earlier, $\log_e(\hat{\text{IRR}}_w) = 0.402$, and using Equation 10.20, we have

$$\hat{\text{Var}}\left\{\log_e\left(\hat{\text{IRR}}_w\right)\right\} = \frac{1}{5.833 + 46.680} = 0.019.$$

Thus, a 95% CI for $\log_e$(IRR) using this method is

$$\log_e(1.495) \pm 1.96\sqrt{0.019} = (0.132, 0.672),$$

from which a 95% CI for the IRR is given by (1.141, 1.958).

**Maximum likelihood method** — As obtained earlier, $\hat{\text{IRR}}_{\text{ML}} = 1.495$. Using Equation 10.25, we have

$$\hat{\text{Var}}\left\{\log_e\left(\hat{\text{IRR}}_{\text{ML}}\right)\right\} = \frac{1}{(1.495)\left[\dfrac{24(1701)/1516}{(1.495 + 1701/1516)^2} + \dfrac{197(2245)/949}{(1.495 + 2245/949)^2}\right]}$$
$$= 0.019.$$

Thus, a 95% CI for $\log_e$(IRR) using this method is

$$\log_e(1.495) \pm 1.96\sqrt{0.019} = (0.132, 0.672),$$

from which a 95% CI for the IRR is given by (1.141, 1.958).

**Mantel-Haenszel method** — $\hat{\text{IRR}}_{\text{MH}} = 1.496$, and, using Equation 10.23, we have

$$\hat{\text{Var}}\left\{\log_e\left(\hat{\text{IRR}}_{\text{MH}}\right)\right\} = \frac{\dfrac{24(1701)(1516)}{(3217)^2} + \dfrac{197(949)(2245)}{(3194)^2}}{\left[\left(\dfrac{1701}{3217}\right)14 + \left(\dfrac{2245}{3194}\right)76\right]\left[\left(\dfrac{1516}{3217}\right)10 + \left(\dfrac{949}{3194}\right)121\right]}$$
$$= 0.019.$$

Thus, a 95% CI for $\log_e$(IRR) using this method is

$$\log_e(1.496) \pm 1.96\sqrt{0.019} = (0.133, 0.673),$$

from which a 95% CI for the IRR is given by (1.142, 1.960).

**Test-based method** — To obtain a 95% CI for the IRR using the test-based method, note that $\chi^2_{\text{MH}} = 8.6229$. Therefore, a 95% CI for $\log_e$(IRR) using this method is obtained as

$$\log_e(1.496) \pm 1.96\sqrt{\{\log_e(1.496)\}^2 / 8.6229} = (0.134, 0.672),$$

from which a 95% CI for the IRR is given by (1.143, 1.958).

**Exact method** — An exact CI for the IRR can be determined using Equations 10.27, 10.28, 10.30, and 10.31. The numerical computations, however, are rather complex. The 95% exact limits using a computer program are $\text{IRR}_{\text{L}} = 1.128$ and $\text{IRR}_{\text{U}} = 1.947$.

Note that all the approximate procedures yield nearly the same result and compare favorably with the limits obtained via exact method.

#### 10.1.2.3 Test for Homogeneity of Incidence Rate Ratios

A test for homogeneity of effect over strata in terms of a uniform IRR can be carried out by the statistic

$$\sum_{i=1}^{k}\left[\frac{\left[\log_e\left(\hat{\text{IRR}}_i\right) - \log_e\left(\hat{\text{IRR}}_w\right)\right]^2}{\hat{\text{Var}}\left\{\log_e\left(\hat{\text{IRR}}_i\right)\right\}}\right],$$

which asymptotically has a chi-square distribution with $k - 1$ degrees of freedom. Note that $\hat{\text{IRR}}_i$, $\hat{\text{Var}}\{\log_e(\hat{\text{IRR}}_i)\}$, and $\log_e(\hat{\text{IRR}}_w)$ are defined by Equations 10.12, 10.13, and 10.14, respectively.

The test statistic for the data in Example 10.2 is calculated as

$$\frac{(0.452 - 0.402)^2}{0.171} + \frac{(0.396 - 0.402)^2}{0.021} = 0.016,$$

and from the chi-square table

$$P\left(\chi^2_1 > 0.016\right) = 0.899.$$

Thus, the hypothesis of the homogeneity of IRR for the two age strata cannot be rejected and we lack the evidence that incidence rate ratios are different for the two age groups under consideration.

## 10.2 OTHER SUMMARY EFFECT MEASURES

The basic feature of all the summary measures of effect considered in this chapter is that they are a weighted average of stratum-specific effect estimates, such as the rate difference or rate ratio. The other approach is to summarize effect estimates as the difference or ratio of weighted averages of stratum-specific estimates, known as standardized difference or ratio, rather than the weighted average of the stratum-specific rate difference or ratio.

### 10.2.1 STANDARDIZED MEASURES OF EFFECT

In this section, we consider standardized rate difference, standardized rate ratio, and standardized mortality ratio as the standardized measures of effect estimates.

#### 10.2.1.1 Standardized Rate Difference

The standardized rate difference (SRD) is the difference of the standardized weighted averages of stratum-specific rates for exposed and unexposed groups. Using the notation of Table 10.1, the SRD can be estimated as

$$\hat{\text{SRD}} = \frac{\sum_{i=1}^{k} W_i \hat{R}_{1i}}{\sum_{i=1}^{k} W_i} - \frac{\sum_{i=1}^{k} W_i \hat{R}_{2i}}{\sum_{i=1}^{k} W_i}, \tag{10.32}$$

where $\hat{R}_{1i} = a_i/\text{PT}_{1i}$, $\hat{R}_{2i} = b_i/\text{PT}_{2i}$, and $W_i$ is the standard weight of the $i$th stratum. Equation 10.32 can be rewritten as

$$\hat{\text{SRD}} = \frac{\sum_{i=1}^{k} W_i \,\hat{\text{IRD}}_i}{\sum_{i=1}^{k} W_i}, \tag{10.33}$$

where $\hat{\text{IRD}}_i = \hat{R}_{1i} - \hat{R}_{2i}$. Thus, $\hat{\text{SRD}}$s are calculated in a manner similar to the pooled (weighted) averages of stratum-specific rate differences, although the choice of standard weights differs.

#### 10.2.1.2 Standardized Rate Ratio

The standardized rate ratio (SRR) is the ratio of the weighted standardized rates in exposed and unexposed groups. Using the notation of Table 10.1, the SRR can be estimated as

$$\hat{\text{SRR}} = \frac{\sum_{i=1}^{k} W_i \hat{R}_{1i} \bigg/ \sum_{i=1}^{k} W_i}{\sum_{i=1}^{k} W_i \hat{R}_{2i} \bigg/ \sum_{i=1}^{k} W_i}, \tag{10.34}$$

where $\hat{R}_{1i} = a_i/\text{PT}_{1i}$, $\hat{R}_{2i} = b_i/\text{PT}_{2i}$, and $W_i$ is the standard weight of the $i$th stratum. Equation 10.34 can be rewritten as

$$\hat{\text{SRR}} = \frac{\sum_{i=1}^{k} W_i \hat{R}_{1i}}{\sum_{i=1}^{k} W_i \hat{R}_{2i}}. \tag{10.35}$$

Note that in Equation 10.34, the numerator and the denominator are the standardized rates of exposed and unexposed groups, respectively.

Two common choices of taking stratum-specific standard weights for computing standardized rates are available. One choice is to take weights based on the distribution of unexposed group (reference population), i.e., $W_i = \text{PT}_{2i}$. Such a measure is simply known as SRR and expression (10.35) reduces to (Miettinen, 1972)

$$\hat{\text{SRR}} = \frac{\sum_{i=1}^{k} (\text{PT}_{2i}) \hat{R}_{1i}}{\sum_{i=1}^{k} b_i}. \tag{10.36}$$

Thus, $\hat{\text{SRR}}$ is the ratio of the number of expected cases in the unexposed group, based on the rates in the exposed group, to the number of observed cases in the reference population.

#### 10.2.1.3 Standardized Mortality Ratio

Another approach of taking weights is to take weights based on the distribution of exposed group, i.e., $W_i = \text{PT}_{1i}$. In the epidemiologic literature such a measure is generally known as *standardized mortality ratio* (SMR). Thus, expression (10.35) reduces to (Miettinen, 1972)

$$\hat{\text{SMR}} = \frac{\sum_{i=1}^{k} a_i}{\sum_{i=1}^{k} (\text{PT}_{1i})\hat{R}_{2i}}. \tag{10.37}$$

Thus, $\hat{\text{SMR}}$ is the sum of the observed cases in the exposed group, relative to the sum of the expected cases in the exposed group, based on the rates in the unexposed group.

### 10.2.2 Confidence Intervals for Standardized Measures of Effect

Confidence intervals for standardized measures of effect can be calculated readily, but the procedure depends on the type of weights assigned for standardization.

#### 10.2.2.1 Standardized Rate Difference

For the SRD (Equation 10.33), an approximate variance estimate is given by

$$\hat{\text{Var}}\left(\hat{\text{SRD}}\right) = \frac{\sum_{i=1}^{k} W_i^2 \, \hat{\text{Var}}\left(\hat{\text{IRD}}_i\right)}{\left(\sum_{i=1}^{k} W_i\right)^2}, \tag{10.38}$$

where $W_i$ is the standard weight and $\hat{\text{Var}}(\hat{\text{IRD}}_i)$ can be obtained from Equation 10.2. An approximate CI for the SRD can be obtained in the usual way, using the standard normal theory.

#### 10.2.2.2 Standardized Rate Ratio

An approximate CI for the SRR can be obtained by using a formula for the approximate variance of the logarithm of the SRR. Assuming a Poisson model for the incidence of disease in the exposed and unexposed categories, an approximate variance estimate for $\log_e(\hat{\text{SRR}})$ is

$$\hat{\text{Var}}\left\{\log_e\left(\hat{\text{SRR}}\right)\right\} \approx \frac{\sum_{i=1}^{k} \text{PT}_{2i}^2\left(a_i/\text{PT}_{1i}^2\right)}{\left[\sum_{i=1}^{k} \text{PT}_{2i}\left(a_i/\text{PT}_{1i}\right)\right]^2} + \frac{1}{\sum_{i=1}^{k} b_i}. \tag{10.39}$$

The resulting CI for the SRR can be obtained in the usual way, using the standard normal theory. (For a discussion of some other available methods of determining CIs for the SRR, refer to papers by Miettinen, 1976; Greenland, 1982; and Flanders, 1984.)

#### 10.2.2.3 Standardized Mortality Ratio

An "exact" CI for the SMR can be obtained by assuming that the number of observed cases in the exposed population, i.e., $D = \sum_{i=1}^{k} a_i$, has Poisson distribution with mean $\lambda = E(D)$. A pair of exact confidence limits for the SMR is then obtained by finding the lower and upper confidence limits of $\lambda$. The lower and upper confidence limits of $\lambda$, $\lambda_L$ and $\lambda_U$, can be determined by solving the following equations involving Poisson probabilities (see, e.g., Sahai and Khurshid, 1993):

$$\sum_{i=D}^{\infty} \frac{e^{-\lambda_L} \lambda_L^i}{i!} = \alpha/2 \tag{10.40}$$

and

$$\sum_{i=0}^{D} \frac{e^{-\lambda_U} \lambda_U^i}{i!} = \alpha/2. \tag{10.41}$$

The solutions to Equations 10.40 and 10.41 are in general obtained using the trial and error method and entail the use of Poisson probability tables. The solutions are, however, more readily obtained in terms of percentiles of the chi-square distribution and are given by (see, e.g., Sahai and Khurshid, 1993)

$$\lambda_L = (1/2)\chi^2_{\nu_1,\alpha/2} \text{ and } \lambda_U = (1/2)\chi^2_{\nu_2,1-\alpha/2}, \tag{10.42}$$

where $\nu_1 = 2D$, $\nu_2 = 2(D + 1)$, $\chi^2_{\nu_1,\alpha/2}$ denotes the $100(\alpha/2)$th percentile of the chi-square distribution with $\nu_1$ degrees of freedom, and $\chi^2_{\nu_2,1-\alpha/2}$ denotes the $100(1 - \alpha/2)$th percentile of the chi-square distribution with $\nu_2$ degrees of freedom. If the denominator of Equation 10.37, i.e., $\sum_{i=1}^{k}(\mathrm{PT}_{1i})\hat{R}_{2i}$, is calculated from the incidence or mortality rate of the whole country or another large population, it can be assumed to be constant. Using Equation 10.42, the confidence limits for the SMR, $\mathrm{SMR}_L$ and $\mathrm{SMR}_U$, are then given by

$$\mathrm{SMR}_L = \frac{(1/2)\chi^2_{\nu_1,\alpha/2}}{\sum_{i=1}^{k}(\mathrm{PT}_{1i})\hat{R}_{2i}} \text{ and } \mathrm{SMR}_U = \frac{(1/2)\chi^2_{\nu_2,1-\alpha/2}}{\sum_{i=1}^{k}(\mathrm{PT}_{1i})\hat{R}_{2i}}. \tag{10.43}$$

The above method of determining confidence limits is fairly simple and straightforward to apply. The tables of percentiles of the chi-square distribution are widely available (including computer programs) to evaluate the desired percentiles. Because the calculations of the SMR are now usually done by a computer (Coleman et al., 1986), the above method can be readily implemented in a computer analysis. In the absence of appropriate chi-square tables or computer software, the confidence limits (Equation 10.43) can be approximated using the Wilson and Hilferty (1931) approximation of the chi-square percentiles, which gives

$$\chi^2_{\nu,\alpha} = \nu\left(1 - \frac{2}{9\nu} + Z_\alpha\sqrt{\frac{2}{9\nu}}\right)^3.$$

The resulting limits for the SMR are

$$\begin{aligned} \text{SMR}_\text{L} &= \frac{D}{\sum_{i=1}^{k}(\text{PT}_{1i})R_{2i}}\left[1 - \frac{1}{9D} - \frac{Z_{\alpha/2}}{3\sqrt{D}}\right]^3 \\ \text{SMR}_\text{U} &= \frac{D+1}{\sum_{i=1}^{k}(\text{PT}_{1i})R_{2i}}\left[1 - \frac{1}{9(D+1)} + \frac{Z_{\alpha/2}}{3\sqrt{D+1}}\right]^3. \end{aligned} \qquad (10.44)$$

Note that the exact limits determined by Equation 10.43 are exact in the sense that we obtain a confidence coefficient of at least 1 – α. Because the Poisson distribution is a discrete distribution, we usually do not obtain a prespecified confidence coefficient exactly equal to 1 – α. Thus, these limits are usually conservative. (For a discussion of some improved procedures to the "exact" limits, including various approximate methods of determining confidence limits, see Sahai and Khurshid, 1993.)

*Example 10.3*

Consider the person-years data on age-specific coronary disease deaths as a result of cigarette smoking among British male doctors, as reported by Doll and Hill (1966) and further discussed by Rothman (1986). The data are summarized in Table 10.3.

To calculate the SRR of incidence rates, one uses weights based on person-years distribution of nonsmoking doctors. The resulting estimate of the SRR, using Equation 10.36, is

**TABLE 10.3**
**Person-Time Data on Age-Specific Coronary Disease Deaths from Cigarette Smoking among British Male Doctors**

| | Smokers | | Nonsmokers | |
|---|---|---|---|---|
| Age | Deaths | Person-years | Deaths | Person-years |
| 35–44 | 32 | 52,407 | 2 | 18,790 |
| 45–54 | 104 | 43,248 | 12 | 10,673 |
| 55–64 | 206 | 28,612 | 28 | 5,710 |
| 65–74 | 186 | 12,663 | 28 | 2,585 |
| 75–84 | 102 | 5,317 | 31 | 1,462 |
| Total | 630 | 142,247 | 101 | 39,220 |

Doll, R. and Hill, A. B. (1966). *Epidemiological Approaches to the Study of Cancer and Other Chronic Diseases,* NCI Monogr. Vol. 19 (Ed. W. Haenszel) pp. 205–255. National Cancer Institute, Bethesda, MA. With permission.

$$\hat{\text{SRR}} = \frac{18790(32/52407) + 10673(104/43248) + \ldots + 1462(102/5317)}{2 + 12 + \ldots + 31}$$

$$= 1.430.$$

To calculate SMR, the choice of standard weights would be the person-years distribution of smoking doctors. The resulting estimate of the SMR, using Equation 10.37, is given by

$$\hat{\text{SMR}} = \frac{32 + 104 + \ldots + 102}{52407(2/18790) + 43248(12/10673) + \ldots + 5317(31/1462)}$$

$$= 1.411.$$

For a CI of the SRR, a variance estimate of $\log_e(\hat{\text{SRR}})$, using Equation 10.39, is given by

$$\hat{\text{Var}}\left\{\log_e\left(\hat{\text{SRR}}\right)\right\}$$

$$\approx \frac{(18790)^2 \dfrac{32}{(52407)^2} + (10673)^2 \dfrac{104}{(43248)^2} + \cdots + (1462)^2 \dfrac{102}{(5317)^2}}{\left[18790(32/52407) + 10673(104/43248) + \ldots + 1462(102/5317)\right]^2} + \frac{1}{101}$$

$$= 0.0115.$$

Thus, a 95% CI for $\log_e$(SRR) is obtained as

$$\log_e(1.430) \pm 1.96\sqrt{0.0115} = (0.148, 0.568),$$

from which a 95% CI for the SRR is given by (1.159, 1.765).

For a CI of the SMR, using Equation 10.44, the 95% confidence limits are determined by

$$\text{SMR}_\text{L} = \frac{630}{444.402}\left[1 - \frac{1}{9 \times 630} - \frac{1.96}{3\sqrt{630}}\right]^3 = 1.309$$

and

$$\text{SMR}_\text{U} = \frac{631}{444.402}\left[1 - \frac{1}{9 \times 631} + \frac{1.96}{3\sqrt{631}}\right]^3 = 1.533.$$

# References

**Breslow, N. E.** (1981). "Odds Ratio Estimators When the Data Are Sparse", *Biometrika,* 68, 73–84.

**Breslow, N. E. and Day, N. E.** (1987). *Statistical Methods in Cancer Research, Vol. 2: The Design and Analysis of Cohort Studies.* International Agency for Research on Cancer, Lyons, France.

**Clayton, D. G.** (1982). "The Analysis of Prospective Studies of Disease Aetiology", *Commun. Stat. Theory Methods,* 11, 2129–2155.

**Coleman, M., Douglas, A., and Hermon, C.** (1986). "Cohort Analysis with a FORTRAN Computer Program", *Int. J. Epidemiol.,* 16, 134–137.

**Doll, R. and Hill, A. B.** (1966). "Mortality in British Doctors in Relation to Smoking: Observations on Coronary Thrombosis", In: *Epidemiological Approaches to the Study of Cancer and Other Chronic Diseases.* NCI Monogr. Vol. 19 (Ed. W. Haenszel), pp. 205–225. National Cancer Institute, Bethesda, MD.

**Flanders, W. D.** (1984). "Approximate Variance Formulas for Standardized Rate Ratios", *J. Chronic Dis.,* 37, 449–453.

**Greenland, S.** (1982). "Interpretation and Estimation of Summary Ratios Under Heterogeneity", *Stat. Med.,* 1, 217–227.

**Greenland, S. and Robins, J. M.** (1985). "Estimation of a Common Effect Parameter from Sparse Follow-Up Data", *Biometrics,* 41, 55–68.

**Haberman, S. J.** (1974). *The Analysis of Frequency Data.* University of Chicago Press, Chicago.

**Miettinen, O. S.** (1972). "Standardization of Risk Ratio", *Am. J. Epidemiol.,* 96, 383–388.

**Miettinen, O. S.** (1975). Principles of Epidemiologic Research, unpublished course text, Department of Epidemiology and Biostatistics, School of Public Health, Harvard University, Cambridge, MA.

**Miettinen, O. S.** (1976). "Estimability and Estimation in Case-Referent Studies", *Am. J. Epidemiol.,* 103, 226–235.

**Rothman, K. J.** (1986). *Modern Epidemiology.* Little, Brown, Boston.

**Rothman, K. J. and Boice, J. D.** (1982). *Epidemiologic Analysis with a Programmable Calculator, New Edition.* Epidemiology Resources, Chestnut Hill, MA. (First edition published by the U.S. Government Printing Office, Washington, D. C., NIH Publ. No. 79–1649, 1979.)

**Rothman, K. J. and Monson, R. R.** (1973). "Survival in Trigeminal Neuralgia", *J. Chronic Dis.,* 26, 303–309.

**Sahai, H. and Khurshid, A.** (1993). "Confidence Intervals for the Mean of a Poisson Distribution: A Review", *Biometrical J.,* 35, 857–867.

**Shore, R. E., Pasternack, B. S., and Curnen, M. C.** (1976). "Relating Influenza Epidemics to Childhood Leukemia in Tumor Registries Without a Defined Population Base: A Critique with Suggestions for Improved Methods", *Am. J. Epidemiol.,* 103, 527–535.

**Tarone, R. E.** (1981). "On Summary Estimators of Relative Risk", *J. Chronic Dis.,* 34, 463–468.

**Walker, A. M.** (1985). "Small Sample Properties of Some Estimators of a Common Hazard Ratio", *Appl. Stat.,* 34, 42–48.

**Wilson, E. B. and Hilferty, M. M.** (1931). "The Distribution of Chi-Square", *Proc. Natl. Acad. Sci. U.S.A.,* 17, 684–688.

**Wolfram, S.** (1991). *Mathematica: A System for Doing Mathematics by Computers,* 2nd ed. Addison-Wesley, Reading, MA.

# 11 Attributable Risk

The risk difference discussed in this volume is commonly known as attributable risk (AR). As noted earlier, the AR is a measure of association that provides information about the absolute effect of the exposure or the excess of risk of disease in those exposed as compared to those who are not exposed. It is the proportion of disease among the exposed that is attributable to the exposure or the proportion of the disease in the exposed group, which could be prevented by eliminating the exposure to an etiologic agent, provided that it is causal. Unlike the risk ratio and odds ratio, AR takes into account the number of exposed individuals in the population. Hence, the AR assesses the public health importance of an exposure or risk factor in a population study. The literature on AR is diverse and voluminous and appears in a variety of journals from different fields. (For a discussion of AR in situations in which exposure is polychotmous and when estimates of AR at specified levels of exposure are of interest, see Miettinen, 1974, and Denman and Schlesselman, 1983. For a historical survey of the concept of AR and an annotated bibliography, see Gefeller, 1992.)

## 11.1 PERCENT ATTRIBUTABLE RISK

The AR is often expressed as a percentage. The percent attributable risk (AR%), also referred to in the epidemiologic literature as *attributable proportion, attributable rate percent,* or *preventive fraction,* is calculated as AR divided by the rate of disease among the exposed:

$$\begin{aligned} \text{AR\%} &= \frac{\text{AR}}{p_e} \times 100 \\ &= \left( \frac{p_e - p_u}{p_e} \right) \times 100, \end{aligned} \tag{11.1}$$

where $p_e$ and $p_u$ denote the rate or risk of disease among exposed and unexposed groups, respectively. A sample estimate of AR% is

$$\hat{\text{AR}}\% = \left(\frac{\hat{p}_e - \hat{p}_u}{\hat{p}_e}\right) \times 100, \tag{11.2}$$

where $\hat{p}_e$ and $\hat{p}_u$ denote the estimates of the risk of disease among exposed and unexposed groups, respectively.

For most case-control studies, AR cannot be calculated because the incidence rates among the exposed and unexposed groups are not estimable. However, by dividing both the numerator and the denominator of the right side of Equation 11.1 by $p_u$, we have

$$\text{AR}\% = \left(\frac{\text{RR} - 1}{\text{RR}}\right) \times 100, \tag{11.3}$$

where RR (risk ratio) = $p_e/p_u$. Thus, an estimate of AR%, as given in Equation 11.3, is

$$\hat{\text{AR}}\% = \left(\frac{\hat{\text{RR}} - 1}{\hat{\text{RR}}}\right) \times 100. \tag{11.4}$$

Although Equation 11.4 requires $\hat{\text{RR}}$ (risk ratio estimate) for its calculation, the odds ratio estimate ($\hat{\text{OR}}$) may be used as a surrogate value for the $\hat{\text{RR}}$ if the disease rarely occurs in the population.

Alternatively, in case-control studies in which rate or risk in the total population of interest is known or can be estimated from other sources, and the distribution of exposure among the controls is assumed to be representative of the whole population, this information can be used to calculate incidence rates in exposed and unexposed groups. Because the overall incidence rate of the disease in a population ($p_t$) may be considered to be the weighted average of the incidence rates in the exposed and unexposed categories, we have

$$p_t = \boldsymbol{P}_e p_e + \boldsymbol{P}_u p_u, \tag{11.5}$$

where $\boldsymbol{P}_e$ and $\boldsymbol{P}_u$ denote the proportion of individuals in the total population representing exposed and unexposed groups, respectively. Noting that RR = $p_e/p_u$, Equation 11.5 can be written as

$$p_t = (\text{RR})\boldsymbol{P}_e p_u + \boldsymbol{P}_u p_u. \tag{11.6}$$

Solving Equation 11.6 for $p_u$, one obtains

$$p_u = \frac{p_t}{(\text{RR})\boldsymbol{P}_e + \boldsymbol{P}_u}. \tag{11.7}$$

A sample estimate of $p_u$ in Equation 11.7 is given by

$$\hat{p}_u = \frac{\hat{p}_t}{(\hat{\mathrm{RR}})\boldsymbol{P}_e + \boldsymbol{P}_u}. \tag{11.8}$$

For case-control studies, the relative risk is estimated by the $\hat{\mathrm{OR}}$ and an estimate of $p_e$ is obtained: $\hat{p}_e = (\hat{\mathrm{OR}})\,\hat{p}_u$. Given an estimate of $p_e$ and $p_u$, the AR or the AR% can then be readily calculated.

## 11.2 POPULATION ATTRIBUTABLE RISK

While it is useful to estimate the rate, proportion, or risk of disease for cases that are attributable to the exposure, it is also of interest to estimate the excess risk of disease in the total study population, comprising exposed and unexposed individuals, which can be attributed to the exposure. This measure, referred to as the population attributable rate or risk (PAR), is defined as the risk of disease in the total population $(p_t)$ minus the risk in the unexposed group $(p_u)$:

$$\mathrm{PAR} = p_t - p_u. \tag{11.9}$$

Alternatively, using Equation 11.5 and noting that $\boldsymbol{P}_e + \boldsymbol{P}_u = 1$, PAR in Equation 11.9 can be obtained by multiplying the AR by the proportion of exposed individuals in the population:

$$\mathrm{PAR} = (\mathrm{AR})\boldsymbol{P}_e. \tag{11.10}$$

Similar to the AR% in the exposed group, the population attributable risk percent (PAR%) is defined as the proportion of the risk to the disease in the study population that is attributable to the exposure, and thus could be avoided by limiting the exposure to the risk factor. The PAR% is obtained by dividing the PAR by the risk of disease in the total population:

$$\begin{aligned} \mathrm{PAR}\% &= \frac{\mathrm{PAR}}{p_t} \times 100 \\ &= \left(\frac{p_t - p_u}{p_t}\right) \times 100. \end{aligned} \tag{11.11}$$

Equation 11.11, used for calculating PAR%, was first reported by Leviton (1973). A sample estimate of PAR% is obtained as

$$\hat{\text{PAR}}\% = \left( \frac{\hat{p}_t - \hat{p}_u}{\hat{p}_t} \right) \times 100 \tag{11.12}$$

where $\hat{p}_t$ and $\hat{p}_u$ denote the estimates of the risk of disease among the total population and the unexposed group, respectively.

In a case-control study the PAR% can be calculated if the proportion of individuals exposed in the control group can be used as an estimate of the proportion of individuals exposed in the total population ($\boldsymbol{P}_e$), or if the prevalence of exposure in the population is obtainable from other sources. This follows from the fact that the PAR% is the number of cases due to association with the risk factor divided by the total number of cases in the population, or equivalently, the proportion of the number of cases in the population due to the risk factor:

$$\text{PAR}\% = \frac{N\boldsymbol{P}_e p_e(\text{AR})}{N\boldsymbol{P}_e p_e + N\boldsymbol{P}_u p_u} \times 100, \tag{11.13}$$

where $N$ is the size of the entire population. Note that $N\boldsymbol{P}_e p_e$(AR) is the number of cases due to the association with the risk factor, $N\boldsymbol{P}_e p_e$ is the number of cases occurring among those exposed to the risk factor and $N\boldsymbol{P}_u p_u$ is the number of cases occurring among those unexposed to the risk factor. Noting that AR = (RR – 1)/RR, Equation 11.13 can be written as

$$\text{PAR}\% = \frac{N\boldsymbol{P}_e p_e[(\text{RR}-1)/\text{RR}]}{N\boldsymbol{P}_e p_e + N\boldsymbol{P}_u p_u} \times 100. \tag{11.14}$$

Dividing the numerator and the denominator of Equation 11.14 by $N\boldsymbol{P}_u p_u$ and simplifying, we get

$$\text{PAR}\% = \frac{\boldsymbol{P}_e(\text{RR}-1)}{1+\boldsymbol{P}_e(\text{RR}-1)} \times 100. \tag{11.15}$$

In the epidemiologic literature, several names and formulas are equivalent to the proportion (fraction) or AR% defined by Equation 11.15 (see, e.g., Leviton, 1973; Markush, 1977). Whereas Cole and MacMahon (1971) term it a *population attributable risk percent,* Walter (1976) and Lillienfeld and Stolley (1994) refer to it simply as *attributable fraction or risk.* Miettinen (1974) used the term *etiologic fraction,* although the concept of etiologic fraction comes from Levin (1953). A sample estimate of PAR% in Equation 11.15 is then given by

**TABLE 11.1**
**A 2 × 2 Display of Count Data in an Epidemiologic Study**

| | Exposed | Unexposed | Total |
|---|---|---|---|
| Cases | $a$ | $b$ | $m_1$ |
| Controls | $c$ | $d$ | $m_2$ |
| Total | $n_1$ | $n_2$ | $n$ |

$$\hat{\text{PAR}}\% = \frac{\hat{P}_e(\hat{\text{RR}} - 1)}{1 + \hat{P}_e(\hat{\text{RR}} - 1)} \times 100. \tag{11.16}$$

Again, in the calculation of $\hat{\text{PAR}}\%$, the $\hat{\text{OR}}$ may be used as a surrogate value for the $\hat{\text{RR}}$ if the disease occurs rarely in the population.
(11.17)

## 11.3 CONFIDENCE INTERVALS

Consider a general 2 × 2 table arising in an epidemiologic study, as shown in Table 11.1. By determining an estimate of the sample variance of $\hat{\text{PAR}}\%$ and assuming that it is normally distributed, an approximate confidence interval (CI) for the $\hat{\text{PAR}}\%$ can be obtained in the usual way. Appropriate formulas for sample variances are available for cohort and case-control studies (Walter, 1978). For prospective cohort data

$$\hat{\text{Var}}(\hat{\text{PAR}}\%) = \frac{bn}{m_1^3 n_2^3}\left[ad(n-b) + b^2 c\right] \times 100, \tag{11.17}$$

and for retrospective case-control data

$$\hat{\text{Var}}(\hat{\text{PAR}}\%) = \left(\frac{bm_2}{dm_1}\right)^2 \left[\frac{a}{bm_1} + \frac{c}{dm_2}\right] \times 100. \tag{11.18}$$

For alternative and related methods to setting confidence limits, see Walter (1975) and Leung and Kupper (1981). Walter (1976) presents interval estimation procedures for other measures of AR for more complex situations.

**TABLE 11.2**
**Data from the Framingham Study of Coronary Heart Disease**

| | Level of serum control | | |
|---|---|---|---|
| | ≥220 | <220 | Total |
| CHD | 72 | 20 | 92 |
| No CHD | 684 | 553 | 1237 |
| Total | 756 | 573 | 1329 |

From Cornfield, J. (1962). *Fed. Proc.*, 21, 58–61. With permission.

*Example 11.1*

Consider a small subset of the data from the Framingham study as reported by Cornfield (1962) and further discussed by Walter (1978). The results summarized in Table 11.2 show the number of cases of coronary heart disease (CHD) which developed after 6 years of follow-up of 1329 men in the age group 40 to 59 years. The subjects are stratified by their initial level of serum cholesterol, which is considered a risk factor.

In order to estimate PAR, we have

$$\hat{p}_t = \frac{92}{1329} = 0.0692 \text{ and } \hat{p}_u = \frac{20}{573} = 0.0349.$$

Therefore, using Equation 11.12, one obtains

$$\hat{\text{PAR}}\% = \frac{0.0692 - 0.0349}{0.0692} \times 100 = 49.6.$$

Alternatively, we can estimate $\hat{\text{PAR}}\%$ using Equation 11.15. First, we estimate the relative risk by

$$\hat{\text{RR}} = \frac{72/756}{20/573} = 2.73.$$

The other quantity needed to estimate $\hat{\text{PAR}}\%$ is the fraction of the exposed population ($\boldsymbol{P}_e$). We may estimate the observed fraction of men exposed to the risk by

$$\hat{\boldsymbol{P}}_e = \frac{756}{1329} = 0.569.$$

**TABLE 11.3**
**Data from a Retrospective Study of Oral Cancer**

| | Smoking status (cigarettes/d) | | |
|---|---|---|---|
| | ≥16 | <16 | Total |
| Cases | 255 | 49 | 304 |
| Controls | 93 | 46 | 139 |
| Total | 348 | 95 | 443 |

From Wynder, E. L., Bross, I. J., and Feldman, R. M. (1957). *Cancer,* 10, 1300. With permission.

However, sampling variability is associated with this estimate, which should be taken into account when estimating the AR. An estimate of the $\hat{PAR}$ % is then given by

$$\hat{PAR}\% = \frac{0.569(2.73-1)}{1+0.569(2.73-1)} \times 100 = 49.6,$$

which is the same value as that obtained earlier using Equation 11.12.

Using Equation 11.17, an estimate of the corresponding sample variance is given by

$$\hat{Var}\left(\hat{PAR}\%\right) = \frac{(20 \times 1329)\left[(72 \times 553)(1329-20) + (20)^2(684)\right]}{(92)^3 (573)^3} \times 100$$

$$= 0.951.$$

An approximate 95% CI for $\hat{PAR}\%$ is given by

$$49.6 \pm 1.96\sqrt{0.951} = (30.5, 68.7).$$

Thus, the percentage of CHD cases associated with, or attributable to, serum cholesterol levels above 220 mg% is between 31 and 69% for men of this age group.

*Example 11.2*

Consider the data from a retrospective case-control study of the association between smoking and oral cancer described by Wynder et al. (1957) and further discussed by Rothman and Keller (1972) and Walter (1978). The results are summarized in Table 11.3.

First, we will obtain a point estimate of the $\hat{\text{PAR}}\%$ using Equation 11.15. As indicated earlier, we will use the OR as an approximation of the RR. An estimate of the OR is

$$\hat{\text{OR}} = \frac{255 \times 46}{49 \times 93} = 2.574.$$

The additional parameter required to estimate the $\hat{\text{PAR}}\%$ is the fraction of the population exposed to the risk ($\boldsymbol{P}_e$). In this study the exposed population comprises the individuals smoking 16 or more cigarettes per day. Assuming that the controls are representative of the general population, we can estimate the fraction of exposed individuals as

$$\hat{\boldsymbol{P}}_e = 93/139 = 0.669.$$

An estimate of the $\hat{\text{PAR}}\%$, using Equation 11.15, is obtained as

$$\hat{\text{PAR}}\% = \frac{0.669(2.574 - 1)}{1 + 0.669(2.574 - 1)} \times 100 = 51.3.$$

Using Equation 11.18, an estimate of the variance is given by

$$\hat{\text{Var}}\left(\hat{\text{PAR}}\%\right) = \left(\frac{49 \times 139}{46 \times 304}\right)^2 \left[\frac{255}{49 \times 304} + \frac{93}{46 \times 139}\right] \times 100 = 0.751.$$

Assuming that $\hat{\text{PAR}}$ is approximately normally distributed, an approximate 95% CI for the PAR% is given by

$$51.3 \pm 1.96\sqrt{0.751} = (34.3, 68.7).$$

## 11.4 ADJUSTMENT FOR CONFOUNDING

Estimates of the PAR that are not adjusted for confounding factors may lead to biased results, even if adjusted estimates of RR are used in Equation 11.16 (see, e.g., Whittemore, 1983). Thus, in an epidemiologic study it is often of interest to adjust for the effects of confounding factors. Similar to the methods of stratified analysis described in Chapter 6 for the RD, RR, and OR, an adjusted PAR may be derived by the weighted average of the individual PAR estimates, where weights may be taken simply as the proportion of cases in each stratum or the reciprocal of the stratum-specific variances. Walter (1976, 1978), Ejigou (1979), and Whittemore (1982, 1983) discuss this approach. The weighted average procedure does not require the assumption of a common OR and can allow for the control of both confounding and effect modification (see, e.g., Benichou, 1991). However, the choice of inverse variances as weights has been shown to be inconsistent and may lead to substantial bias if the data are sparse and the probability of exposure is large (see Whittemore, 1982; Benichou, 1991). Alternative estimation procedures for the control of confounding, including methods for CIs, were proposed by Greenland (1987) and Kuritz and Landis (1987, 1988) which, for the case-control data, make use of the Mantel-Haenszel estimator of the common OR. The Greenland (1987) method also can be employed with the conditional maximum likelihood estimate of the OR in place of the Mantel-Haenszel estimate. In contrast to the weighted average approach, Mantel-Haenszel procedure is suitable for sparse data and can also be used for matched-pair data (see Benichou, 1991).

Multivariate methods to control confounding that utilize the logistic regression model to estimate the PAR for a given factor, while simultaneously controlling for other factors included in the model, also were proposed. Such models were first suggested by Walter (1976) and Sturmans et al. (1977) for case-control data. Deubner et al. (1980) subsequently used a logistic model for prospective data from a mortality study investigating cardiovascular disease risk factors. A detailed description of the use of the logistic regression model to obtain adjusted PAR estimates from case-control data was provided by Bruzzi et al. (1985). Methods of CIs associated with PAR estimates obtained using the logistic regression were discussed by Benichou and Gail (1990). Kooperberg and Petitti (1991) used a bootstrap technique to construct CIs for adjusted PAR estimates from unmatched case-control data using the logistic regression model. An alternative approach for obtaining CIs under an unconditional logistic regression model is discussed by Drescher and Schill (1991). In addition, Greenland and Drescher (1993) provide an extension for the previous method to allow for the control of multiple and continuous confounders, and also present results of a simulation study comparing various methods of CIs. Additional discussion and details of various adjustment procedures of interest to epidemiologists can be found in reviews by Walter (1976), Whittemore (1983), Benichou (1991), and Coughlin et al. (1994).

# References


**Benichou, J.** (1991). "Methods of Adjustment for Estimating the Attributable Risk in Case-Control Studies: A Review", *Stat. Med.,* 10, 1753–1773.

**Benichou, J. and Gail, M. H.** (1990). "Variance Calculations and Confidence Intervals for Estimates of the Attributable Risk Based on Logistic Models", *Biometrics,* 46, 991–1003.

**Bruzzi, P., Green, S. B., Byar, D. P., Brinton, L. A., and Schairer, C.** (1985). Estimating the Population Attributable Risk for Multiple Risk Factors Using Case-Control Data", *Am. J. Epidemiol.,* 122, 904–914.

**Cole, P. and MacMahon, B.** (1971). "Attributable Risk Percent in Case-Control Studies", *Br. J. Prevent. Soc. Med.,* 25, 242–244.

**Cornfield, J.** (1962). "Joint Dependence of Risk of Coronary Heart Disease on Serum Cholesterol and Systolic Blood Pressure: A Discriminant Function Analysis", *Fed. Proc.,* 21, 58–61.

**Coughlin, S. S., Benichou, J., and Weed, D. L.** (1994). "Attributable Risk Estimation in Case-Control Studies", *Epidemiol. Rev.,* 16, 51–63.

**Denman, D. W. and Schlesselman, J. J.** (1983). "Interval Estimation of the Attributable Risk for Multiple Exposure Levels in Case-Control Studies", *Biometrics,* 39, 185–192.

**Deubner, D. C., Wilkinson, W. E., Helms, M. J., Tyroler, H. A., and Hames, C. G.** (1980). "Logistic Model Estimation of Death Attributable to Risk Factors for Cardiovascular Disease in Evans County, Georgia", *Am. J. Epidemiol.,* 112, 135–143.

**Drescher, K. and Schill, W.** (1991). "Attributable Risk Estimation from Case-Control Data Via Logistic Regression", *Biometrics,* 47, 1247–1256.

**Ejiguo, A.** (1979). "Estimation of the Attributable Risk in the Presence of Confounding", *Biometrical J.,* 21, 155–165.

**Gefeller, O.** (1992). "An Annotated Bibliography on the Attributable Risk", *Biometrical J.,* 34, 1007–1012.

**Greenland, S.** (1987). "Variance Estimators for Attributable Fraction Estimates, Consistent in Both Large Strata and Sparse Data", *Stat. Med.,* 6, 701–708.

**Greenland, S. and Drescher, K.** (1993). "Maximum Likelihood Estimation of the Attributable Fraction from Logistic Models", *Biometrics,* 49, 865–872.

**Kooperberg, C. and Petitti, D. B.** (1991). "Using Logistic Regression to Estimate the Adjusted Attributable Risk of Low Birthweight in an Unmatched Case-Control Study", *Epidemiology,* 2, 363–366.

**Kuritz, S. J. and Landis, J. R.** (1987). "Attributable Risk Ratio Estimation from Matched-Pairs Case-Control Data", *Am. J. Epidemiol.,* 125, 324–328.

**Kuritz, S. J. and Landis, J. R.** (1988). "Summary Attributable Risk Estimation from Matched-Pairs Case-Control Data", *Biometrics,* 44, 355–367.

**Leung, H. M. and Kupper, L. L.** (1981). "Comparisons of Confidence Intervals for Attributable Risk", *Biometrics,* 37, 293–302.

**Levin, M. L.** (1953). "The Occurrence of Lung Cancer in Man", *Acta U. Int. Contra Cancer,* 9, 531–541.

**Leviton, A.** (1973). "Definitions of Attributable Risk", *Am. J. Epidemiol.,* 98, 231.

**Lillienfeld, A. M. and Stolley, P. D.** (1994). *Foundations of Epidemiology,* 3rd ed. Oxford University Press, New York.

**Markush, R. E.** (1977). "Levin's Attributable Risk Statistic for Analytic Studies and Vital Statistics", *Am. J. Epidemiol.,* 105, 401–406.

**Miettinen, O. S.** (1974). "Proportion of Disease Caused or Prevented by a Given Exposure", *Am. J. Epidemiol.,* 96, 168–172.

**Rothman, K. J. and Keller, A.** (1972). "The Effect of Joint Exposure to Alcohol and Tobacco on Risk of Cancer of the Mouth and Pharynx", *J. Chronic Dis.,* 25, 711–716.

**Sturmans, F., Mulder, P. G. H., and Valkenburg, H. A.** (1977). "Estimation of the Possible Effect of Interventive Measures in the Area of Ischemic Heart Diseases by the Attributable Risk Percentage", *Am. J. Epidemiol.,* 105, 281–289.

**Walter, S. D.** (1975). "The Distribution of Levin's Measure of Attributable Risk", *Biometrika,* 62, 371–374.

**Walter, S. D.** (1976). "The Estimation and Interpretation of Attributable Risk in Health Research", *Biometrics,* 32, 830–849.

**Walter, S. D.** (1978). "Calculation of Attributable Risks from Epidemiologic Data", *Int. J. Epidemiol.,* 7, 175–182.

**Whittemore, A. S.** (1982). "Statistical Methods for Estimating Attributable Risk from Retrospective Data", *Stat. Med.,* 1, 229–243.

**Whittemore, A. S.** (1983). "Estimating Attributable Risk from Case-Control Studies", *Am. J. Epidemiol.,* 117, 76–85.

**Wynder, E. L., Bross, I. J., and Feldman, R. M.** (1957). "A Study of the Etiologic Factors in Cancer of the Mouth", *Cancer,* 10, 1300.

# A Pearson Chi-Square vs. Mantel-Haenszel Chi-Square

Consider the following 2 × 2 table:

| | Column | | |
|---|---|---|---|
| | $a$ | $b$ | $m_1$ |
| **Row** | $c$ | $d$ | $m_2$ |
| | $n_1$ | $n_2$ | $n$ |

The Pearson or ordinary chi-square statistic ($\chi_P^2$) is defined as

$$\chi_P^2 = \Sigma \frac{(\text{Obs - Exp})^2}{\text{Exp}}$$

$$= \frac{(a - m_1 n_1/n)^2}{m_1 n_1/n} + \frac{(b - m_1 n_2/n)^2}{m_1 n_2/n} + \frac{(c - m_2 n_1/n)^2}{m_2 n_1/n} + \frac{(d - m_2 n_2/n)^2}{m_2 n_2/n}$$

$$= \frac{n(ad - bc)^2}{n_1 n_2 m_1 m_2}.$$

The Mantel-Haenszel chi-square statistic ($\chi_{MH}^2$) is based on the large sample approximation of the hypergeometric distribution of $a$ by a normal distribution with mean and variance given by

$$E(a) = \frac{m_1 n_1}{n} \text{ and } \text{Var}(a) = \frac{m_1 m_2 n_1 n_2}{n^2(n-1)}.$$

That is,

$$\chi^2_{\mathrm{MH}} = \frac{\left(a - m_1 n_1/n\right)^2}{n_1 n_2 m_1 m_2 / n^2 (n-1)}$$

$$= \frac{(n-1)(ad - bc)^2}{n_1 n_2 m_1 m_2}.$$

Note that $\chi^2_{\mathrm{MH}}$ differs from $\chi^2_{\mathrm{P}}$ by the multiple of $(n - 1)/n$. The difference between the two statistics is negligible when $n$ is moderately large.

Both $\chi^2_{\mathrm{P}}$ and $\chi^2_{\mathrm{MH}}$ are approximate chi-square statistics and the approximation* is reasonably well behaved when all the cell frequencies exceed 5 (although less stringent criteria involving a minimum expected value of 3.5 and 1 also have been proposed). Cochran's commonly quoted guideline is that the expected value should exceed 1.00 in all cells and at least 80% of the cells should exceed 5.00. Larntz (1978) and Koehler and Larntz (1980) have shown that the chi-square approximation can be very good, even for smaller expected frequencies.

For the purpose of test-based confidence interval, the Mantel-Haenszel chi-square statistic is preferred over the Pearson chi-square statistic. The advantages of using the Mantel-Haenszel chi-square statistic are more apparent in a stratified analysis (Chapter 6) and in matching (Chapter 7) (see Appendix J). The principle advantage is the accuracy of the large sample chi-square approximation, which is determined by the amount of information accumulated over all strata rather than stratum-specific sample sizes. Thus, the large sample chi-square approximation is generally adequate as long as the total sample size is sufficiently large, even though individual strata may have very few cases.

The "corrected for continuity" versions of the two chi-square statistics are

$$\chi^2_{\mathrm{P}} = \frac{n\left[|ad - bc| - n/2\right]^2}{n_1 n_2 m_1 m_2}$$

and

$$\chi^2_{\mathrm{MH}} = \frac{(n-1)\left[|ad - bc| - n/2\right]^2}{n_1 n_2 m_1 m_2}.$$

* Under most conditions, the approximation used in the Mantel-Haenszel chi-square is a slightly better approximation.

The use of continuity correction for the Pearson chi-square statistic has been the subject of considerable debate in the statistical literature. The most recent consensus seems to be that its use results in the actual probability of type I errors to be substantially lower than the nominal alpha levels for the common chi-square tests of independence (both sets of marginals free to vary) and homogeneity (one set of marginal frequencies fixed and the other free to vary). (For a discussion of the pros and cons of the appropriateness of the Yates' correction, see Grizzle, 1967; Mantel and Greenhouse, 1968; Conover, 1974; Camilli and Hopkins, 1978, 1979; Upton, 1982, 1992; Yates, 1984; D'Agostino et al., 1988; Haviland, 1990; and Sahai and Khurshid, 1995, among others. For a discussion of the appropriateness of the continuity correction with respect to the Mantel-Haenszel chi-square, see Li et al., 1979.)

# References

**Camilli, G. and Hopkins, K. D.** (1978). "Applicability of Chi-Square to 2 × 2 Contingency Tables with Small Expected Cell Frequencies", *Psychol. Bull.,* 85, 163–167.

**Camilli, G. and Hopkins, K. D.** (1979). "Testing for Association in 2 × 2 Contingency Tables with Very Small Sample Sizes", *Psychol. Bull.,* 86, 1011–1014.

**Conover, W. J.** (1974). "Some Reasons for Not Using the Yates Continuity Correction on 2 × 2 Contingency Tables", *J. Am. Stat. Assoc.,* 69, 374–376.

**D'Agostino, R. B., Chase, W., and Belanger, A.** (1989). "The Appropriateness of Some Common Procedures for Testing the Equality of Two Independent Binomial Parameters", *Am. Stat.,* 42, 198–202.

**Grizzle, J. E.** (1967). "Continuity Correction in the $\chi^2$-test for 2 × 2 Tables", *Am. Stat.,* 21, 28–32.

**Haviland, M. G.** (1990). "Yates' Correction for Continuity and the Analysis of 2 × 2 Contingency Tables (with Comments and Rejoinder)", *Stat. Med.,* 9, 363–382 (see also *ibid.,* 1992, 11, 845–846).

**Koehler, K. J. and Larntz, K.** (1980). "An Empirical Investigation of Goodness-of-Fit Statistics for Sparse Multinomials", *J. Am. Stat. Assoc.,* 75, 336–344.

**Larntz, K.** (1978). "Small-Sample Comparison of Exact Levels of Chi-Square Goodness-of-Fit Statistics", *J. Am. Stat. Assoc.,* 73, 253–263.

**Li, S.-H., Simon, R. M., and Gart, J. J.** (1979). "Small Sample Properties of the Mantel-Haenszel Test", *Biometrika,* 66, 181–183.

**Mantel, N. and Greenhouse, S. W.** (1968). "What is the Continuity Correction?", *Am. Stat.,* 22, 27–30.

**Sahai, H. and Khurshid, A.** (1995). "On Analysis of Epidemiologic Data Involving a $2 \times 2$ Contingency Table: An Overview of Fisher's Exact Test and Yates' Correction for Continuity", *J. Biopharm. Stat.,* 5, 1, 43–70.

**Upton, G. J. G.** (1982). "A Comparison of Alternative Tests for the $2 \times 2$ Comparative Trial", *J. R. Stat. Soc.,* A, 145, 86–105.

**Upton, G. J. G.** (1992). "Fisher's Exact Test", *J. R. Stat. Soc.,* A, 155, 395–402.

**Yates, F.** (1984). "Tests of Significance for $2 \times 2$ Contingency Tables (with discussion)", *J. R. Stat. Soc.,* A, 147, 426–463.

# B Variance of a Function of a Random Variable

For any random variable *X*, the Taylor series approximation to the function *f(x)* can be written as

$$f(x) = f(\mu_x) + (x - \mu_x)\frac{d}{dx}f(\mu_x) + (x - \mu_x)^2 \frac{d^2}{dx^2}f(\mu_x) + \ldots .$$

Taking only the first order (or linear) Taylor series approximation, we have

$$f(x) = f(\mu_x) + (x - \mu_x)\frac{d}{dx}f(\mu_x).$$

Then

$$\begin{aligned}\text{Var}\{f(x)\} &= \text{E}\{f(x) - f(\mu_x)\}^2 \\ &= \left\{\frac{d}{dx}f(\mu_x)\right\}^2 \text{E}(x - \mu_x)^2 \\ &= \left\{\frac{d}{dx}f(\mu_x)\right\}^2 \text{Var}(x).\end{aligned}$$

For a logarithmic function, $f(x) = \log_e(x)$, we have

$$\text{Var}\{\log_e(x)\} = \left\{\frac{d}{dx}\log_e(\mu_x)\right\}^2 \text{Var}(x) = \frac{\text{Var}(x)}{\mu_x^2}.$$

We will illustrate the application of this result to obtain approximate expressions for the variance of the ratio of two binomial sample proportions and two Poisson sample means. Thus, let $\hat{p}_1$ and $\hat{p}_2$ be the estimates of $p_1$ and $p_2$ based on $n_1$ and $n_2$ trials. Then

$$\begin{aligned}\mathrm{Var}\{\log_e(\hat{p}_1/\hat{p}_2)\} &= \mathrm{Var}\{\log_e(\hat{p}_1) - \log_e(\hat{p}_2)\} \\ &= \mathrm{Var}\{\log_e(\hat{p}_1)\} + \mathrm{Var}\{\log_e(\hat{p}_2)\} \\ &= \frac{\mathrm{Var}(\hat{p}_1)}{\{\mu(\hat{p}_1)\}^2} + \frac{\mathrm{Var}(\hat{p}_2)}{\{\mu(\hat{p}_2)\}^2}.\end{aligned}$$

Because

$$\mu(\hat{p}_1) = \boldsymbol{E}(\hat{p}_1) = p_1, \ \mathrm{Var}(\hat{p}_1) = \frac{p_1(1-p_1)}{n_1},$$

$$\mu(\hat{p}_2) = \boldsymbol{E}(\hat{p}_2) = p_2, \text{ and } \mathrm{Var}(\hat{p}_2) = \frac{p_2(1-p_2)}{n_2},$$

it follows that

$$\mathrm{Var}\{\log_e(\hat{p}_1/\hat{p}_2)\} = \frac{(1-p_1)}{n_1 p_1} + \frac{(1-p_2)}{n_2 p_2}.$$

Similarly, let $\hat{\lambda}_1$ and $\hat{\lambda}_2$ be the estimates of the Poisson parameters $\lambda_1$ and $\lambda_2$ based on $n_1$ and $n_2$ trials. Then

$$\begin{aligned}\mathrm{Var}\{\log_e(\hat{\lambda}_1/\hat{\lambda}_2)\} &= \mathrm{Var}\{\log_e(\hat{\lambda}_1) - \log_e(\hat{\lambda}_2)\} \\ &= \mathrm{Var}\{\log_e(\hat{\lambda}_1)\} + \mathrm{Var}\{\log_e(\hat{\lambda}_2)\} \\ &= \frac{\mathrm{Var}(\hat{\lambda}_1)}{\{\mu(\hat{\lambda}_1)\}^2} + \frac{\mathrm{Var}(\hat{\lambda}_2)}{\{\mu(\hat{\lambda}_2)\}^2}.\end{aligned}$$

Because

$$\mu(\hat{\lambda}_1) = \boldsymbol{E}(\hat{\lambda}_1) = \lambda_1, \ \ \mathrm{Var}(\hat{\lambda}_1) = \frac{\lambda_1}{n_1},$$

$$\mu(\hat{\lambda}_2) = \boldsymbol{E}(\hat{\lambda}_2) = \lambda_2, \ \text{and} \ \ \mathrm{Var}(\hat{\lambda}_2) = \frac{\lambda_2}{n_2},$$

it follows that

$$\mathrm{Var}\left\{\log_e\left(\hat{\lambda}_1/\hat{\lambda}_2\right)\right\} = \frac{1}{n_1\lambda_1} + \frac{1}{n_2\lambda_2}.$$

# C The Odds Ratio*

The odds ratio (OR) plays a central role in many epidemiologic studies. However, it is not the simplest measure of association to understand and interpret. This appendix describes some additional details and properties of the OR not covered in the main text.

The OR is defined as the mathematical quotient of two sets of odds calculated under two different conditions.** For example, let $p_1$ be the probability that an event occurs under a set of conditions A and $p_2$ be the probability that the same event occurs under a set of conditions B. Then

$$\text{Odds (under set of conditions A)} = \frac{p_1}{1-p_1}$$

and

$$\text{Odds (under set of conditions B)} = \frac{p_2}{1-p_2}.$$

The OR is defined by

$$\text{OR} = \frac{p_1/(1-p_1)}{p_2/(1-p_2)}.$$

The range of all the possible values of an OR is from zero to infinity. The OR is symmetric about the value 1 in the sense that the OR represents the same degree of association as 1/OR.

* Appendix C of Selvin (1991) served as resource material for much of this appendix.

** Odds are a quotient of two probabilities: the probability that an event occurs divided by the probability that it does not occur. (The word *odds* denotes a single number, although the tradition and usage of formal English requires that it be considered a plural noun.) If an event has probability $p$, then the odds of the event are $p/(1-p)$. If a sequence of $n$ Bernoulli trials are performed in which an outcome of interest occurs $a$ times and it does not occur $b$ times ($n = a + b$), then the odds of the outcome of interest are defined by $a/b$. Figure C.1 depicts the mathematical relationship between odds and probability.

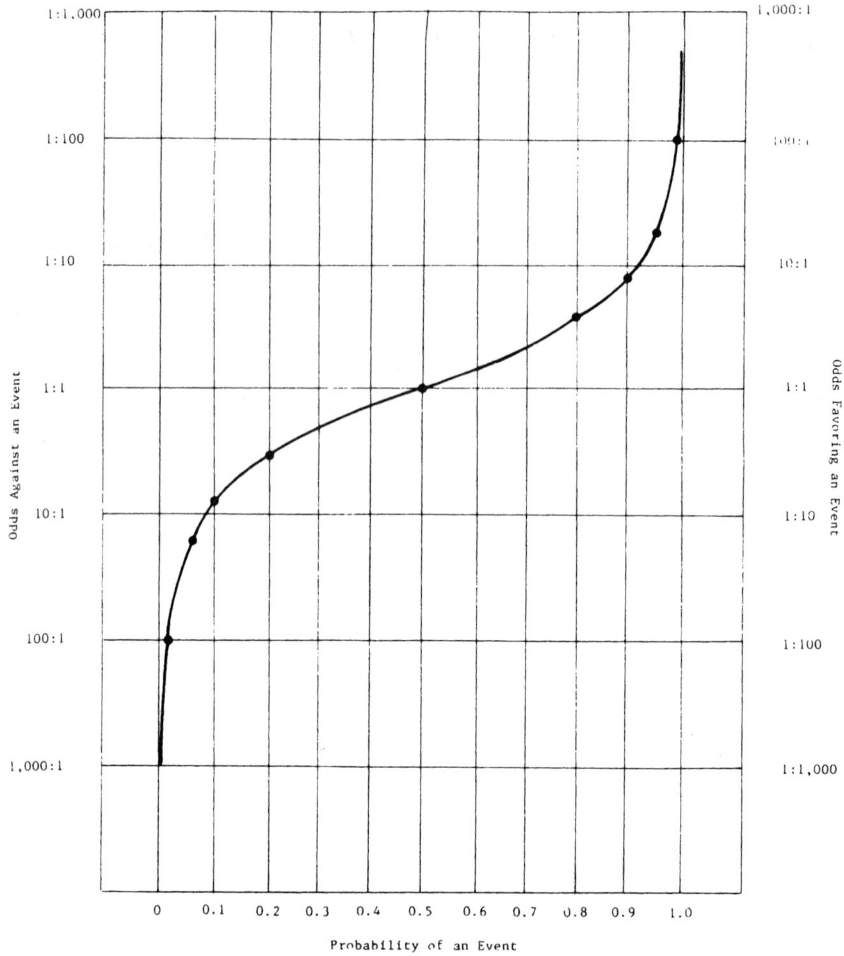


**FIGURE C.1** The relationship between odds and probability. (From Weinstein, M. C. and Fineberg, H. V. [1980]. *Clinical Decision Analysis,* W. B. Saunders, Philadelphia, p. 106. With permission.)

The concept of OR as a measure of association in a contingency table was first introduced by Cornfield (1951) as measure of relative risk for a retrospective study. Because of the nature of its definition involving quotient of diagonal products of cell entries in a $2 \times 2$ table, Fisher (1962) and Mosteller (1968) referred to it as the cross-product ratio. Numerous other measures of association for contingency tables are available, some of which may be found in papers by Goodman and Kruskal (1954, 1959) and Mosteller (1968).

The sample data for the calculation of an OR are usually arranged in the form of a $2 \times 2$ table (see Table C.1). From Table C.1, an estimate of the OR is

**TABLE C.1**
**A 2 × 2 Table Relating Outcome and Conditions**

| | Occurrence | Nonoccurrence | Total |
|---|---|---|---|
| Conditions A | $a$ | $b$ | $a + b$ |
| *Conditions B* | $c$ | $d$ | $c + d$ |
| *Total* | $a + c$ | $b + d$ | $n$ |

$$\hat{OR} = \frac{a/b}{c/d} = \frac{ad}{bc}.$$

Because the OR is generally calculated from a set of sample values, it will assume different values from different samples. An approximate estimate of the sampling variance of the sample OR ( $\hat{OR}$ ) is given by

$$\hat{Var}(\hat{OR}) \simeq (\hat{OR})^2 \left(\frac{1}{a} + \frac{1}{b} + \frac{1}{c} + \frac{1}{d}\right).$$

Figure C.2a shows a sampling distribution of 500 values of the OR calculated from samples of size $n = 50$, generated under two sets of conditions ($p_1 = 0.8$ and $p_2 = 0.6$) using Monte Carlo simulation. The sampling distribution of these estimated ORs is skewed to the right. The mean of the distribution is 3.170, indicating that the estimated OR is biased [the expected OR is (0.8)(0.4)/ (0.2)(0.6) = 2.667].

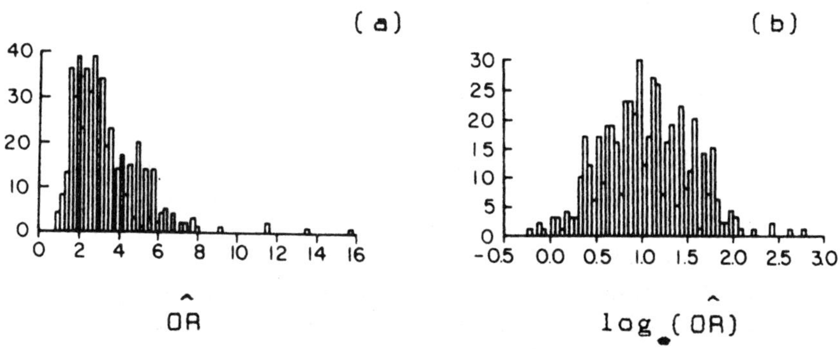


**FIGURE C.2** Histograms of $\hat{OR}$ (a) and $\log_e(\hat{OR})$ (b) for two sets of conditions ($p_1 = 0.8$, $p_2 = 0.6$). (From Selvin, S. [1991]. *Statistical Analysis of Epidemiologic Data,* Oxford University Press, New York, p. 345. With permission.)

To reduce the bias by making the distribution more symmetric, the logarithmic transformation of the OR is generally employed. The values of $\log_e(\text{OR})$ range from $-\infty$ to $\infty$. An approximate estimate of the sample variance of $\log_e(\hat{\text{OR}})$ is given by

$$\hat{\text{Var}}\left\{\log_e\left(\hat{\text{OR}}\right)\right\} \simeq \left(\frac{1}{a}+\frac{1}{b}+\frac{1}{c}+\frac{1}{d}\right).$$

A simulated distribution of $\log_e(\hat{\text{OR}})$ (also for $p_1 = 0.8$ and $p_2 = 0.6$) is shown in Figure C.2b. In addition, Figure C.3 shows the simulated distributions of $\hat{\text{OR}}$ and $\log_e(\hat{\text{OR}})$ for the case when the two odds are same with $p_1 = p_2 = 0.4$.

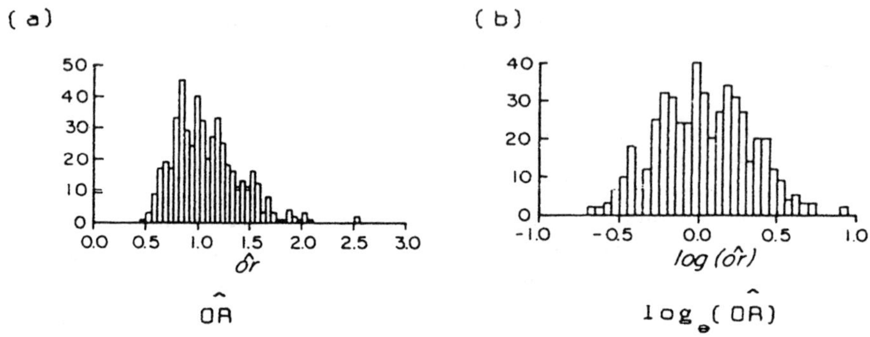


**FIGURE C.3** Histograms of $\hat{\text{OR}}$ (a) and $\log_e(\hat{\text{OR}})$ (b) for two sets of conditions ($p_1 = 0.4$, $p_2 = 0.4$). (From Selvin, S. [1991]. *Statistical Analysis of Epidemiologic Data,* Oxford University Press, New York, p. 345. With permission.)

Some of the properties of the OR obtained from a 2 × 2 table are

1. The OR is invariant to the interchange of rows and columns (interchanging a row only or a column only changes OR to 1/OR).
2. The value of the OR is not changed by multiplying the rows and/or the columns by a positive constant.
3. The OR yields a probabilistic interpretation in terms of odds.
4. The OR is approximated by the risk ratio when the probability of the outcome is very low among those with and without the risk factor.
5. The logarithm of the OR follows approximately a symmetric distribution that can be approximated generally by a normal distribution.

For a discussion of some other properties of the OR, see Mosteller (1968).

The estimator $\hat{\text{OR}} = ad/bc$ is also the maximum likelihood estimate (MLE) of the OR. This follows from the fact that the MLE of $p_1$ is $a/(a + b)$, so by the invariance the MLE of $p_1/(1 - p_1)$ is $a/b$. Similarly, the MLE of $p_2/(1 - p_2)$ is $c/d$. Hence, the MLE of the OR is $ad/bc$. This MLE of the OR is commonly known as the unconditional MLE (UMLE).

In the derivation of the UMLE, only the row marginals $(a + b)$ and $(c + d)$ were assumed to be fixed by virtue of the binomial sampling design. In contrast, the conditional maximum likelihood estimate (CMLE) also fixes the other marginal totals $(a + c)$ and $(b + d)$. The reason usually put forth for also conditioning the column marginals is that the marginals do not contain information relevant to statistical inference, for example, on the difference between two outcome proportions, $p_1$ and $p_2$. Hence, the conditioning is a useful device for eliminating the nuisance parameter, which in this case is the common probability of success in the combined sample. In fact, the margins contain information on the association between the row and column factors of the table (Berkson, 1978). However, the amount of information thus conveyed is sufficiently small and thus the conditioning on the second margins is still considered to be appropriate. This issue has been considered at great length by Yates (1984) and by discussants of his paper.

The CMLE of the OR, which conditions on the second margin of the table, is obtained by solving the following likelihood equation:

$$a - E\left(a \mid \text{OR}\right) = 0,$$

where $a$ is the observed value of one of the cell frequencies and $E(a|\text{OR})$ is the expected value of the noncentral hypergeometric distribution with the noncentrality parameter OR (see Birch, 1964; Breslow and Day, 1980). The determination of the CMLE in general involves a polynomial of high order in the OR which requires an iterative approach for its solution.

Note that if $b$ and $c$ are zero in any particular sample, the UMLE of the OR is undefined. Similarly, if any of the cell frequency is zero, then $\log_e(\hat{\text{OR}})$ and the CMLE are undefined. To circumvent this problem, a positive constant $\varepsilon$ is usually added to each cell, leading to the estimator

$$\hat{\text{OR}} = \frac{(a+\varepsilon)(d+\varepsilon)}{(b+\varepsilon)(c+\varepsilon)}.$$

Haldane (1955), commenting on a paper by Woolf (1955), proposed using $\varepsilon = 1/2$, basing his argument on a Taylor series expansion of $\log_e(\hat{\text{OR}})$, which shows that the first-order bias term (in the statistical sense of expectation) can be eliminated with this choice of $\varepsilon$. It was also suggested that a similar modification should be made to the expression of the estimated standard error of $\hat{\text{OR}}$ and $\log_e(\hat{\text{OR}})$ (Gart and Zweifel, 1967). Thus, a commonly employed bias reducing estimator of the OR is $\hat{\text{OR}}_{\text{H}}$(H stands for Haldane) given by

$$\hat{\text{OR}}_{\text{H}} = \frac{(a+1/2)(d+1/2)}{(b+1/2)(c+1/2)},$$

with estimated variance

$$\hat{\text{Var}}\left(\hat{\text{OR}}_{\text{H}}\right) \simeq \left(\hat{\text{OR}}_{\text{H}}\right)^2 \left(\frac{1}{(a+1/2)} + \frac{1}{(b+1/2)} + \frac{1}{(c+1/2)} + \frac{1}{(d+1/2)}\right)$$

and

$$\hat{\text{Var}}\left\{\log_e\left(\hat{\text{OR}}_{\text{H}}\right)\right\} \simeq \left(\frac{1}{(a+1/2)} + \frac{1}{(b+1/2)} + \frac{1}{(c+1/2)} + \frac{1}{(d+1/2)}\right).$$

Other values of $\varepsilon$ have been considered in the context of logistic regression and for the combination of sets of $2 \times 2$ tables. Hitchcock (1962) suggested the use of $\varepsilon = 1/4$ for a bioassay logistic model at three dose levels. Gart et al. (1985) and Davis (1985) showed that the optimal value of $\varepsilon$ for the $2 \times k$ table depends on $k$. Hauck et al. (1982) suggested the use of $\varepsilon = 1/4$ in a $k$ set of $2 \times 2$ tables. (The interested reader is referred to Walter (1987) for a discussion of such estimators and their properties.)

Jewell (1986) proposed an estimator $\hat{\text{OR}}_{\text{J}}$(J stands for Jewell) given by

$$\hat{\text{OR}}_{\text{J}} = \frac{ad}{(b+1)(c+1)}.$$

The addition of $\varepsilon = 1$ to the $b$ and $c$ cells in $\hat{\text{OR}}_{\text{J}}$ is intended to reduce the positive bias of the UMLE and to define it for all possible tables. It has been shown that $\hat{\text{OR}}_{\text{J}}$ has better bias and mean square error properties. For a further discussion of the properties of this estimator vis-á-vis the maximum likelihood estimator, see Becker (1989), Jewell (1991), Walter and Cook (1991), and Mantel (1992).

# References

**Becker, S.** (1989). "A Comparison of Maximum Likelihood and Jewell's Estimator of the Odds Ratio and Relative Risk in Single 2 × 2 Tables", *Stat. Med.,* 8, 987–996.

**Berkson, J.** (1978). "In Dispraise of the Exact Test: Do the Marginal Totals of the 2 × 2 Table Contain Relevant Information Respecting the Total Proportions", *J. Stat. Planning Inference,* 2, 27–42.

**Birch, M. W.** (1964). "The Detection of Partial Association, I: The 2 × 2 Case", *J. R. Stat. Soc.,* B, 26, 313–324.

**Breslow, N. E. and Day, N. E.** (1980). *Statistical Methods in Cancer Research, Vol. 1: The Analysis of Case-Control Studies.* International Agency for Research on Cancer, Lyons, France.

**Cornfield, J.** (1951). "A Method of Estimating Comparative Rates from Clinical Data: Application to Cancer of the Lung, Breast and Cervix", *J. Nat. Cancer Inst.,* 11, 1269–1275.

**Davis, L. J.** (1985). "Modification of the Empirical Logit to Reduce Bias in Simple Linear Logistic Regression", *Biometrika,* 72, 199–202.

**Fisher, R. A.** (1962). "Confidence Limits for a Cross-Product Ratio", *Aust. J. Stat.,* 4, 41–45.

**Gart, J. J. and Zwiefel, J. R.** (1967). "On the Bias of Various Estimators of the Logit and Its Variance, with Application to Quantal Bioassay", *Biometrika,* 54, 181–187.

**Gart, J. J., Pettigrew, H. M., and Thomas, D. G.** (1985). "The Effect of Bias, Variance Estimation, Skewness and Kurtosis of the Empirical Logit on Weighted Least Squares Analysis", *Biometrika,* 72, 179–190.

**Goodman, L. A. and Kruskal, W. H.** (1954). "Measures of Association for Cross Classification", *J. Am. Stat. Assoc.,* 49, 732–764.

**Goodman, L. A. and Kruskal, W. H.** (1959). "Measures of Association for Cross Classification, II: Further Discussion and References", *J. Am. Stat. Assoc.,* 54, 123–163.

**Haldane, J. B. S.** (1955). "The Estimation and Significance of the Logarithm of a Ratio of Frequencies", *Ann. Human Gen.,* 20, 309–311.

**Hauck, W. W., Anderson, S., and Leahy, F. J., III** (1982). "Finite-Sample Properties of Some Old and Some New Estimators of a Common Odds Ratio from Multiple 2 × 2 Tables", *J. Am. Stat. Assoc.,* 77, 145–152.

**Hitchcock, S. E.** (1962). "A Note on the Estimation of Parameters of the Logistic Function, Using the Minimum Logit $\chi^2$ Method", *Biometrika,* 49, 250–252.

**Jewell, N. P.** (1986). "Small-Sample Bias of Point Estimators of the Odds Ratio from Matched Sets", *Biometrics,* 40, 421–435.

**Jewel, N. P.** (1991). "Letter to the Editor", *Stat. Med.,* 10, 151–153.

**Mantel, N.** (1992). "An Invalid Comparison of Several Point Estimators of the Odds Ratio in a Single 2 × 2 Contingency Table", *Biometrics,* 48, 1289–1295.

**Mosteller, F.** (1968). "Association and Estimation in Contingency Tables", *J. Am. Stat. Assoc.,* 63, 1–28.

**Selvin, S.** (1991). *Statistical Analysis of Epidemiologic Data.* Oxford University Press, New York.

**Walter, S. D.** (1987). "Point Estimator of the Odds Ratio in Sparse 2 × 2 Contingency Tables", In: *Biostatistics: Advances in the Statistical Sciences,* Vol. 5. pp. 71–102 (Eds. I. B. MacNeill and G. J. Umphrey). D. Reidel Publishing, Dordrecht.

**Walter, S. D. and Cook, R. J.** (1991). "A Comparison of Several Point Estimators of the Odds Ratio in a Single 2 × 2 Contingency Table", *Biometrics,* 47, 795–811.

**Weinstein, M. C. and Fineberg, H. V.** (1980). *Clinical Decision Analysis.* W. B. Saunders, Philadelphia.

**Woolf, B.** (1955). "On Estimating the Relation between Blood Group and Disease", *Ann. Human Gen.,* 19, 251–253.

**Yates, F.** (1984). "Tests of Significance for 2 × 2 Contingency Tables (with Discussion)", *J. R. Stat. Soc.,* A, 147, 426–463.

# D More Confidence Intervals for the Risk Ratio

This appendix constitutes a brief summary of some additional methods of determining confidence intervals (CIs) for the risk ratio (RR) proposed in the literature.

For the first method, consider a $2 \times 2$ table with fixed marginals, as shown in Table D.1. Note that the specification of a single cell frequency automatically determines the value in other cells. In the notation of Table D.1 the sample estimates of the odds ratio (OR) and the RR are given by

$$\hat{\text{OR}} = \frac{x(n_2 - m_1 + x)}{(m_1 - x)(n_1 - x)} \tag{D.1}$$

and

$$\hat{\text{RR}} = \frac{x/n_1}{(m_1 - x)/n_2}. \tag{D.2}$$

Let $\text{OR}_\text{L}$ and $\text{OR}_\text{U}$ be the lower and upper $100(1 - \alpha)\%$ confidence limits for the OR, defined by Equations 4.14 and 4.15. Let $\text{RR}_\text{L}$ and $\text{RR}_\text{U}$ be the corresponding $100(1 - \alpha)\%$ confidence limits for the RR. Thomas and Gart (1977) suggested that on substituting $\text{OR}_\text{L}$ and $\text{OR}_\text{U}$ in Equation D.1, one can solve the equation for $x_\text{L}$ and $x_\text{U}$, respectively. The substitution of the respective values of $x_\text{L}$ and $x_\text{U}$ in Equation D.2 yields the corresponding limits for the RR:

$$\text{RR}_\text{L} = \frac{x_\text{L}/n_1}{(m_1 - x_\text{L})/n_2}$$

and

$$\text{RR}_\text{U} = \frac{x_\text{U}/n_1}{(m_1 - x_\text{U})/n_2}.$$

**TABLE D.1**
**A 2 × 2 Table for Count Data in an Epidemiologic Study**

| | **Exposed** | **Unexposed** | **Total** |
|---|---|---|---|
| Cases | $x$ | $m_1 - x$ | $m_1$ |
| Controls | $n_1 - x$ | $n_2 - m_1 + x$ | $m_2$ |
| Total | $n_1$ | $n_2$ | $n$ |

Thomas and Gart claimed that the procedure is "exact" in the sense that it produces a confidence coefficient of at least $1 - \alpha$. A simulation study of Katz et al. (1978) showed, however, that this method only produces approximate confidence intervals.

In the first method the determination of the limits $OR_L$ and $OR_U$, by Equations 4.14 and 4.15, is computationally complex and generally requires the use of a computer program. However, the approximate values of $x_L$ and $x_U$ may be determined by Cornfield's method, with the help of Equations 4.22 and 4.23. The simulation study of Katz et al. (1978) showed that this method yields results similar to those of the first method.

In the third method let $\hat{p}_1$ and $\hat{p}_2$ be the sample probabilities denoting risks for developing cases in the population of exposed and unexposed groups, respectively. A sample estimate of the RR is $\widehat{RR} = \hat{p}_1/\hat{p}_2$. Because $\widehat{RR}$ can be considered approximately normally distributed with mean RR, the variate $\hat{p}_1 - RR\,\hat{p}_2$ is approximately normally distributed with zero mean and the approximate variance estimator

$$\frac{\hat{p}_1(1-\hat{p}_1)}{n_1} + (RR)^2\frac{\hat{p}_2(1-\hat{p}_2)}{n_2}.$$

Thus, a pair of approximate $100(1 - \alpha)\%$ confidence limits for the RR, $RR_L$ and $RR_U$, are determined by solving the equations

$$\frac{\hat{p}_1 - RR_L\hat{p}_2}{\sqrt{\dfrac{\hat{p}_1(1-\hat{p}_1)}{n_1} + \dfrac{RR_L^2\hat{p}_2(1-\hat{p}_2)}{n_2}}} = Z_{\alpha\,2}$$

and

$$\frac{\hat{p}_1 - \text{RR}_\text{U}\hat{p}_2}{\sqrt{\frac{\hat{p}_1(1-\hat{p}_1)}{n_1} + \frac{\text{RR}_\text{U}^2\hat{p}_2(1-\hat{p}_2)}{n_2}}} = -Z_{\alpha\ 2},$$

where $Z_{\alpha/2}$ is the upper $100(\alpha/2)$th percentile of the standard normal distribution. This method may, however, lead to negative or complex values for the confidence limits. The simulation study of Katz et al. (1978) showed that the method is "erratic" and should not be used.

Noether (1957) proposed another method based on the variate $\hat{p}_1 - \text{RR}\,\hat{p}_2$. However, the method is asymmetric with respect to which sample proportion appears in the numerator of $\hat{\text{RR}}$, and therefore is not recommended.

# References

**Katz, D., Baptista, J., Azen, S. P., and Pike, M. C.** (1978). "Obtaining Confidence Intervals for the Risk Ratios in Cohort Studies", *Biometrics,* 34, 469–474.

**Noether, G. E.** (1957). "Two Confidence Intervals for the Ratio of Two Probabilities and Some Measures of Effectiveness", *J. Am. Stat. Assoc.,* 52, 36–45.

**Thomas, D. G. and Gart, J. J.** (1977). "A Table of Exact Confidence Limits for Differences and Ratios of Two Proportions and Their Odds Ratio", *J. Am. Stat. Assoc.,* 72, 73–76.

# E Maximum Likelihood Estimation

Maximum likelihood estimation is a general method of estimation developed by Sir Ronald A. Fisher, who ranks among the great scientists of the 20th century. The method is based on the concept of likelihood function, which represents the probability of obtaining the data as a function of the unknown parameter(s). The maximum likelihood estimate of a parameter is that value that maximizes the likelihood function. In other words, it is the value of the parameter that is most likely to occur for the observed data.

The usual method of maximizing a likelihood function, with respect to a parameter, is to differentiate the function with respect to that parameter and equate the derivative to zero. In maximizing the likelihood function, however, it is generally more convenient to maximize its logarithm for ease of algebraic manipulation. The value of the parameter that maximizes the logarithm of the likelihood also maximizes the likelihood function.

The mathematical task of finding maximum likelihood estimates becomes more tedious as the number of parameters in the model increases, but the principle remains the same. Thus, in estimating the $k$ parameters of a model, for example, $\theta_1,\theta_2,...,\theta_k$, the maximum likelihood estimates of the parameters are values, for example, $\hat{\theta}_1, \hat{\theta}_2,..., \hat{\theta}_k$, such that the likelihood function is maximum.

In most situations involving several parameters the maximum likelihood estimates can be obtained only when using computer algorithms. Initial estimates of the unknown parameters, for example, $\hat{\theta}_1^0, \hat{\theta}_2^0,..., \hat{\theta}_k^0$, are obtained and these are substituted into the likelihood function to derive new estimates that increase the value of the likelihood function. The process is repeated iteratively until estimates are found that maximize the likelihood function. These are the maximum likelihood estimates of the unknown parameters.

Maximum likelihood estimators have several desirable properties such as being consistent, asymptotically normal, and asymptotically efficient, for large samples, under fairly general conditions. Maximum likelihood estimators are often biased, but the bias can be corrected frequently by a simple adjustment. Another attractive property of maximum likelihood estimators is that a function of a maximum likelihood estimate is a maximum likelihood estimate of the function itself. Maximum likelihood estimates of parameters in many statistical models can frequently be obtained using standard statistical packages.

In stratified analysis, unlike the logit and Mantel-Haenszel estimators, the maximum likelihood estimators do not involve any directly weighted average of the stratum-specific estimates, although they are similar to the weighted averages in the sense that the larger strata effectively exercise more weight. The maximum likelihood estimation usually yields standard errors associated with estimated parameters that can be used to calculate confidence intervals.

# F Variance of the Conditional Maximum Likelihood Estimator of the Odds Ratio and the Log Odds Ratio

Consider the conditional likelihood function (Equation 4.11) given by

$$L\left(x \mid n_1, n_2, m_1, m_2, \text{OR}\right) = \frac{\binom{n_1}{x}\binom{n_2}{m_1 - x}(\text{OR})^x}{\sum_{\delta_1 \le k \le \delta_2} \binom{n_1}{k}\binom{n_2}{m_1 - k}(\text{OR})^k},$$

for $\delta_1 = \max(0, m_1 - n_2) \le x \le \min(n_1, m_1) = \delta_2$.

The derivative of the log likelihood with respect to $\log_e(\text{OR})$ is

$$\frac{\delta\{\log_e(\text{L})\}}{\delta\{\log_e(\text{OR})\}} = x - \frac{\sum_{\delta_1 \le x \le \delta_2} x\binom{n_1}{x}\binom{n_2}{m_1 - x}(\text{OR})^x}{\sum_{\delta_1 \le k \le \delta_2} \binom{n_1}{k}\binom{n_2}{m_1 - k}(\text{OR})^k}.$$

Note that the second term in the above expression represents the expected value of the noncentral hypergeometric distribution. If we take the second derivative of the log likelihood with respect to $\log_e(\text{OR})$, we obtain

$$\frac{\delta^2\{\log_e(\text{L})\}}{\delta\{\log_e(\text{OR})\}^2} = E^2(x) - E\left(x^2\right) = -\text{Var}(x).$$

Thus, the asymptotic variance of $\log_e(\hat{\text{OR}})$ is given by

$$\text{Var}\left\{\log_e\left(\hat{\text{OR}}\right)\right\} = -\frac{1}{E\left[\dfrac{\delta^2\{\log_e(\text{L})\}}{\delta\{\log_e(\text{OR})\}^2}\right]}$$

$$= \frac{1}{\text{Var(x)}}.$$

Similarly,

$$\frac{\delta^2\{\log_e(\text{L})\}}{\delta\{(\text{OR})^2\}} = \frac{1}{(\text{OR})^2}\left[E^2(x) - E\left(x^2\right) + E(x) - x\right],$$

so that the asymptotic variance of $\hat{\text{OR}}$ is given by

$$\text{Var}\left(\hat{\text{OR}}\right) = -\frac{1}{E\left[\dfrac{\delta^2\{\log_e(\text{L})\}}{\delta\{(\text{OR})^2\}}\right]}$$

$$= \frac{(\text{OR})^2}{\text{Var(x)}}.$$

Although the exact expression of Var*(x)* is not readily obtainable, under large sample conditions, an estimate of the asymptotic variance is

$$\hat{\text{Var}}(\text{x}) \simeq \left[\frac{1}{x} + \frac{1}{m_1 - x} + \frac{1}{m_2 - x} + \frac{1}{n_2 - m_1 + x}\right]^{-1}.$$

Thus, the sample estimates of Var( $\hat{\text{OR}}$ ) and Var{log$_e$( $\hat{\text{OR}}$ )} are

$$\hat{\text{Var}}\left(\hat{\text{OR}}\right) \approx \left(\hat{\text{OR}}\right)^2\left[\frac{1}{x} + \frac{1}{m_1 - x} + \frac{1}{m_2 - x} + \frac{1}{n_2 - m_1 + x}\right]$$

and

$$\hat{\text{Var}}\left\{\log_e\left(\hat{\text{OR}}\right)\right\} \approx \left[\frac{1}{x} + \frac{1}{m_1 - x} + \frac{1}{m_2 - x} + \frac{1}{n_2 - m_1 + x}\right].$$

# G Variance of the Unconditional Maximum Likelihood Estimator of the Common Odds Ratio in a Stratified Analysis

Consider the unconditional likelihood function given by

$$\mathrm{L} = \prod_{i=1}^{k} (p_{1i})^{a_i} (1 - p_{1i})^{b_i} (p_{2i})^{c_i} (1 - p_{2i})^{d_i}.$$

In order to find the asymptotic variance of the unconditional maximum likelihood estimator of the odds ratio ($\widehat{\mathrm{OR}}_{\mathrm{UML}}$), we reparametrize the likelihood function, eliminating the $k$ parameters, which are made redundant due to the restriction of the common OR, $\widehat{\mathrm{OR}}_i = \widehat{\mathrm{OR}}_j = \mathrm{OR}$ ($i, j = 1,\ldots,k,\ i \neq j$). Letting

$$p_{2i} = \frac{p_{1i}}{p_{1i} + \mathrm{OR}(1 - p_{1i})},$$

we have $k + 1$ parameters, $p_{11}, p_{12},\ldots,p_{1k}$, and OR, to be estimated.

The likelihood function can now be written as

$$\mathrm{L} = \prod_{i=1}^{k} (p_{1i})^{a_i} (1 - p_{1i})^{b_i} \frac{(p_{1i})^{c_i} (\mathrm{OR})^{d_i} (1 - p_{1i})^{d_i}}{\{p_{1i} + \mathrm{OR}(1 - p_{1i})\}^{c_i} \{p_{1i} + \mathrm{OR}(1 - p_{1i})\}^{d_i}}.$$

The elements of the information matrix are

$$E\left\{-\frac{\partial^2(\log_e \mathrm{L})}{\partial(\mathrm{OR})^2}\right\} = (\mathrm{OR})^{-2}\sum_{i=1}^{k} n_{2i}\, p_{2i}\left(1 - p_{2i}\right),$$

$$E\left\{-\frac{\partial^2(\log_e \mathrm{L})}{\partial(\mathrm{OR})\,\partial\left(p_{1i}\right)}\right\} = -(\mathrm{OR})^{-1}\,\frac{n_{2i}\, p_{2i}\left(1 - p_{2i}\right)}{p_{1i}\left(1 - p_{1i}\right)}, \quad i = 1,\ldots,k$$

$$E\left\{-\frac{\partial^2(\log_e \mathrm{L})}{\partial\left(p_{1i}^2\right)}\right\} = \frac{n_{1i}\, p_{1i}\left(1 - p_{1i}\right) + n_{2i}\, p_{2i}\left(1 - p_{2i}\right)}{p_{1i}^2\left(1 - p_{1i}\right)^2}, \quad i = 1,\ldots,k$$

$$E\left\{-\frac{\partial^2(\log_e \mathrm{L})}{\partial\left(p_{1i}\right)\partial\left(p_{1j}\right)}\right\} = 0, \quad i = 1,\ldots,k; \; j = 1,\ldots,k; \; i \neq j.$$

On inverting the information matrix, the asymptotic variance of $\hat{\mathrm{OR}}_{\mathrm{ML}}$ is determined:

$$\mathrm{Var}\left(\hat{\mathrm{OR}}_{\mathrm{ML}}\right) = \frac{(\mathrm{OR})^2}{\sum_{i=1}^{k}\left\{\frac{1}{n_{1i}\, p_{1i}\left(1 - p_{1i}\right)} + \frac{1}{n_{2i}\, p_{2i}\left(1 - p_{2i}\right)}\right\}^{-1}}.$$

# H Some Important Probability Distributions

The binomial, Poisson, hypergeometric, noncentral hypergeometric, and multinomial distributions are basic to many aspects of epidemiologic data analysis. This appendix provides a brief review of these distributions and some of their properties. Further details on these distributions can be found in many introductory statistics texts or specialized publications such as Haight (1967), Johnson et al. (1992), and Takeuchi and Fujino (1981).

The *binomial distribution* arises in many different contexts whenever a random variable can be hypothesized to have arisen as the number of occurrences of a certain characteristic or property in a series of independent trials of the random phenomenon. It has been utilized for statistical inferences about dichotomous data for more than 250 years. In the early 18th century, British physician Arbuthnott used binomial probability calculations as an argument for the sexual balance maintained by Divine Providence and against the practice of polygamy. In modern biomedical and epidemiologic applications binomial distribution is the source of many statistical properties calculated from mortality or disease data. The binomial distribution is also used to derive expressions for the variance of more complicated measures of mortality such as the standardized mortality ratio and the directly adjusted standardized mortality rate. Undoubtedly, the statistical procedures based on binomial distribution remain one of the easiest and most useful kinds of procedures in the statistical repertoire of the epidemiologic researcher.

In general, the binomial distribution arises under the following conditions:

1. There is a sequence of $n$-independent trials.
2. Each trial may result in one of the two mutually exclusive outcomes, which are denoted as "success" and "failure" (e.g., head or tail, diseased or nondiseased, exposed or unexposed, etc.).
3. The probability of success is constant from trial to trial and is denoted by the letter $p$.

The probability distribution of the number of successes in $n$-independent trials, in which the probability of success for each trial is $p$, is known as the binomial distribution. Let $X$ denote the number of successes in $n$ trials. Then the probability distribution of $X$ is given by the formula:

$$P(X = x) = \binom{n}{x} p^x (1-p)^{n-x}, \quad x = 0, 1, \ldots, n$$

The binomial distribution depends on two parameters, $n$ and $p$. Note that $\binom{n}{x} = n!/x!\,(n-x)!$, where $\binom{n}{x}$ is the number of combinations of $n$ things taken $x$ at a time. The mean and variance of the binomial distribution are given by $\mu = np$ and $\sigma^2 = np(1-p)$ respectively. The binomial distribution can be approximated by a normal distribution if $np \geq 5$ and $n(1-p) \geq 5$.

The *Poisson distribution* is the second most frequently used discrete distribution after the binomial distribution. In many epidemiologic studies the distribution is usually associated with rare diseases and plays an important role in analyzing discrete data. The Poisson distribution has found an extensive and varied application in formulating probability models for a wide variety of phenomena dealing with counts of rare events. In biomedical and epidemiologic applications the Poisson probability model is often used to describe successfully such diverse phenomena as radioactive counts per unit time; the number of plankton per aliquot of seawater; the number of bacterial colonies per petri plate; the number of photons reaching the retina; the number of birth defects; or the number of victims with various specific diseases. In epidemiology the inferences on the standard mortality ratio (SMR) are based on the Poisson probability model. The probability distribution of a Poisson random variable $X$ is given by the formula

$$P(X = x) = \frac{e^{-\lambda} \lambda^x}{x!}, \quad x = 0, 1, \ldots, \infty$$

The mean and variance of the Poisson distribution are $\mu = \lambda$ and $\sigma^2 = \lambda$, respectively. It is assumed that $\lambda > 0$. If in the binomial distribution $n$ is very large and $p$ is very small, the distribution of the number of successes is approximated by a Poisson distribution with mean $\lambda = np$. That the Poisson distribution is useful for modeling certain types of health count data is usually justified on the basis of the Poisson approximation to the binomial distribution. For many health outcomes (e.g., the development of rare diseases) the length $T_i$ of follow-up time (analogous to $n$) is large and the probability of occurrence of the health outcome in question (analogous to $p$) is small, thus suggesting the application of the Poisson model. For example, the probability of the number of cases of leukemia occurring in a specific geographic area has been modeled by a Poisson distribution. Here, $n$ is all possible persons at risk for leukemia (which is very large) and $p$ is the probability that any one person is diagnosed with leukemia (which is very small).

For the application of Poisson distribution, the knowledge of $n$ and $p$ is not necessary; only the value of the parameter $\lambda$ is required to evaluate the probabilities of interest. That the Poisson distribution may be derived as an approximation to the binomial distribution can be shown as follows. We have

$$P(X=k)=\binom{n}{k}p^k(1-p)^{n-k}=\frac{n(n-1)(n-2)\ldots(n-k+1)}{k!}p^k\left(1-\frac{np}{n}\right)^{n-k}.$$

Dividing the numerator and denominator by $n^k$, we obtain

$$P(X=k)=\frac{1\left(1-\frac{1}{n}\right)\left(1-\frac{2}{n}\right)\cdots\left(1-\frac{k-1}{n}\right)}{k!}(np)^k\left(1-\frac{np}{n}\right)^{n-k}.$$

If $n$ is large and $p$ is small, then $(1-np/n)^{n-k}\approx e^{-np}$, yielding

$$P(X=k)=\frac{(np)^k e^{-np}}{k!}=\frac{\lambda^k e^{-\lambda}}{k!}.$$

Although the Poisson distribution may be considered as an approximation to the binomial distribution, as described above, it also arises more directly as follows. Suppose that a time period or interval of space exists which can be thought of as divisible into small intervals of time (minutes or seconds) or space (centimeters or millimeters), and during this interval the number of occurrences of a certain event is to be observed. Suppose also that the following assumptions are satisfied:

1. The probability of occurrence of any one event in a very small interval is proportional to the size of the interval (i.e., $P$[one event in the interval $(t, t+h)$] $\approx \alpha h$, where $h$ is the size of the interval and $\alpha$ is the rate parameter).
2. The probability of occurrence of two or more events in a very small interval is very low.
3. The occurrences of events during any interval are independent of those in any other interval.
4. The average number of occurrences over a fixed interval of time or space is constant.

Letting $X$ be the number of events over the entire time period $(0,T)$, the probability distribution of $X$ is

$$P(X=k)=\frac{(\alpha T)^k e^{-\alpha T}}{k!},\quad k=0,1,2\ldots.$$

which is the Poisson distribution with $\lambda = \alpha T$.

The Poisson distribution can be approximated by the normal distribution or other probability distributions depending on the value of the parameter $\lambda$. In general, if $\lambda$ is sufficiently large, a normal distribution with $\mu = \lambda$ and standard deviation $\sigma = \sqrt{\lambda}$ can be used to approximate a Poisson probability distribution.

*Hypergeometric distribution* frequently arises from a random experiment in which a random sample of $n$ units is selected without replacement from a population of $N$ units. In such experiments, each unit in the population can be classified into one of two categories (which we arbitrarily designate as "success" and "failure") according to whether the unit does or does not possess a certain property of interest. The random variable $X$, denoting the number of successes in the sample, is said to follow a hypergeometric distribution. Let $M$ denote the number of units in the population of $N$ units which possess the property of interest. Assuming that each of the $\binom{N}{n}$ samples has the same probability of being selected, the probability of obtaining $x$ successes in a sample of $n$ units without replacement is

$$P(X = x) = \frac{\binom{M}{x}\binom{N-M}{n-x}}{\binom{N}{n}}, \quad x = \max(0, n-(N-M)), \ldots, \min(n, M).$$

The mean and variance of the hypergeometric distribution are

$$\mu = \frac{nM}{N} \text{ and } \sigma^2 = \frac{nM}{N}\left(1-\frac{M}{N}\right)\left(1-\frac{n-1}{N-1}\right),$$

respectively.

The hypergeometric distribution is very important in the analysis of opinion surveys, in which the interviewer is interested in the number of people, for example, in the sample who answer his question in a certain way, because the value of $x$ allows him to make inferences about the proportion $p$ of people in the population of interest. Another application of the hypergeometric distribution arises in the area of quality control in which from an inventory of $N$ items a random sample of $n$ items without replacement is sampled and one is interested in making inferences concerning the proportion of defective items in the inventory based on the knowledge of the number of defectives in the sample. In many epidemiologic applications the hypergeometric distribution plays an important role in the analysis of a $2 \times 2$ contingency table, in which both row and column marginal totals are fixed. For example, consider a standard $2 \times 2$ contingency table of a particular sample of $N$ individuals, classified according to a dichotomous risk factor (present or absent) and a dichotomous outcome measure (positive or negative), with cell frequencies and marginals as shown below.

| | | Risk Factor | | |
|---|---|---|---|---|
| | | **Positive** | **Negative** | **Total** |
| | Present | $a$ | $b$ | $m_1$ |
| **Outcome Measure** | Absent | $c$ | $d$ | $m_2$ |
| | Total | $n_1$ | $n_2$ | $N$ |

Assuming that all marginal totals $n_1$, $n_2$, $m_1$, and $m_2$ are fixed, knowing any cell frequency, $a$, for example, implies that we know all other cell frequencies. The probability of obtaining a particular value of $a$, or more correctly any pattern of cell frequencies, is then given by the hypergeometric distribution:

$$p(a) = \frac{\binom{n_1}{a}\binom{n_2}{b}}{\binom{N}{n_1}}.$$

*Noncentral Hypergeometric Distribution* — Consider two independent binomial variables with parameters $(n_1,p_1)$ and $(n_2,p_2)$, respectively. The distribution of one of the binomial variable, $X_1$, conditional on the sum of the two has a probability distribution given by

$$P(X_1 = x_1 \mid X_1 + X_2 = m_1) = \frac{\binom{n_1}{x_1}\binom{n_2}{m_1 - x_1}(\text{OR})^{x_1}}{\sum_{\delta_1 \le i \le \delta_2}\binom{n_1}{i}\binom{n_2}{m_1 - i}(\text{OR})^{i}},$$

where

$$\text{OR} = \frac{p_1/(1-p_1)}{p_2/(1-p_2)}, \quad \delta_1 = \max(0, m_1 - n_2) \text{ and } \delta_2 = \min(m_1, n_1).$$

The distribution is known as the noncentral hypergeometric distribution. Note that for the special case with $p_1 = p_2$, the distribution reduces to the (central) hypergeometric distribution. This distribution plays an important role in the statistical inference of the odds ratio.

The *multinomial distribution* is the natural generalization of the binomial distribution. This distribution arises when $k$ ($k \ge 2$) mutually exclusive and exhaustive categories of outcomes exist. For example, a psychological state of degree of anxiety may be diagnosed as none, mild, moderate, or severe; then each person falls into exactly one of these four ($k = 4$) categories.

The multinomial distribution is an appropriate model under the conditions: there are $n$-independent trials; each trial must result in one of the $k$ mutually exclusive outcome categories called category 1, category 2,..., category $k$; and the probability of a category $i$ outcome is $p_i$ and is constant from trial to trial ($\sum_{i=1}^{k} p_i = 1$).

Define a set of $k$ random variables:

$X_1$ = number of trials resulting in category 1 outcomes,

$X_2$ = number of trials resulting in category 2 outcomes,

$\vdots$

and

$X_k$ = number of trials resulting in category $k$ outcomes.

The event $\{X_1 = x_1, X_2 = x_2, ..., X_k = x_k\}$ is the event that $x_1$ of outcomes are of category 1, $x_2$ are of category 2, and $x_k$ are of category $k$. The multinomial distribution is the distribution of the set of $k$ random variables, $X_1,...,X_k$, which are the number of category 1,2,..., $k$ outcomes, respectively, in a sequence of $n$ trials. The probability distribution of $(X_1, X_2, ..., X_k)$ is given by

$$P(X_1 = x_1, \ldots, X_k = x_k) = \frac{n!}{x_1!x_2!\ldots x_k!}(p_1)^{x_1}(p_2)^{x_2}\ldots(p_k)^{x_k},$$

where $x_1, x_2, ..., x_k$ are non-negative integers satisfying $\sum_{i=1}^{k} x_i = n$.

The mean and variance of each $X_i$ are given by $\mu_i = np_i$ and $\sigma_i^2 = np_i(1 - p_i)$, respectively. The correlation between $x_i$ and $x_j$ is

$$\text{Corr}(x_i, x_j) = -\sqrt{p_i p_j / (1 - p_i)(1 - p_j)}.$$

# References

**Haight, F. A.** (1967). *Handbook of the Poisson Distribution.* John Wiley & Sons, New York.

**Johnson, N. L., Kotz, S., and Kemp, A.** (1992). *Discrete Distributions,* 2nd ed. John Wiley & Sons, New York.

**Takeuchi, K. and Fujino, Y.** (1981). *Binomial and Poisson Distributions.* University of Tokyo Press, Tokyo (in Japanese).

# I Randomized and Mid-$p$ Tests and Mid-$p$ Confidence Intervals

Exact test procedures based on discrete distributions (e.g., binomial, Poisson, and hypergeometric) compute the individual probabilities of the observed outcomes and the more extreme outcomes that could have been obtained. Thus, the $p$-value of an exact test is calculated as

$$p = P(T \geq t) \text{ for the upper-tail probability}$$

or

$$p = P(T \leq t) \text{ for the lower-tail probability,}$$

where $T$ denotes the random variable of a particular discrete distribution and $t$ is the observed number of outcomes. However, because of the discreteness of the problem, these tests usually do not attain a prespecified nominal level $\alpha$ and tend to be somewhat conservative.

To maximize the power of a test with discrete data and still maintain the probability level exactly equal to the prescribed level $\alpha$, statistical theory uses *randomized tests* (Lehmann, 1959, 1986; Cox and Hinkley, 1974). To explain the randomized test for a $2 \times 2$ table entailing the nonrandomized Fisher's exact test, let $X$ be the random variable denoting the frequency in the upper-left cell. If $x$ is the corresponding observed cell frequency and $P(X \geq x) \leq \alpha$, the randomized test rejects the null hypothesis just as the nonrandomized test does. If, however, $P(X \geq x) > \alpha$, but $P(X \geq x + 1) \leq \alpha$, then a randomized experiment is conducted which rejects the null hypothesis with probability $\gamma$ determined such that

$$\alpha = \gamma P(X = x) + P(X \geq x + 1).$$

This makes the overall probability of rejection exactly equal to $\alpha$.

The *mid-p* ("median probability" or "middle probability") *test* was originally introduced by Lancaster (1949, 1952, 1961) (see also Miettinen, 1974, 1985;

Pratt and Gibbons, 1981) as an approximation to the randomized test. For the mid-$p$-value, only half of the probability of the observed event is counted, so the mid-$p$-value is always less than or equal to the conventional $p$-value. In the notation of the $2 \times 2$ table introduced previously

$$\text{mid-}p = \frac{1}{2} P(X = x) + P(X \geq x + 1).$$

In other words, mid-$p$ averages the exact $p$-values for the observed cell frequency $x$ and $x + 1$. The mid-$p$ tests usually can reduce the conservativeness; however, the true level can exceed the nominal level.

The *mid-p confidence intervals* (CIs) are based on the concept of the mid-$p$-value. For example, to obtain the mid-$p$ CI of the odds ratio (OR) in a single $2 \times 2$ table, Equations 4.14 and 4.15 are replaced by

$$\frac{\frac{1}{2}\binom{n_1}{x}\binom{n_2}{m_1 - x}(\mathrm{OR_L})^x + \sum_{k=x+1}^{\delta_2}\binom{n_1}{k}\binom{n_2}{m_1 - k}(\mathrm{OR_L})^k}{\sum_{\delta_1 \leq u \leq \delta_2}\binom{n_1}{u}\binom{n_2}{m_1 - u}(\mathrm{OR_L})^u} = \alpha/2$$

and

$$\frac{\sum_{k=\delta_1}^{x-1}\binom{n_1}{k}\binom{n_2}{m_1 - k}(\mathrm{OR_U})^k + \frac{1}{2}\binom{n_1}{x}\binom{n_2}{m_1 - x}(\mathrm{OR_U})^x}{\sum_{\delta_1 \leq u \leq \delta_2}\binom{n_1}{u}\binom{n_2}{m_1 - u}(\mathrm{OR_U})^u} = \alpha/2.$$

For a stratified analysis involving several $2 \times 2$ tables, Equations 6.51 and 6.52 can be modified similarly to obtain the mid-$p$ CI for the common OR.

The exact CIs based on the discrete distributions usually do not attain a prespecified confidence coefficient exactly equal to $1 - \alpha$, but rather $1 - \alpha'$, where $\alpha' < \alpha$. Thus, these intervals usually tend to be conservative. The mid-$p$ intervals can reduce the conservativeness. Unfortunately, its coverage at the $100(1 - \alpha)\%$ level is generally not guaranteed.

Mehta and Walsh (1992) compared the exact, mid-$p$ and Mantel-Haenszel CIs for the common OR across several $2 \times 2$ tables in terms of the length and the probability of coverage. It was found that the mid-$p$ method, in addition to producing shorter intervals, also preserves the empirical coverage probability. In small samples with large values of the OR, the Mantel-Haenszel interval was often degenerate; however, a modified Mantel-Haenszel approach involving exact intervals at the boundary values, in addition to preserving nominal coverage, produced shorter coverage length than either the exact or mid-*p* intervals. (For further discussion and comments involving the comparison of exact and mid-*p* CIs, including several other methods of interval estimation of the common OR and log OR in a stratified analysis, see Sato, 1990; Takagi, 1991; Mantel, 1993; and Sato and Takagi 1993.)

# References

**Cox, D. R. and Hinkley, D. V.** (1974). *Theoretical Statistics.* Chapman & Hall, London.

**Lancaster, H. O.** (1949). "The Combination of Probabilities Arising from Data in Discrete Distributions", *Biometrika,* 36, 370–382.

**Lancaster, H. O.** (1952). "Statistical Control of Counting Experiments", *Biometrika,* 39, 419–422.

**Lancaster, H. O.** (1961). "The Combination of Probabilities: An Application of Orthonormal Functions", *Aust. J. Stat.,* 3, 20–33.

**Lehmann, E. L.** (1959, 1986). *Testing Statistical Hypotheses,* 1st and 2nd eds. John Wiley & Sons, New York.

**Mantel, N.** (1993). "Letter to the Editor", *Am. Stat.,* 47, 86.

**Mehta, C. R. and Walsh, S. J.** (1992). "Comparison of Exact, Mid-p, and Mantel-Haenszel Confidence Intervals for the Common Odds Ratio Across Several Contingency Tables", *Am. Stat.,* 46, 146–150.

**Miettinen, O. S.** (1974). "Comment on 'Some Reasons for Not Using the Yates' Continuity Correction on 2 × 2 Contingency Tables' by W. J. Conover", *J. Am. Stat. Assoc.*, 69, 380–382.

**Miettinen, O. S.** (1985). *Theoretical Epidemiology: Principles of Occurrence Research in Medicine.* John Wiley & Sons, New York.

**Pratt, J. W. and Gibbons, J. D.** (1981). *Concepts of Nonparametric Theory.* Springer-Verlag, New York.

**Sato, T.** (1990). "Confidence Limits for the Common Odds Ratio Based on the Asymptotic Distribution of the Mantel-Haenszel Estimator", *Biometrics,* 46, 71–80.

**Sato, T. and Takagi, H.** (1993). "Letter to the Editor", *Am. Stat.,* 47, 86–87.

**Takagi, H.** (1991). "Approximate and Exact Methods for Computing Confidence Limits for the Common Odds Ratio in a Series of 2 × 2 Tables", Paper presented at the 1991 Annual Meeting of the Japanese Region of the Biometric Society.

# J Mantel-Haenszel Chi-Square Statistic for Stratified 2 × 2 Tables

The Mantel-Haenszel chi-square statistic ($\chi^2_{\text{MH}}$), based on stratified 2 × 2 tables, is

$$\chi^2_{\text{MH}} = \frac{\left[\sum_{i=1}^{k} a_i - E\left(\sum_{i=1}^{k} a_i\right)\right]^2}{\text{Var}\left(\sum_{i=1}^{k} a_i\right)}, \tag{J.1}$$

which has a chi-square distribution with one degree of freedom. To compute $E\left(\sum_{i=1}^{k} a_i\right)$ and $\text{Var}\left(\sum_{i=1}^{k} a_i\right)$, consider a 2 × 2 table for the $i$th level of the confounding factor:

| | Risk Factor | | |
|---|---|---|---|
| **Disease** | **+** | **–** | **Total** |
| Case | $a_i$ | $b_i$ | $m_{1i}$ |
| Control | $c_i$ | $d_i$ | $m_{2i}$ |
| Total | $n_{1i}$ | $n_{2i}$ | $n_i$ |

Under the null hypothesis of no association between the disease and the risk factor, it can be proven that (see, e.g., Ross, 1987; Giri, 1992)

$$E(a_i) = \frac{m_{1i} n_{1i}}{n_i} \tag{J.2}$$

and

$$\text{Var}(a_i) = \frac{m_{1i} m_{2i} n_{1i} n_{2i}}{n_i^2 (n_i - 1)}. \tag{J.3}$$

Noting that $E(\sum_{i=1}^{k} a_i) = \sum_{i=1}^{k} E(a_i)$ and $\text{Var}(\sum_{i=1}^{k} a_i) = \sum_{i=1}^{k} \text{Var}(a_i)$ and substituting the values of $E(a_i)$ and $\text{Var}(a_i)$, from Equations J.2 and J.3 into Equation J.1, the Mantel-Haenszel chi-square statistic is*

$$\chi^2_{\text{MH}} = \frac{\left[\sum_{i=1}^{k} a_i - \sum_{i=1}^{k} \frac{m_{1i} n_{1i}}{n_i}\right]^2}{\sum_{i=1}^{k} \frac{m_{1i} m_{2i} n_{1i} n_{2i}}{n_i^2 (n_i - 1)}}. \tag{J.4}$$

The statistic (J.4) was initially proposed by Mantel and Haenszel (1959) for the test of significance across all strata. Under the null hypothesis of no association between the presence of disease and the risk factor, the statistic has asymptotically a chi-square distribution with 1 degree of freedom. The statistic was also shown to be optimal for the alternative hypothesis, stating a constant practical association across all strata between the condition and the exposure (Birch, 1964). The statistic (J.4) provides the uniformly most powerful unbiased test against logistic alternative (Birch, 1964; Day and Byar, 1979). Bennett and Kaneshiro (1974) studied some small sample properties of power and size of the test using Monte Carlo methods and Wittes and Wallenstein (1987) have derived large sample approximations to the power. Mantel (1966) also showed how the test statistic may be used in comparing independent life tables, and Mantel (1977) employed the statistic (J.4) to derive approximate confidence limits for the common odds ratio.

A rule of thumb for ascertaining the validity of the Mantel-Haenszel chi-square statistic (J.4) was prescribed by Mantel and Fleiss (1980). They recommend that for a satisfactory interpretation, the sum of the minimum value be 5, or larger than the sum of the expected values for $a_i$. Note also that the test statistic (J.4) does not include a correction for continuity. Mantel and Haenszel (1959) also suggested the use of Yates' correction for continuity, leading to the statistic

$$\chi^2_{\text{MH}} = \frac{\left[\left|\sum_{i=1}^{k} a_i - \sum_{i=1}^{k} \frac{m_{1i} n_{1i}}{n_i}\right| - 1/2\right]^2}{\sum_{i=1}^{k} \frac{m_{1i} m_{2i} n_{1i} n_{2i}}{n_i^2 (n_i - 1)}}. \tag{J.5}$$

* The test statistic is calculated by adding the differences between the observed and expected values of $a_i$ over the subsets. Because these subsets are independent, the variance of the sum is equal to the sum of the separate variances.

Much controversy has arisen in the statistical literature over the use of the continuity correction for a single 2 × 2 table (see Appendix A). The use of continuity correction in statistic (J.5) is subject to the same controversy and leads to a $p$-value that is conservative (Levin, 1982). (For a discussion of the appropriateness of the continuity correction with respect to the Mantel-Haenszel chi-square statistic [J.4], see Li et al., 1979; and Wittes and Wallenstein, 1987.)

Although the Mantel-Haenszel chi-square statistic is based on an asymptotic distribution, the large sample requirements are pertinent to the information accumulated from all strata and are not needed for each 2 × 2 table. This highlights the principal advantage of using the Mantel-Haenszel chi-square statistic over Pearson chi-square in a stratified analysis. The Pearson chi-square, which has asymptotically a chi-square distribution with $k$ degrees of freedom, has an advantage over the Mantel-Haenszel statistic in that it is appropriate for all alternatives to the null hypothesis; however, it is less powerful in detecting a consistent difference that shows up in most of the individual strata.

The Mantel-Haenszel chi-square statistic can be extended for the more general situation involving several disease states and exposure categories. Mantel (1963) also has developed a procedure for comparing cases and controls when the exposure factor is ordinally scaled (dose-response relationship) and for the situation in which disease states are also ordinally scaled.

Finally, Cochran (1954) proposed calculating a unit normal deviate equivalent to the square root of 1 degree of freedom chi-square for each stratum and then summing those $Z_i$ values to obtain a normal deviate with variance equal to the number of strata, across which the unit normal deviates $Z_i$ were summed. The statistic $\chi = \sum_{i=1}^{k} Z_i / \sqrt{k}$ is thus a unit normal deviate that is essentially the square root of the Mantel-Haenszel chi-square statistic without the correction for continuity. The rationale of these two approaches for controlling the effects of a confounding factor on binary response probabilities in two treatment groups is the same.

# References

**Bennett, B. M. and Kaneshiro, C.** (1974). "On the Small-Sample Properties of the Mantel-Haenszel Test for Relative Risk", *Biometrika,* 61, 233–236.

**Birch, M. W.** (1964). "The Detection of Partial Association, I: The 2 × 2 Case", *J. R. Stat. Soc.,* B, 26, 313–324.

**Cochran, W. G.** (1954). "Some Methods of Strengthening the Common $\chi^2$ Tests", *Biometrics,* 10, 417–451.

**Day, N. E. and Byar, D. P.** (1979). "Testing Hypotheses in Case-Control Studies — Equivalence of Mantel-Haenszel Statistic and Logit Score Tests", *Biometrics,* 35, 623–630.

**Giri, N. C.** (1992). *Introduction to Probability and Statistics, Part I: Probability,* 2nd ed. Marcel Dekker, New York.

**Levin, B.** (1982). "On the Accuracy of a Normal Approximation to the Power of the Mantel-Haenszel Procedure", *J. Stat. Comp. Stim.,* 14, 201–218.

**Li, S-H., Simon, R. M., and Gart, J. J.** (1979). "Small Sample Properties of the Mantel-Haenszel Test", *Biometrika,* 66, 181–183.

**Mantel, N.** (1963). "Chi-Square Tests with One Degree of Freedom, Extensions of the Mantel-Haenszel Procedure", *J. Am. Stat. Assoc.,* 58, 690–700.

**Mantel, N.** (1966). "Evaluation of Survival Data and Two New Rank Order Statistics Arising in Its Consideration", *Cancer Chemother. Rep.,* 50, 163–170.

**Mantel, N.** (1977). "Tests and Limits for the Common Odds Ratio of Several 2 × 2 Contingency Tables: Methods in Analogy with the Mantel-Haenszel Procedure", *J. Stat. Planning Inference,* 1, 179–189.

**Mantel, N. and Fleiss, J.** (1980). "Minimum Expected Cell Size Requirements for the Mantel-Haenszel One Degree of Freedom Chi-Square Test and a Related Rapid Procedure", *Am. J. Epidemiol.,* 112, 129–139.

**Mantel, N. and Haenszel, W. M.** (1959). "Statistical Aspects of the Analysis of Data from Retrospective Studies of Disease", *J. Nat. Cancer Inst.,* 22, 719–748.

**Ross, S. M.** (1987). *Introduction to Probability and Statistics for Engineers and Scientists.* John Wiley & Sons, New York.

**Wittes, J. and Wallenstein, S.** (1987). "The Power of the Mantel-Haenszel Test", *J. Am. Stat. Assoc.,* 82, 1104–1109.

# K Analysis of a 2 × $l$ Table

In many epidemiologic studies it is frequently of interest to include exposure involving three or more levels in order to describe the manner in which an effect changes with varying levels of exposure. This is particularly of interest in the evaluation of dose-response relationships to investigate the increasing or decreasing trends with increasing levels of exposure. One simple and common approach is to analyze the data as a series of 2 × 2 tables, relating each level to the lowest level of exposure, using the Mantel-Haenszel procedure. However, odds ratios (ORs) involving each pairwise comparison levels will be different usually, and their estimates for the different levels will not be comparable across all the strata.

Mantel (1963) extended the Mantel-Haenszel procedure to provide a chi-square test for trend and also to combine a number of subsets of the data. Consider a 2 × $l$ contingency table involving $l$ levels of an exposure variable $X$. If the exposure levels are assigned the values $x_1, x_2, \ldots, x_l$ with corresponding cell counts for cases as $r_1, r_2, \ldots, r_l$, the data can be summarized as follows:

| **Level** | **1** | **2** | **...** | $l$ | |
|---|---|---|---|---|---|
| **Exposure values** | $x_1$ | $x_2$ | **...** | $x_l$ | **Total** |
| Cases (+) | $r_1$ | $r_2$ | ... | $r_l$ | $R$ |
| Noncases (–) | $n_1 - r_1$ | $n_2 - r_2$ | ... | $n_l - r_l$ | $N - R$ |
| Total | $n_1$ | $n_2$ | ... | $n_l$ | $N$ |

The crude analysis of the data to test the hypothesis that no differences exist in the risks of becoming a case between $l$ exposure levels can be performed by the statistic

$$\frac{\sum_{i=1}^{l} r_i^2/n_i - R^2/N}{\frac{R}{N}\left(1-\frac{R}{N}\right)},$$

which is approximately distributed as a chi-square with $l - 1$ degrees of freedom. Note that this is a test of the differences between the proportions without taking into account the ordering of the exposure levels.

The Mantel chi-square statistic for trend is based on the statistic $\sum_{j=1}^{l} r_j x_j$, which is the total of exposure values ($x$) for all the cases. Under the null hypothesis of no association, the statistic

$$\frac{\left[\sum_{j=1}^{l} r_j x_j - E_0\left(\sum_{j=1}^{l} r_j x_j\right)\right]^2}{\mathrm{Var}_0\left(\sum_{j=1}^{l} r_j x_j\right)},$$

where

$$E_0\left(\sum_{j=1}^{l} r_j x_j\right) = \frac{R\left(\sum_{j=1}^{l} n_j x_j\right)}{N}$$

and

$$\mathrm{Var}_0\left(\sum_{j=1}^{l} r_j x_j\right) = \frac{R(N-R)}{N^2(N-1)}\left\{N\left(\sum_{j=1}^{l} n_j x_j^2\right) - \left(\sum_{j=1}^{l} n_j x_j\right)^2\right\}$$

is approximately distributed as chi-square with 1 degree of freedom.

The Mantel chi-square statistic for trend relies on the assignment of values to each exposure level and is derived from a linear regression. This statistic is, however, still valid for nonlinear trends because the derivation of expectation and variance of $\sum_{j=1}^{l} r_j x_j$ makes no assumption of a linear trend. When two or more strata involve a confounding variate, the statistic is summed across all the strata and its null mean and variance, $E_0(\sum_{j=1}^{l} r_j x_j)$ and $\mathrm{Var}_0(\sum_{j=1}^{l} r_j x_j)$, are also summed separately in a manner analogous to that for the Mantel-Haenszel chi-square statistic. A test of the uniformity of the linear component of trend can be obtained by subtracting the above test statistic from the sum of the chi-squares for linear trend in each table.

One may wish to estimate a regression coefficient in many applications of the extended Mantel-Haenszel procedure. Mantel (1963) proposed two weighted regression coefficients. For a stratified analysis involving *k* strata, these coefficients are

$$b = \frac{\sum_{i=1}^{k}\left\{\sum_{j=1}^{l} r_j x_j - E_0\left(\sum_{j=1}^{l} r_j x_j\right)\right\}}{\sum_{i=1}^{k}\left\{\frac{\left(\sum_{j=1}^{l} r_j\right)\left(\sum_{j=1}^{l}(n_j - r_j)\right)}{\sum_{j=1}^{l} n_j}\right\}}$$

and

$$b' = \frac{\sum_{i=1}^{k}\left\{\sum_{j=1}^{l} r_j x_j - E_0\left(\sum_{j=1}^{l} r_j x_j\right)\right\}}{\sum_{i=1}^{k}\left\{\sum_{j=1}^{l} n_j x_j^2 - \frac{\left(\sum_{j=1}^{l} n_j x_j\right)^2}{\sum_{j=1}^{l} n_j}\right\}}.$$

Interval estimation involving confidence bands appropriate for the regression coefficient also may be calculated.

Mantel (1963) extended the test of trend for the case involving stratified data to adjust for confounding (see also Tarone and Gart, 1980). Mantel (1963) also proposed a test for trend involving several levels of both the disease and the exposure. Yates (1948), Cochran (1954), and Armitage (1955) proposed tests of trend in proportions which are related to the test given by Mantel (1963). (Further details and discussion of tests of trend in proportions can be found in Fleiss, 1981; Armitage and Berry, 1994; and Snedecor and Cochran, 1989.)

# References

**Armitage, P.** (1955). "Tests for Linear Trends in Proportion and Frequencies", *Biometrics,* 11, 375–386.

**Armitage, P. and Berry, G.** (1994). *Statistical Methods in Medical Research,* 3rd ed. Blackwell Scientific, Oxford.

**Cochran, W. G.** (1954). "Some Methods of Strengthening the Common $\chi^2$ Tests", *Biometrics,* 10, 417–418.

**Fleiss, J. L.** (1981). *Statistical Methods for Rates and Proportions,* 2nd ed. John Wiley & Sons, New York.

**Mantel, N.** (1963). "Chi-Square Tests with One Degree of Freedom, Extensions of the Mantel-Haenszel Procedure", *J. Am. Stat. Assoc.,* 58, 690–700.

**Snedecor, G. W. and Cochran, W. G.** (1989). *Statistical Methods,* 8th ed. Iowa State University Press, Ames, IA.

**Tarone, R. R. and Gart, J. J.** (1980). "On the Robustness of Combined Tests for Trends in Proportions", *J. Am. Stat. Assoc.,* 75, 110–116.

**Yates, F.** (1948). "The Analysis of Contingency Tables with Groupings Based on Quantitative Characteristics", *Biometrika,* 35, 176–181.

# L Maximum Likelihood Estimation for the Logistic Regression Model

Given a sample of $n$ subjects, let $Y_j$ denote the binary response variate of interest and $\boldsymbol{X}_j = (X_{1j}, X_{2j}, \ldots, X_{kj})$ be the vector of explanatory variables corresponding to the $j$th individual selected in the sample. Let the conditional probability that the response outcome is present, $P\{Y_j = 1 | \boldsymbol{X}_j = \boldsymbol{x}_j\}$, be denoted by $p(\boldsymbol{x}_j)$. Then the logistic regression model (8.3) can be written as

$$p(\boldsymbol{x}_j) = \frac{\exp\left(\beta_0 + \sum_{i=1}^{k} \beta_i x_{ij}\right)}{1 + \exp\left(\beta_0 + \sum_{i=1}^{k} \beta_i x_{ij}\right)}. \tag{L.1}$$

The quantity $1 - p(\boldsymbol{x}_j)$ gives the conditional probability that the outcome is absent, $P\{Y_j = 0 | \boldsymbol{X}_j = \boldsymbol{x}_j\}$. Thus, when $y_j = 1$, the contribution of the $j$th observation to the likelihood function is $p(\boldsymbol{x}_j)$, and when $y_j = 0$, the contribution of the $j$th observation to the likelihood function is $1 - p(\boldsymbol{x}_j)$. Hence, the likelihood function *(L)* for a sample of size $n$ is obtained as the product of the $n$ terms, $[p(x_j)]^{y_j} [1 - p(\boldsymbol{x}_j)]^{1-y_j}$, $j = 1,2,\ldots,n$, as follows:

$$L = \prod_{j=1}^{n} \left[p(\boldsymbol{x}_j)\right]^{y_j} \left[1 - p(\boldsymbol{x}_j)\right]^{1-y_j}, \tag{L.2}$$

where $p(\boldsymbol{x}_j)$ is determined from Equation L.1.

The log likelihood function obtained as the log of Equation L.2 is

$$\begin{aligned}\log_e L &= \sum_{j=1}^{n} y_j \log_e\left[p(\boldsymbol{x}_j)\right] + \sum_{j=1}^{n}(1-y_j)\log_e\left[1-p(\boldsymbol{x}_j)\right]\\ &= \sum_{j=1}^{n} y_j \log_e\left(\frac{p(\boldsymbol{x}_j)}{1-p(\boldsymbol{x}_j)}\right) + \sum_{j=1}^{n}\log_e\left[1-p(\boldsymbol{x}_j)\right]\\ &= \sum_{j=1}^{n} y_j\left[\beta_0 + \sum_{i=1}^{k}\beta_i x_{ij}\right] - \sum_{j=1}^{n}\log_e\left(1+\exp\left[\beta_0+\sum_{i=1}^{k}\beta_i x_{ij}\right]\right).\end{aligned}$$

To derive the maximum likelihood estimates, the normal equations, obtained by equating the first-order partial derivatives of the log likelihood equation to zero, are

$$\frac{\partial \log_e L}{\partial \beta_0} = \sum_{j=1}^{n} y_j - \sum_{j=1}^{n}\frac{\exp\left[\beta_0+\sum_{i=1}^{k}\beta_i x_{ij}\right]}{1+\exp\left[\beta_0+\sum_{i=1}^{k}\beta_i x_{ij}\right]} = 0 \qquad \text{(L.3)}$$

$$\frac{\partial \log_e L}{\partial \beta_l} = \sum_{j=1}^{n} y_j x_{lj} - \sum_{j=1}^{n}\frac{x_{lj}\exp\left[\beta_0+\sum_{i=1}^{k}\beta_i x_{ij}\right]}{1+\exp\left[\beta_0+\sum_{i=1}^{k}\beta_i x_{ij}\right]} = 0 \qquad \text{(L.4)}$$

for $l = 1, 2, \ldots, k$.

We now show there exists a unique solution to the normal equations for maximum likelihood estimators of $\beta_0, \beta_1, \ldots, \beta_k$. Letting $x_{0j} = 1$, for $j = 1,2,\ldots,n$, in normal Equation L.3, both normal Equations L.3 and L.4 can be written as a single equation:

$$\frac{\partial \log_e L}{\partial \beta_l} = \sum_{j=1}^{n} y_j x_{lj} - \sum_{j=1}^{n} \frac{x_{lj} \exp\left[\beta_0 + \sum_{i=1}^{k} \beta_i x_{ij}\right]}{1 + \exp\left[\beta_0 + \sum_{i=1}^{k} \beta_i x_{ij}\right]} = 0$$

$$\text{for } l = 0, 1, \ldots, k$$

Taking the second-order partial derivatives, we obtain:

$$\begin{aligned}
\frac{\partial^2 \log_e L}{\partial \beta_l \, \partial \beta_m} &= -\sum_{j=1}^{n} \frac{x_{lj} x_{mj} \exp\left[\beta_0 + \sum_{i=1}^{k} \beta_i x_{ij}\right]}{\left(1 + \exp\left[\beta_0 + \sum_{i=1}^{k} \beta_i x_{ij}\right]\right)^2} = 0 \\
&= -\sum_{j=1}^{n} x_{lj} x_{mj} p(\boldsymbol{x}_j)\left[1 - p(\boldsymbol{x}_j)\right] \\
&= -\sum_{j=1}^{n} x_{lj} x_{mj} V_j \quad \text{for } l, m = 0, 1, \ldots, k
\end{aligned}$$

where $V_j = p(\boldsymbol{x}_j)\,[1 - p(\boldsymbol{x}_j)]$ denotes the conditional variance of $Y_j$ given $\boldsymbol{X}_j = \boldsymbol{x}_j$. The matrix of the second-order partial derivatives can be written as

$$\begin{bmatrix}
-\sum_{j=1}^{n} x_{0j}^2 V_j & -\sum_{j=1}^{n} x_{0j} x_{1j} V_j & \cdots & -\sum_{j=1}^{n} x_{0j} x_{kj} V_j \\
\cdots\cdots & -\sum_{j=1}^{n} x_{1j}^2 V_j & \cdots & -\sum_{j=1}^{n} x_{1j} x_{kj} V_j \\
\cdots\cdots\cdots & \cdots\cdots\cdots & \cdots\cdots & -\sum_{j=1}^{n} x_{kj}^2 V_j
\end{bmatrix},$$

which is clearly negative definite. Hence, there exists a unique solution to the maximum likelihood estimators of the parameters $\beta_0, \beta_1, \ldots, \beta_k$.

The solution to the normal equations for determining the maximum likelihood estimates is obtained iteratively. Various iterative procedures are available to obtain approximate maximum likelihood estimates to any degree accuracy. The most commonly used procedure is the Newton-Raphson technique (see Atkinson, 1989; Ralston and Wilf, 1967). The matrix containing the negative terms of the second-order partial derivatives given above is called the *information matrix.* The variances and covariances of the estimated coefficients are obtained from the inverse of this matrix. However, except in very special cases, it is not possible to write an explicit expression for the elements of this matrix. In practice, variances and covariances of maximum likelihood estimates are usually estimated from the observed information matrix, replacing the unknown parameters by their estimates.

# References

**Atkinson, K. E.** (1989). *An Introduction to Numerical Analysis,* 2nd ed. John Wiley & Sons, New York.

**Ralston, A. and Wilf, H.** (1967). *Mathematical Methods for Digital Computers.* John Wiley & Sons, New York.

# M Logistic Regression Model for a Case-Control Design

In a case-control study the sampling is performed conditional on the outcome being a case or control. However, the odds ratio (OR) is invariant under the case-control design. We define the following random variables:

$$S_j = \begin{cases} 1 \text{ if the } j\text{th individual is selected in the sample} \\ 0 \text{ if the } j\text{th individual is not selected in the sample} \end{cases}$$

and

$$Y_j = \begin{cases} 1 \text{ if the } j\text{th individual is a case} \\ 0 \text{ if the } j\text{th individual is a control} \end{cases}$$

Also, let $\boldsymbol{X}_j = (X_{1j}, X_{2j}, \ldots, X_{kj})$ be the vector of explanatory variables or covariates corresponding to $j$th individual and consider the following probabilities:

$$\tau_1 = P\{S_j = 1 \mid Y_j = 1, \boldsymbol{X}_j = \boldsymbol{x}_j\}$$

and

$$\tau_0 = P\{S_j = 1 \mid Y_j = 0, \boldsymbol{X}_j = \boldsymbol{x}_j\}.$$

Note that $\tau_1$ and $\tau_0$ represent the probabilities of selection of the $j$th individual with covariates $\boldsymbol{x}_j$ as a case or control, respectively. Define the following probabilities:

$$p^*(\boldsymbol{x}_j) = P\{Y_j = 1 \mid S_j = 1, \boldsymbol{X}_j = \boldsymbol{x}_j\}$$

and

$$p(\boldsymbol{x}_j) = P\{Y_j = 1 \mid \boldsymbol{X}_j = \boldsymbol{x}_j\}.$$

Here, $p^*(\boldsymbol{x}_j)$ denotes the probability that the $j$th individual in the sample, with characteristics $\boldsymbol{x}_j$, is a case and $p(\boldsymbol{x}_j)$ denotes the probability that the $j$th individual in the population with characteristics $\boldsymbol{x}_j$, is a case.

Let $A = \{Y_j = 1\}$, $B = \{S_j = 1\}$, $C = \{\boldsymbol{X}_j = \boldsymbol{x}_j\}$ be three events and consider the following form of the Bayes theorem:

$$P(A \mid B \cap C) = \frac{P(A \cap B \cap C)}{P(A \cap B \cap C) + P(A' \cap B \cap C)}$$

$$= \frac{P(B \mid A \cap C)P(A \mid C)P(C)}{P(B \mid A \cap C)P(A \mid C)P(C) + P(B \mid A' \cap C)P(A' \mid C)P(C)}.$$

Hence, applying the Bayes theorem to the events defined above, we have

$$p^*(\boldsymbol{x}_j) = P\{Y_j = 1 \mid S_j = 1, \boldsymbol{X}_j = \boldsymbol{x}_j\}$$

$$= \frac{P\{S_j = 1 \mid Y_j = 1, \boldsymbol{X}_j = \boldsymbol{x}_j\}P\{Y_j = 1 \mid \boldsymbol{X}_j = \boldsymbol{x}_j\}}{\left[P\{S_j = 1 \mid Y_j = 1, \boldsymbol{X}_j = \boldsymbol{x}_j\}P\{Y_j = 1 \mid \boldsymbol{X}_j = \boldsymbol{x}_j\} + P\{S_j = 1 \mid Y_j = 0, \boldsymbol{X}_j = \boldsymbol{x}_j\}P\{Y_j = 0 \mid \boldsymbol{X}_j = \boldsymbol{x}_j\}\right]}$$

$$= \frac{\tau_1 \, p(\boldsymbol{x}_j)}{\tau_1 \, p(\boldsymbol{x}_j) + \tau_0 \left(1 - p(\boldsymbol{x}_j)\right)}.$$

Furthermore, it follows that

$$\frac{p^*(\boldsymbol{x}_j)}{1 - p^*(\boldsymbol{x}_j)} = \frac{\tau_1}{\tau_0} \frac{p(\boldsymbol{x}_j)}{\left(1 - p(\boldsymbol{x}_j)\right)}. \tag{M.1}$$

The above result states that the odds in a case-control design are equal to the odds in the population multiplied by $(\tau_1/\tau_0)$, which represents the theoretical probability of an individual being selected in the sample. It, therefore, follows that the OR in a case-control design is invariant because the factor $(\tau_1/\tau_0)$ is canceled out.

Suppose we have $n_1$ cases and $n_0$ controls in a sample of size $n$. The likelihood function ($L^*$) under the case-control design is

$$L^* = \prod_{j=1}^{n_1} P\{\boldsymbol{X}_j = \boldsymbol{x}_j \mid Y_j = 1, S_j = 1\} \prod_{j=1}^{n_0} P\{\boldsymbol{X}_j = \boldsymbol{x}_j \mid Y_j = 0, S_j = 1\}.$$

Let $A' = \{\boldsymbol{X}_j = \boldsymbol{x}_j\}$, $B' = \{Y_j = 1\}$, and $C' = \{S_j = 1\}$ be three events and consider the following form of the Bayes theorem:

$$P(A' \mid B' \cap C') = \frac{P(A' \cap B' \cap C')}{P(B' \cap C')} = \frac{P(B' \mid A' \cap C')P(A' \mid C')}{P(B' \mid C')}.$$

Hence, applying the Bayes theorem to the events defined above, we have

$$L^* = \prod_{j=1}^{n_1} \frac{P\{Y_j = 1 \mid S_j = 1, \boldsymbol{X}_j = \boldsymbol{x}_j\} P\{\boldsymbol{X}_j = \boldsymbol{x}_j \mid S_j = 1\}}{P\{Y_j = 1 \mid S_j = 1\}}$$

$$\times \prod_{j=1}^{n_0} \frac{P\{Y_j = 0 \mid S_j = 1, \boldsymbol{X}_j = \boldsymbol{x}_j\} P\{\boldsymbol{X}_j = \boldsymbol{x}_j \mid S_j = 1\}}{P\{Y_j = 0 \mid S_j = 1\}}.$$

Furthermore, noting that $p^*(\boldsymbol{x}_j) = P\{Y_j = 1 \mid S_j = 1, \boldsymbol{X}_j = \boldsymbol{x}_j\}$ and $P\{\boldsymbol{X}_j = \boldsymbol{x}_j \mid S_j = 1\} = P(\boldsymbol{X}_j = \boldsymbol{x}_j)$ (because the sampling is independent of the covariate values), the likelihood function $L^*$ can be written:

$$\begin{aligned} L^* &= \prod_{j=1}^{n_1} \frac{p^*(\boldsymbol{x}_j) P(\boldsymbol{X}_j = \boldsymbol{x}_j)}{P\{Y_j = 1 \mid S_j = 1\}} \prod_{j=1}^{n_0} \frac{(1 - p^*(\boldsymbol{x}_j)) P(\boldsymbol{X}_j = \boldsymbol{x}_j)}{P\{Y_j = 0 \mid S_j = 1\}} \\ &= \prod_{j=1}^{n} [p^*(\boldsymbol{x}_j)]^{y_j} [1 - p^*(\boldsymbol{x}_j)]^{1-y_j} \prod_{j=1}^{n} \frac{P(\boldsymbol{X}_j = \boldsymbol{x}_j)}{P\{Y_j = y_j \mid S_j = 1\}}. \end{aligned} \tag{M.2}$$

The first term in Equation M.2 represents the likelihood function, assuming that the data for a case-control study were obtained as in a cohort design, in which the response variable $Y_j$ denotes a dependent variable. Furthermore, assuming that the probability distribution $P(\boldsymbol{X}_j = \boldsymbol{x}_j)$ contains no information about the parameters in the logistic regression model, the maximization of $L^*$ with respect to the coefficients in the logistic model depends only on the constraint that $P\{Y_j = 1|S_j = 1\} = n_1/n$ and $P\{Y_j = 0|S_j = 1\} = n_0/n$. It can be seen that for the likelihood equation obtained by differentiating with respect to $\beta_0^*$ this condition is satisfied. Thus, in the maximization of the likelihood (M.2), one need only consider the first term which represents the likelihood function corresponding to a cohort design. Using Equation M.1, we obtain

$$\log_e\left(\frac{p^*(\boldsymbol{x}_j)}{1-p^*(\boldsymbol{x}_j)}\right) = \log_e\left(\frac{\tau_1}{\tau_0}\right) + \log_e\left(\frac{p(\boldsymbol{x}_j)}{(1-p(\boldsymbol{x}_j))}\right).$$

It, therefore, follows that in a logistic regression model the coefficients remain unchanged under the case-control design, while the intercept parameter $\beta_0^*$ is related to the $\beta_0$ by the relation

$$\beta_0^* = \log_e\left(\frac{\tau_1}{\tau_0}\right) + \beta_0.$$

In a case-control design the parameters $\tau_1$, $\tau_0$, and $\beta_0$ cannot generally be estimated; only the parameter $\beta_0^*$ can be estimated.

# N Odds Ratio as an Approximation to Risk Ratio

This appendix shows that in a retrospective study involving a rare condition, the risk ratio (RR) is approximately estimated by the odds ratio (OR). Define the events $D$, $D'$, $E$, and $E'$ as follows:

$D$: The person has the disease.
$D'$: The person does not have the disease.
$E$: The person is exposed to the risk factor.
$E'$: The person is not exposed to the risk factor.

In terms of conditional probabilities, the RR can be expressed as

$$\text{RR} = \frac{P(D \mid E)}{P(D \mid E')}.$$

Using Bayes' theorem, the conditional probabilities can be written as follows (see Neutra and Drolette, 1978):

$$P(D \mid E) = \frac{P(D)P(E \mid D)}{P(D)P(E \mid D) + P(D')P(E \mid D')}$$

and

$$P(D \mid E') = \frac{P(D)P(E' \mid D)}{P(D)P(E' \mid D) + P(D')P(E' \mid D')}.$$

Substituting these values in the formula for the RR, we have

$$\mathrm{RR} = \frac{P(E \mid D)}{P(E' \mid D)} \left[ \frac{P(D)P(E' \mid D) + P(D')P(E' \mid D')}{P(D)P(E \mid D) + P(D')P(E \mid D')} \right].$$

If the risk of the disease is low, so that $P(D) \simeq 0$, the above expression simplifies to

$$\mathrm{RR} = \frac{P(E \mid D) \div P(E' \mid D)}{P(E \mid D') \div P(E' \mid D')}.$$

Note that the numerator of the above expression represents the odds of being exposed for a case and the denominator represents the odds of being exposed for a noncase. Thus, the RR is approximately equal to the exposure OR.

# Reference

**Neutra, R. R. and Drolette, M. E.** (1978). "Estimating Exposure-Specific Disease Rates from Case-Control Studies Using Bayes' Theorem", *Am. J. Epidemiol.*, 108, 214–222.

# Exercises

## CHAPTER 3

1. Consider the data from the Framingham Heart Study as described by Shurtleff (1970, 1974). The following table gives the 16-year incidence of myocardial infarction (MI) in Framingham, MA, for men aged 35 to 44 years, by level of serum cholesterol (SC):

| SC (mg%) | MI (+) | MI (–) | Total |
|---|---|---|---|
| >250 | 10 | 125 | 135 |
| ≤250 | 21 | 449 | 470 |
| Total | 31 | 574 | 605 |

   Carry out the chi-square test of significance to evaluate the possible association between SC level and the incidence of MI and calculate 95% confidence intervals (CIs) for the risk difference (RD), risk ratio (RR), and odds ratio (OR) using the methods described in the text.

2. The following table gives Framingham data relating systolic blood pressure (SBP) to coronary heart disease (CHD) after 18 years among those who were free of the disease on the first examination:

| SBP (mmHg) | CHD Yes | CHD No | Total |
|---|---|---|---|
| ≥165 | 95 | 201 | 296 |
| <165 | 173 | 894 | 1067 |
| Total | 268 | 1095 | 1363 |

   Carry out the chi-square test of significance to evaluate the possible association between SBP and the incidence of CHD and calculate

95% CIs for the RD, RR, and OR, using the methods described in the text.

3. The following table gives Framingham data on the total number of cancer deaths during the 18-year period according to smoking history:

| Smoker | Cancer deaths Yes | No | Total |
|---|---|---|---|
| Yes | 40 | 593 | 633 |
| No | 39 | 733 | 772 |
| Total | 79 | 1326 | 1405 |

Carry out the chi-square test of significance, comparing cancer mortality between smokers and nonsmokers and calculate 95% CIs for the RD, RR, and OR using the methods described in the text. Do the OR and the associated CIs provide adequate approximations for the estimates of the RR?

4. Lewak et al. (1979) conducted a study of the age of the mother at the birth of the child as a risk factor in the development of sudden infant death syndrome (SIDS). A total of 7330 women, who were under the age of 25 when the child was born, were selected for the study. Of these, 29 bore children who died from SIDS. Of the 11,256 women selected for the study who were 25 years of age or older when their children were born, 15 had children affected with SIDS. Carry out the chi-square test of significance to evaluate the possible association between SIDS and the age of the mother at the birth of the child as a risk factor. Calculate 95% CIs for RD, RR, and OR using the methods described in the text. Do the OR and the estimated CIs provide adequate approximations for the estimates of the RR?
5. Consider the data from a cohort study to determine the risk of urethral strictures in the male offspring of diethylstilbestrol-exposed pregnant woman, as reported by Henderson et al. (1976). From a sample of 111 unexposed pregnancies, 17 offspring with symptoms of urogenital tract abnormalities and two offspring with problems in passing urine were found. From another sample of 225 exposed pregnancies, the numbers of offspring with the above two symptoms are 55 and 29, respectively. Carry out the chi-square test of significance to evaluate the possible association between the risk of urethral strictures in male offspring and exposure to diethylstilbestrol in pregnant women. Calculate 95% CIs for the RD, RR, and OR using the methods described in the text.
6. Consider a randomized double-blind multicenter clinical trial, as described in the Report of the Sixty-Plus Reinfarction Study

Research Group (1980). The purpose of the trial was to determine whether continuation of well-controlled oral anticoagulant therapy in elderly patients who received this therapy since their primary MI, would result in a substantial decrease in total mortality over a period of 2 years. Half of the 878 patients, all over 60 years of age, were randomly assigned to the placebo group instead of the anticoagulant group and the others continued anticoagulant therapy. The results on the distribution of deaths after 2 years of follow-up in two groups of patients are shown below:

| Group | No. dead | No. alive | Total |
|---|---|---|---|
| Placebo | 49 | 390 | 439 |
| Anticoagulant | 28 | 411 | 439 |
| Total | 77 | 801 | 878 |

Carry out the chi-square test of significance, comparing mortality rates between the two groups of patients and calculate 95% CIs for the RD, RR, and OR, using the methods described in the text.

## CHAPTER 4

7. Consider a case-control study of the possible association between menopausal estrogen therapy and breast cancer described by Ross et al. (1980). Only women with intact ovaries, which comprise 80% of the cases, were included in the study. All the subjects were divided by dose level (total milligram accumulated dose, TMD), and the individual matches were ignored. The data are shown below:

| TMD | Cases | Controls | Total |
|---|---|---|---|
| >1500 | 28 | 23 | 51 |
| 0–1499 | 71 | 159 | 230 |
| Total | 99 | 182 | 281 |

Carry out the chi-square test of significance to evaluate the possible association between estrogen therapy and breast cancer. Calculate 95% CIs of the OR using logit, test-based, and Cornfield's methods. Compare the results to the limits obtained via the exact method.

8. Cantor et al. (1988) reported a study of the relationship between the regular use of hair dye and the development of leukemia. The study

entailed 577 leukemia patients and 1245 persons free from the disease (controls) who were questioned concerning their use of hair dye. Forty-three patients and 55 controls claimed to have had significant exposure to hair dye. Carry out the chi-square test of significance for the possible association between the use of hair dye and the development of leukemia. Calculate 95% CIs of the OR using logit, test-based, and Cornfield's methods. Compare the results to the limits obtained via the exact method.

9. Consider the data from a case-control study on the relationship of cataracts to diabetes reported by Hiller and Kahn (1976). The results are summarized in the following table:

| Diabetes | Cases | Controls | Total |
|---|---|---|---|
| Present | 56 | 84 | 140 |
| Absent | 552 | 1927 | 2479 |
| Total | 608 | 2011 | 2619 |

Carry out the chi-square test of significance for the possible association between diabetes and cataracts. Calculate 95% CIs of the OR using logit, test-based and Cornfield's methods. Compare the results to the limits obtained via the exact method. (*Note:* For the $2 \times 2$ table with cells of such large magnitude, all three methods should give virtually the same interval.)

10. Consider a case-control study of smoking tobacco and oral cancer described by Graham et al. (1977), which is illustrative of a study with very large, approximately equal sample sizes and a larger relative risk. The data are summarized in the table below:

| Tobacco used | Cases | Controls | Total |
|---|---|---|---|
| Ever | 399 | 414 | 813 |
| Never | 20 | 102 | 122 |
| Total | 419 | 516 | 935 |

Carry out the chi-square test of significance for the possible association between tobacco use and oral cancer. Calculate 95% CIs of the OR using the logit, test-based and Cornfield's methods. Compare the results to the limits obtained via the exact method.

11. Consider the Hoover and Strasser (1979) study on the possible association between the use of artificial sweeteners and bladder cancer. The following data on diet drink consumption for nonsmoking women are extracted from Table 19 of the study:

| Diet drinks | Cases | Controls | Total |
|---|---|---|---|
| Ever used | 75 | 240 | 315 |
| Never used | 151 | 441 | 592 |
| Total | 226 | 681 | 907 |

Carry out the chi-square test of significance for the possible association between the use of artificial sweeteners and bladder cancer. Calculate 95% CIs of the OR using logit, test-based and Cornfield's methods. Compare the results to the limits obtained via the exact method. (*Note:* As would be expected from a study involving large numbers, all three methods should yield quite similar results.)

12. Consider Mintz's (1980) study on possible birth defects in children born to mothers who have used benedictine. The study, reported to the Food and Drug Administration by Dr. Herschel Jick of the Boston Drug Surveillance Program, was done in collaboration with the Group Health Cooperative of Puget Sound, Washington. The survey included 2966 mothers who used the drug in pregnancy and 4663 mothers who did not. Six relatively severe limb disorders were found in each group. Carry out the chi-square test of significance for the possible association between the use of benedictine by mothers and birth defects in children. Calculate 95% confidence limits of the OR using logit, test-based and Cornfield's methods. Compare the results to the limits obtained via the exact method. (*Hint:* For such low proportions, the RR and the OR are virtually identical, and the data may be analyzed similar to a case-control study.)
13. Suppose a population of 10 million were classified as follows:

| | Lung cancer | No lung cancer | Total |
|---|---|---|---|
| Smokers | 900 | 999,700 | 1,000,600 |
| Nonsmokers | 2100 | 8,997,300 | 8,999,400 |
| Total | 3000 | 9,997,000 | 10,000,000 |

Carry out the chi-square test of significance for the possible association between smoking and lung cancer. Calculate 95% CIs for the RR using various methods described in the text. (*Hint:* For such low proportions, the RR and OR are nearly identical, and the data may be analyzed similar to a case-control study.)

14. Consider the data from a case-control study of the association between current postmenopausal hormone use and risk of nonfatal MI described by Bain et al. (1981). The study entailed 88 women reporting a diagnosis of MI and 1873 healthy control subjects

identified from a large population of married female registered nurses, aged 30 to 55 years. The data are given below:

| Hormone use | Cases | Controls | Total |
|---|---|---|---|
| Current use | 32 | 825 | 857 |
| Never used | 56 | 1048 | 1104 |
| Total | 88 | 1873 | 1961 |

Carry out the chi-square test of significance for the possible association between hormone use and the risk of MI. Calculate 95% CIs of the OR using logit, test-based and Cornfield's methods. Compare the results to the limits obtained via the exact method.

15. Consider the data from a case-control study of cancer of the nasal cavity and paranasal sinuses and formaldehyde exposures reported by Hayes et al. (1986). The data are summarized below:

| | Exposed | Unexposed | Total |
|---|---|---|---|
| Cases | 31 | 60 | 91 |
| Controls | 34 | 161 | 195 |
| Total | 65 | 221 | 286 |

Carry out the chi-square test of significance to evaluate the possible association between the cancer of the nasal cavity and paranasal sinuses and formaldehyde exposures. Calculate 95% CIs of the OR using logit, test-based and Cornfield's methods. Compare the results to the limits obtained via the exact method.

16. Consider a case-control study of the possible association between alcohol consumption and the risk of esophageal cancer as reported by Tyns et al. (1977). The study entailed 200 males diagnosed with esophageal cancer in one of the regional hospitals between the years 1972 and 1974, and controls were a sample of 775 adult males selected from electoral lists in each community. The data on alcohol consumption dichotomized at a value of 80 g/d for cases and controls are summarized below:

| Av. daily alcohol consumption (g) | Disease status Cases | Controls | Total |
|---|---|---|---|
| ≥80 | 96 | 109 | 205 |
| <80 | 104 | 666 | 770 |
| Total | 200 | 775 | 975 |

Carry out the chi-square test of significance to evaluate the possible association between the average daily alcohol consumption and the risk of esophageal cancer. Calculate 95% CIs of the OR using logit, test-based and Cornfield's methods. Compare the results to the limits obtained via the exact method.

## CHAPTER 5

17. It is known that AIDS patients often develop tuberculosis. Cot et al. (1990) reported a study of the risk factors associated with the development of tuberculosis in these patients. A primary risk factor of interest was the abuse of intravenous drugs. Of the 1992 patients in the study, 307 abused intravenous drugs; 46 of the patients had tuberculosis, and of these 11 abused intravenous drugs. Carry out the chi-square test of significance for the possible association between the development of tuberculosis and the intravenous drug abuse rate among AIDS patients. Calculate 95% CIs for the RD, RR, and OR using the methods described in the text. Analyze and interpret the data as a cross-sectional study.

## CHAPTER 6

18. Stewart et al. (1958) conducted a retrospective study of childhood malignancies by investigating the history of abdominal X-ray during pregnancy. The following data show distributions of cases and controls according to the number of films of the abdomen taken during pregnancy. The relative risks have been calculated and are shown in the adjacent column. (The relative risks relate the risk of malignant disease among fetuses exposed in utero to the risk among those with no exposure.)

| No. of films | Cases | Controls | Relative risks |
|---|---|---|---|
| 4+ | 32 | 10 | 3.44 |
| 3 | 23 | 10 | 2.47 |
| 2 | 60 | 26 | 2.48 |
| 1 | 37 | 27 | 1.47 |
| 0 | 1121 | 1206 | 1.00 |

Note that with 4+ films relative risks = (32/1121) ÷ (10/1206) = 3.44. These results indicate that the risk of malignant disease in childhood is associated with abdominal X-ray; indeed, there seems to be some evidence of a dose-response relationship. Analyze the above data, ignoring the dose of exposure, and carry out the chi-square test of significance for the possible association between exposure to abdominal X-ray and childhood malignancies. Calculate 95% CIs for the OR using logit and test-based methods.

19. Hills (1974) reported the findings of four case-control studies of the effect of smoking on lung cancer. The following data show the distribution of the number of cases and controls among smokers and nonsmokers:

| | Cases | | | Controls | | |
|---|---|---|---|---|---|---|
| Study | Smokers *(a)* | Non-Smokers *(b)* | Total | Smokers *(c)* | Non-Smokers *(d)* | Total |
| 1 | 83 | 3 | 86 | 72 | 14 | 86 |
| 2 | 129 | 7 | 136 | 81 | 19 | 100 |
| 3 | 499 | 19 | 518 | 462 | 56 | 518 |
| 4 | 412 | 32 | 444 | 299 | 131 | 430 |

Apply the chi-square test of homogeneity to determine whether these studies yield significantly different relative risks. Use logit, Mantel-Haenszel, and maximum likelihood methods to combine the results of these studies and obtain point estimates of the overall relative risk (OR). Obtain 95% CIs of the common OR using logit, Mantel-Haenszel, maximum likelihood, test-based, Birch, and Cornfield's methods. Compare the results to the limits obtained via the exact method.

20. The following hypothetical data show the results of three case-control studies of the association between the use of oral contraceptives and breast cancer:

**Study 1**

| | Cases | Controls | Total |
|---|---|---|---|
| Used | 31 | 73 | 104 |
| Never Used | 59 | 107 | 166 |
| Total | 90 | 180 | 270 |

**Study 2**

| | Cases | Controls | Total |
|---|---|---|---|
| Used | 84 | 85 | 169 |
| Never Used | 148 | 147 | 295 |
| Total | 232 | 232 | 464 |

**Study 3**

| | Cases | Controls | Total |
|---|---|---|---|
| Used | 9 | 170 | 179 |
| Never Used | 112 | 672 | 784 |
| Total | 121 | 842 | 963 |

Apply the chi-square test of homogeneity to determine whether these studies yield significantly different relative risks. Use logit, Mantel-Haenszel, and maximum likelihood methods to combine the relative risk of these studies and obtain point estimates of the overall relative risk (OR). Calculate 95% CIs of the common OR using logit, Mantel-Haenszel, maximum likelihood, test-based, Birch, and Cornfield's methods. Compare the results to the limits obtained via the exact method.

21. Gart (1970) and Vollset and Hirji (1991) analyzed the data of Gordon and Foss (1966), given by Cox (1966), in which the re-

sponse is the presence or absence of crying babies in a nursery. The data, consisting of 18 sparse $2 \times 2$ tables, are given below:

| Control | | Treated | |
|---|---|---|---|
| **Not Crying** | **Crying** | **Not Crying** | **Crying** |
| 3 | 5 | 1 | 0 |
| 2 | 4 | 1 | 0 |
| 1 | 4 | 1 | 0 |
| 1 | 5 | 0 | 1 |
| 4 | 1 | 1 | 0 |
| 4 | 5 | 1 | 0 |
| 5 | 3 | 1 | 0 |
| 4 | 4 | 1 | 0 |
| 3 | 2 | 1 | 0 |
| 8 | 1 | 0 | 1 |
| 5 | 1 | 1 | 0 |
| 8 | 1 | 1 | 0 |
| 5 | 3 | 1 | 0 |
| 4 | 1 | 1 | 0 |
| 4 | 2 | 1 | 0 |
| 7 | 1 | 1 | 0 |
| 4 | 2 | 0 | 1 |
| 5 | 3 | 1 | 0 |

Note that in this example, $n_{1i}$ and $n_{2i}$ $(i = 1, 2, \ldots, 18)$ take various values from 5 to 9. The number of crying babies in the test group is $\sum a_i = 3$. The point and interval estimates of the OR using different procedures are summarized as follows:

| Method | Point estimates |
|---|---|
| Logit | 0.7254 |
| Mantel-Haenszel | 0.3002 |
| Exact conditional maximum likelihood | 0.2848 |
| Asymptotic conditional maximum likelihood | 0.2387 |
| Conditional median unbiased | 0.2956 |
| Birch | 0.3562 |
| Goodman | 0.3175 |

| Method | Confidence coefficient | Lower limit | Upper limit |
|---|---|---|---|
| Exact method | 95 | 0.468 | 1.157 |
| | 99 | 0.250 | 1.615 |
| Cornfield (exact | 95 | 0.570 | 1.209 |
| moments) | 99 | 0.398 | 1.708 |
| Cornfield (asymptotic | 95 | 0.412 | 1.136 |
| moments) | 99 | 0.276 | 1.645 |
| Logit method | 95 | 0.125 | 1.684 |
| | 99 | 0.398 | 2.195 |
| Birch | 95 | 0.234 | 1.028 |
| | 99 | 0.885 | 1.434 |
| Goodman | 95 | 0.095 | 0.921 |
| | 99 | 0.784 | 1.286 |

Carry out independent computations to determine the point and interval estimates reported here and check results against those given in the table.

22. Consider the coronary disease data from the Framingham Heart Study (Shurtleff, 1970, 1974). The data relating SBP and the incidence of CHD are summarized below by age-sex category:

**18-Year Coronary Heart Disease Incidence**

**Men, Age ≥55**

| SBP | CHD + | CHD − | Total |
|---|---|---|---|
| SBP <165 | 49 | 139 | 188 |
| SBP ≥165 | 21 | 24 | 45 |

**Men, Age <50**

| SBP | CHD + | CHD − | Total |
|---|---|---|---|
| SBP <165 | 36 | 147 | 183 |
| SBP ≥165 | 9 | 17 | 26 |

**Women, Age ≥55**

| SBP | CHD + | CHD − | Total |
|---|---|---|---|
| SBP <165 | 25 | 148 | 173 |
| SBP ≥165 | 28 | 59 | 87 |

**Women, Age <50**

| SBP | CHD + | CHD − | Total |
|---|---|---|---|
| SBP <165 | 13 | 176 | 189 |
| SBP ≥165 | 7 | 35 | 42 |

Apply the chi-square test of homogeneity to determine whether the relative risks are significantly different among age-sex categories reported. Use pooled, Mantel-Haenszel, and maximum likelihood methods to obtain point estimates of the overall RD and RR. Calculate 95% CIs for the common RD and RR using pooling, Mantel-Haenszel, and test-based procedures.

23. Consider the data from the Western Collaborative Group Study, as given in Selvin (1991). The study assessed the relationship between behavior pattern and the risk of developing CHD among middle-aged men from employees of ten California companies and collected data on 3154 individuals. The table below shows the study participants divided into five age groups to examine the relationship between the behavior type and CHD:

| | Type A | | Type B | | |
|---|---|---|---|---|---|
| | CHD | No CHD | CHD | No CHD | Total |
| Age | $a_i$ | $c_i$ | $b_i$ | $d_i$ | $n_i$ |
| <40 | 20 | 241 | 11 | 271 | 543 |
| 40–44 | 34 | 462 | 21 | 574 | 1091 |
| 45–49 | 49 | 337 | 21 | 343 | 750 |
| 50–54 | 38 | 209 | 17 | 184 | 448 |
| 54+ | 37 | 162 | 9 | 114 | 322 |
| Total | 178 | 1411 | 79 | 1486 | 3154 |

Apply the chi-square test of homogeneity to determine whether the relative risks are significantly different among age categories reported. Use pooled, Mantel-Haenszel, and maximum likelihood methods to obtain point estimates of the overall RD and RR. Calculate 95% CIs for the common RD and RR using pooling, Mantel-Haenszel, maximum likelihood, and test-based procedures.

24. In a study of the relation of blood type to various diseases Woolf (1955) reported data on incidence of peptic ulcer in two communities from London and Manchester. The results are summarized below:

**London**

| Blood type | Peptic ulcer | Control |
|---|---|---|
| Group A | 4219 | 579 |
| Group B | 4578 | 911 |

**Manchester**

| Blood type | Peptic ulcer | Control |
|---|---|---|
| Group A | 3775 | 246 |
| Group B | 4532 | 361 |

Does a relationship exist between blood type and propensity to peptic ulcer in the two communities analyzed above? If so, evaluate the strength of the association for each table. Are the data from London and Manchester comparable in terms of strength of association? Carry out appropriate tests of significance. Use logit, Mantel-Haenszel, and maximum likelihood methods to combine the results of these studies and obtain point estimates of the overall relative risk (OR). Obtain 95% CIs of the common OR using logit, Mantel-Haenszel, maximum likelihood, test-based, Birch, and Cornfield's methods. Compare the results to the limits obtained via the exact method.

25. Consider the Boston Area Health Study, a matched case-control study, described in Problem 32, concerning the association between the level of physical activity and the risk of MI. Cigarette smoking was considered a potential confounder for the association because it is an independent risk factor for MI, and may be related to the level of physical activity. To control this variable, data were first stratified (ignoring matching) by history of cigarette smoking, and the results for each stratum are summarized in the table below:

| Smoking history | Physical activity index | Cases | Controls | Total |
|---|---|---|---|---|
| Never smoked | 2500+ kcal | 41 | 84 | 125 |
| | <2500 kcal | 46 | 52 | 98 |
| | Total | 87 | 136 | 223 |
| Ex-smoker 10+ years | 2500+ kcal | 41 | 80 | 121 |
| | <2500 kcal | 30 | 39 | 69 |
| | Total | 71 | 119 | 190 |
| Ex-smoker <10 years | 2500+ kcal | 22 | 34 | 56 |
| | <2500 kcal | 21 | 26 | 47 |
| | Total | 43 | 60 | 103 |
| Current smoker | 2500+ kcal | 86 | 68 | 154 |
| | <2500 kcal | 79 | 40 | 119 |
| | Total | 165 | 108 | 273 |
| Total | 2500+ kcal | 190 | 266 | 456 |
| | <2500 kcal | 176 | 157 | 333 |
| | Total | 366 | 423 | 789 |

Apply the chi-square test of homogeneity to determine whether the relative risks are significantly different among different smoking history categories. Calculate 95% CIs of the common relative risk (OR) using logit, Mantel-Haenszel, test-based, Birch, and Cornfield's methods. Compare the results to the limits obtained via the exact method.

26. Refer to Problem 25. As with cigarette smoking, gender is a potential confounder because it may be associated with the degree of physical activity and is independently associated with the risk of MI. To control for this variable, the data were stratified by gender, and the results for each stratum are summarized in the table below:

| Gender | Physical activity index | Cases | Controls | Total |
|---|---|---|---|---|
| Men | 2500+ kcal | 141 | 208 | 349 |
| | <2500 kcal | 144 | 112 | 256 |
| | Total | 285 | 320 | 605 |
| Women | 2500+ kcal | 49 | 58 | 107 |
| | <2500 kcal | 32 | 45 | 77 |
| | Total | 81 | 103 | 184 |
| | 2500+ kcal | 190 | 266 | 456 |
| Total | <2500 kcal | 176 | 157 | 333 |
| | Total | 366 | 423 | 789 |

Apply the chi-square test of homogeneity to determine whether the relative risks are significantly different among men and women. Calculate 95% CIs of the common relative risk (OR) using logit, Mantel-Haenszel, test-based, Birch, and Cornfield's methods. Compare the results to the limits obtained via the exact method.

27. Consider the problem of obtaining a combined relative risk (OR) estimate involving strata with a zero cell frequency. The tables below, taken from Kleinbaum et al. (1982), contain a zero cell frequency in stratum one:

**Stratum 1**

| | Exposed | Unexposed | Total |
|---|---|---|---|
| Cases | 7 | 3 | 10 |
| Noncases | 0 | 10 | 10 |
| Total | 7 | 13 | 20 |

**Stratum 2**

| | Exposed | Unexposed | Total |
|---|---|---|---|
| Cases | 5 | 5 | 10 |
| Noncases | 1 | 9 | 10 |
| Total | 6 | 14 | 20 |

Use a modified logit method (Haldane, 1955), which adds the quantity 0.5 to each cell, to calculate the point estimate and the associated

CI of the OR. Compare results with point and interval estimates using other methods described in the text.

28. Consider the data on nonmelanoma skin cancer for women stratified by age in two metropolitan areas: Dallas-Forthworth and Minneapolis-St. Paul, reported by Scott et al. (1974) and also referred to by Gart (1979) and Tarone (1981). The table below shows the numbers of cases and sizes of the populations at risk:

| | Dallas-Fort Worth | | Minneapolis-St. Paul | | |
|---|---|---|---|---|---|
| Age | Cases | Population size | Cases | Population size | Relative risk |
| 15–24 | 4 | 181,343 | 1 | 172,675 | 3.81 |
| 25–34 | 38 | 146,207 | 16 | 123,065 | 2.00 |
| 35–44 | 119 | 121,374 | 30 | 96,216 | 3.14 |
| 45–54 | 221 | 111,353 | 71 | 92,051 | 2.57 |
| 55–64 | 259 | 83,004 | 102 | 72,159 | 2.21 |
| 65–74 | 310 | 55,932 | 130 | 54,722 | 2.33 |
| 75–84 | 226 | 29,007 | 133 | 32,185 | 1.89 |
| 85+ | 65 | 7,538 | 40 | 8,328 | 1.80 |

Carry out the chi-square test for the hypothesis of no difference in incidence of nonmelanoma cancer rates for women in two communities using the method of Armitage (1966). Calculate point estimates and the associated 95% CIs of the overall summary RD and RR between two communities using the methods described in the text.

29. Consider the data on cancer of the nasal cavity and paranasal sinuses and formaldehyde exposures given in Exercise 15. The data given below are stratified on the confounding factor of wood dust exposure:

| Exposure | Exposed | Nonexposed | Total |
|---|---|---|---|
| Low wood dust exposure | | | |
| Cases | 15 | 48 | 63 |
| Noncases | 18 | 143 | 161 |
| Total | 33 | 191 | 224 |
| High wood dust exposure | | | |
| Cases | 16 | 12 | 28 |
| Noncases | 16 | 18 | 34 |
| Total | 32 | 30 | 62 |

Apply the chi-square test of homogeneity to determine whether the relative risks are significantly different among the two dust exposure categories. Use logit, Mantel-Haenszel, and maximum likelihood methods to obtain point estimates of the overall relative risk (OR).

Calculate 95% CIs for the common OR using logit, Mantel-Haenszel, maximum likelihood, test-based, Birch, and Cornfield's methods. Compare the results with the limits obtained via exact method.

30. Consider the data compiled by Cornfield (1956) from ten retrospective studies in which patients with lung cancer and control subjects were classified as smokers or nonsmokers. The studies were culled from a series of 14 studies given by Dorn (1954) and determined by Cornfield to have relative risk homogeneity at the 5% level. The data from these studies were also analyzed by Gart (1962) and Armitage and Berry (1994). The relevant results are summarized below:

| Study | Lung cancer patients | | Control patients | | Relative |
|---|---|---|---|---|---|
| no. | Smokers | Nonsmokers | Smokers | Nonsmokers | risk |
| 1 | 83 | 3 | 72 | 14 | 5.38 |
| 2 | 90 | 3 | 227 | 43 | 5.68 |
| 3 | 129 | 7 | 81 | 19 | 4.32 |
| 4 | 412 | 32 | 299 | 131 | 5.64 |
| 5 | 1350 | 7 | 1296 | 61 | 9.08 |
| 6 | 60 | 3 | 106 | 27 | 5.09 |
| 7 | 459 | 18 | 534 | 81 | 3.87 |
| 8 | 499 | 19 | 462 | 56 | 3.18 |
| 9 | 451 | 39 | 1729 | 636 | 4.25 |
| 10 | 260 | 5 | 259 | 28 | 5.62 |
| Total | 3793 | 136 | 5065 | 1096 | |

Does a relationship exist between smoking and lung cancer in ten studies analyzed separately? If so, evaluate the strength of the association for each study. Are the data from separate studies comparable in terms of strength of association? Carry out appropriate tests of significance. Use logit, Mantel-Haenszel and maximum likelihood methods to combine the results of these studies and obtain point estimates of the overall relative risk (OR). Calculate 95% CIs of the common OR using logit, Mantel-Haenszel, maximum likelihood, test-based, Birch, and Cornfield's methods. Compare the results to the limits obtained via the exact method.

31. Consider the case-control study described in Problem 16, concerning the association between alcohol consumption and the risk of esophagael cancer. The investigators were particularly interested in assessing the association of alcohol consumption with the risk of cancer in different age groups. The following table relates the average daily alcohol consumption to disease status for six strata defined by 10-year age intervals:

| Age group (years) | Av. daily alcohol consumption (g) | Disease status | | Total |
|---|---|---|---|---|
| | | Case | Control | |
| 25–34 | ≥80 | 1 | 9 | 10 |
| | <80 | 0 | 106 | 106 |
| | Total | 1 | 115 | 116 |
| 35–44 | ≥80 | 4 | 26 | 30 |
| | <80 | 5 | 164 | 169 |
| | Total | 9 | 190 | 199 |
| 45–54 | ≥80 | 25 | 29 | 54 |
| | <80 | 21 | 138 | 159 |
| | Total | 46 | 167 | 213 |
| 55–64 | ≥80 | 42 | 27 | 69 |
| | <80 | 34 | 139 | 173 |
| | Total | 76 | 166 | 242 |
| 65–74 | ≥80 | 19 | 18 | 37 |
| | <80 | 36 | 88 | 124 |
| | Total | 55 | 106 | 161 |
| ≥75 | ≥80 | 5 | 0 | 5 |
| | <80 | 8 | 31 | 39 |
| | Total | 13 | 31 | 44 |
| Total | ≥80 | 96 | 109 | 205 |
| | <80 | 104 | 666 | 770 |
| | Total | 200 | 775 | 975 |

Apply the chi-square test of homogeneity to determine whether the relative risks are significantly different among different age groups. Calculate 95% CIs of the common relative risk (OR) using logit, Mantel-Haenszel, maximum likelihood, test-based, Birch, and Cornfield's methods. Compare the results to the limits obtained via the exact method.

## CHAPTER 7

32. Consider the data from the Boston Area Health Study (Gaziano et al., 1993), a matched case-control study of risk factors for myocardial infarction (MI). Cases of first MI from six Boston area hospitals were matched to controls of the same age (within 5 years), sex and neighborhood of residence. One hypothesis of interest was the relationship of the level of physical activity, represented by an index that measures total kilo calories of energy expended from stairs climbed, blocks walked, and recreational/leisure-time activities with risk of

MI. High level exercise was defined as a physical activity index of 2500 Kcal or more per day. The results are summarized below:

| | Controls | | |
|---|---|---|---|
| Cases | Exposed[a] | Unexposed | Total |
| Exposed[a] | 115 | 59 | 174 |
| Unexposed | 99 | 67 | 166 |
| Total | 214 | 126 | 340 |

[a] Exposed: physical activity index ≥2500/kcal/d.

Apply the McNemar's chi-square test of matched proportions to test for the possible association between the level of physical activity and risk of MI. Calculate 95% CIs for the relative risk (OR) using the formulas based on binomial proportion, maximum likelihood, and test-based procedures. Compare the results to the limits obtained via the exact method.

33. A retrospective case-control study was undertaken to examine the association between endometrial carcinoma and the use of estrogens in postmenopausal women (Smith et al., 1975). There were 317 diagnosed cases of endometrial carcinoma obtained from two hospitals which were individually matched with 317 controls from the same hospital. The matching criteria were age at diagnosis (within 4 years) and year of diagnosis (within 2 years). The 317 controls were patients with cervical carcinoma, ovarian cancer, or carcinoma of the vulva. The table below shows the numbers of cases and controls (ignoring matching) who had previously taken estrogens for at least 6 months prior to the diagnosis of cancer:

| | Cases | Controls |
|---|---|---|
| Estrogen used | 152 | 54 |
| Estrogen not used | 165 | 263 |
| Total | 317 | 317 |

In order to allow for the matching it is necessary to construct a 2 × 2 table of the distribution of the pairs and the results of the above case-control study are shown below:

| Cases | Controls: Estrogen used | Controls: Estrogen not used | Total |
|---|---|---|---|
| Estrogen used | 39 | 113 | 152 |
| Estrogen not used | 15 | 150 | 165 |
| Total | 54 | 263 | 317 |

Apply the McNemar's chi-square test of matched proportions to test for the possible association between endometrial carcinoma and the use of estrogens in postmenopausal women. Calculate 95% CIs for the relative risk (OR) using the formulas based on binomial proportion, maximum likelihood, and test-based procedures. Compare the results to the limits obtained via the exact method.

34. It has been hypothesized that tonsils act as a protective barrier in some fashion against Hodgkin's disease. Johnson and Johnson (1972) selected 85 Hodgkin's patients who had a sibling of the same sex, free of the disease, and whose age was within 5 years of the patient's. They summarized their results in the form of the following table:

| Tonsillectomy | Hodgkin's disease: Yes | Hodgkin's disease: No | Total |
|---|---|---|---|
| Yes | 41 | 44 | 85 |
| No | 33 | 52 | 85 |
| Total | 74 | 96 | 170 |

They reported a chi-square statistic of 1.53, which is not statistically significant. These findings appeared to be at odds with the results of an earlier study by Vianna et al. (1971), who found that 66% of the Hodgkin's patients had a tonsillectomy as compared to 40% of the control group, and the difference was highly significant. Several letters to the editor of the *New England Journal of Medicine,* where Johnson and Johnson published their results, pointed out that the data were incorrectly analyzed by ignoring the matchings of the siblings. In order to allow for the pairing, it is necessary to construct a $2 \times 2$ table of the distribution of the pairs of siblings. Johnson and Johnson's data take the form of the following table:

| Patients | Siblings: Tonsillectomy | Siblings: No tonsillectomy | Total |
|---|---|---|---|
| Tonsillectomy | 15 | 7 | 22 |
| No Tonsillectomy | 37 | 26 | 63 |
| Total | 52 | 33 | 85 |

Apply the McNemar's chi-square test of matched proportions to test for the possible association between Hodgkin's disease and tonsillectomy. Calculate 95% CIs for the relative risk (OR) using the formulas based on binomial proportion, maximum likelihood, and test-based procedures. Compare the results to the limits obtained via the exact method.

35. Consider the data from a registry-based matched case-control study of soft tissue sarcoma and farming occupations reported by Smith et al. (1982). The data are summarized below:

| Cases | Controls: Farmers | Controls: Nonfarmers | Total |
|---|---|---|---|
| Farmers | 1 | 11 | 12 |
| Nonfarmers | 8 | 82 | 90 |
| Total | 9 | 93 | 102 |

Apply the McNemar's chi-square test of matched proportions to test for the possible association between soft tissue sarcoma and farming occupations. Calculate 95% CIs for the relative risk (OR) using the formulas based on binomial proportion, maximum likelihood, and test-based procedures. Compare the results to the limits obtained via the exact method.

36. Fleiss (1984) analyzed the data from a case-control study comparing the odds of endometrial cancer for those exposed to conjugated estrogen to those not exposed. The study entailed matched controls with 4 matched sets having 3 controls per case and 55 sets having 4 controls per case. The resulting data, consisting of 4 matched triplets and 55 matched quadruplets, are summarized as follows:

**Number of Controls Exposed**

| Status of case | Matched triplets ($M$ = 3) | | | |
|---|---|---|---|---|
| | **0** | **1** | **2** | **3** |
| Exposed | 1 | 3 | 0 | 0 |
| Unexposed | 0 | 0 | 0 | 0 |

| Status of case | Matched quadruplets ($M$ = 4) | | | | |
|---|---|---|---|---|---|
| | **0** | **1** | **2** | **3** | **4** |
| Exposed | 4 | 17 | 11 | 9 | 2 |
| Unexposed | 1 | 6 | 3 | 1 | 1 |

Obtain point estimates of the relative risk (OR) using the Mantel-Haenszel and maximum likelihood methods. Calculate 95% CIs for the OR using Mantel-Haenszel, maximum likelihood, and test-based procedures. Compare the results to limits obtained via exact method.

37. Consider a nested case-control study of lung cancer and asbestos exposure, based on the cohort of 1261 white male asbestos workers from one textile manufacturing plant, as reported by Dement et al. (1983). The case group included all 35 lung cancer deaths generated by the cohort during the period 1940 to 1975 and the controls were chosen by sampling from the entire cohort. Because all exposure data were calculated prospectively, no potential problems occurred with regard to comparability of information between cases and controls. In view of the small number of cases, four controls were matched to each case, thus yielding a control group of 140 workers. The controls were selected by incidence density matching on age at risk, and other factors were not considered necessary to match. The initial analysis used a dichotomous exposure classification ignoring matching where cases and controls were classified as to whether their cumulative asbestos exposure was greater or less than 10,000 fibers/cc × d. The following table shows the exposure distribution of cases and controls:

| | Asbestos exposure | | |
|---|---|---|---|
| | **<10,000** | **≥10,000** | **Total** |
| Cases | 15 | 20 | 35 |
| Controls | 92 | 48 | 140 |
| Total | 107 | 68 | 175 |

A further analysis involved stratification by age. The following table shows the exposure distribution of cases and controls stratified by age:

| Age | Cases' exposure | | Controls' exposure | |
|---|---|---|---|---|
| group | <10,000 | ≥10,000 | <10,000 | ≥10,000 |
| 45–49 | 5 | 1 | 17 | 7 |
| 50–54 | 3 | 7 | 29 | 11 |
| 55–59 | 0 | 6 | 18 | 6 |
| 60–64 | 1 | 4 | 13 | 7 |
| 65–69 | 4 | 2 | 11 | 13 |
| 70–74 | 2 | 0 | 4 | 4 |
| Total | 15 | 20 | 92 | 48 |

The final analysis incorporated the matching in the analysis and the distribution of matched sets classified according to asbestos exposure is shown below:

| | No. of controls with 10,000 or more fibers/cc × d | | | | |
|---|---|---|---|---|---|
| | 0 | 1 | 2 | 3 | 4 |
| Cases | | | | | |
| ≥10,000 | 3 | 7 | 9 | 1 | 0 |
| <10,000 | 4 | 4 | 6 | 0 | 1 |

For example, 15 cases were classified as unexposed, each of which had four matched controls. In one of them all four matched controls were exposed, in six of them two of the four matched controls were exposed, and so on. Using matched-set analysis involving four controls per case, obtain point estimates of the relative risk (OR) using Mantel-Haenszel and maximum likelihood methods. Calculate 95% CIs for the OR using Mantel-Haenszel, maximum likelihood, and test-based procedures as well as the exact method. Compare results to the corresponding results obtained using crude and stratified analyses.

## CHAPTER 8

38. Health researchers have been increasingly concerned with the possible role of the use of marijuana among pregnant women on the incidence of congenital malformations. Since a host of socioeco-

nomic, sociodemographic, and other lifestyle variables, in addition to being related to marijuana use, are also associated with unfavorable pregnancy developments, it is important that they be simultaneoulsy controlled for in a multivariate analysis. Linn et al. (1983) analyzed data from the Delivery Interview Program (DIP) of 12,424 women and used a multiple logistic regression analysis relating the occurrence of major congenital malformations to several maternal risk factors. The results are given in the table below:

**Multiple Logistic Regression Analysis Relating the Occurrence of Major Congential Malformations to Several Risk Factors, Using 12,424 Women in the DIP Study**

| Variable[a] | Regression coefficient ($\hat{\beta}_i$) | Standard error ($\hat{SE}(\hat{\beta}_i)$) |
|---|---|---|
| Marijuana use (any frequency) | 0.307 | 0.173 |
| Any previous miscarriage | 0.239 | 0.140 |
| Caucasian race | 0.191 | 0.161 |
| Alcohol use in pregnancy | 0.174 | 0.145 |
| Age 35+ | 0.174 | 0.186 |
| Any previous stillbirths | 0.049 | 0.328 |
| On welfare | 0.030 | 0.182 |
| Smoking 3+ cigarettes per day at delivery | –0.174 | 0.144 |
| Any previous induced abortions | –0.198 | 0.168 |
| Parity >1[b] | –0.301 | 0.113 |

[a] All variables are coded as 1 if yes and 0 if no.

[b] Women with at least one previous pregnancy.

From Rosner, B. (1990). *Fundamentals of Biostatistics*, 3rd ed., Duxbury Press, Belmont, CA. p. 471. With permission.

1. Carry out statistical tests of significance for each of the risk factors after controlling for the other risk factors and state results. Let $\alpha = 0.05$.
2. What do the statistical tests carried out in part (1) mean in this instance? State functional conclusions clearly and concisely.
3. Compute the OR and the associated 95% CI relating the presence or absence of each significant independent variable to the risk of malformations.

4. How do you interpret the effect of marijuana usage on congenital malformations based on your findings in part (3)?

39. Several studies have investigated the association between the incidence of sudden death and a host of potential risk factors such as age, blood pressure, cholesterol level, and cigarette smoking, among others. However, most of these studies have been carried out among men. Schatzkin et al. (1984) analyzed data from the Framingham Heart Study for 2-year incidence rates among women. Several potential risk factors were of interest and controlled simultaneously. A multiple logistic regression analysis was performed and the results are shown below:

**Multiple Logistic Regression Model Relating 2-Year Incidence of Sudden Death in Females Without Prior Coronary Heart Disease**

| Risk factor | Regression coefficient ($\hat{\beta}_i$) | Standard error ($SE(\hat{\beta}_i)$) |
|---|---|---|
| Constant | −15.3 | |
| SBP (mmHg) | 0.0019 | 0.0070 |
| Framingham relative weight (%) | −0.0060 | 0.0100 |
| Cholesterol (mg/100 ml) | 0.0056 | 0.0029 |
| Glucose (mg/100 ml) | 0.0066 | 0.0038 |
| Cigarette smoking (cigarettes/d) | 0.0069 | 0.0199 |
| Hematocrit (%) | 0.111 | 0.049 |
| Vital capacity (cl) | −0.0098 | 0.0036 |
| Age (years) | 0.0686 | 0.0225 |

From Rosner, B. (1990). *Fundamentals of Biostatistics*, 3rd ed., Duxbury Press, Belmont, CA, p. 477. With permission.

1. Carry out statistical tests of significance for each individual risk factor after controlling for other variables and state results. Let $\alpha = 0.05$.
2. What do the statistical tests carried out in part (1) mean in this instance? State functional conclusions clearly and concisely.
3. Compute the OR, relating the additional risk of sudden death per 100 cl decrease in vital capacity after adjustment for other risk factors.
4. Calculate a 95% CI associated with the OR estimate in part (3).

40. Rosner (1994) reported data on a study conducted among 234 people who tried to stop smoking. The subjects were followed up for 1 year and for each person, the number of days they were able to abstain from smoking was recorded as well as information on risk factors (e.g., number of cigarettes smoked and serum CO concentration just prior to quitting). The SAS PHGLM (Proportional Hazards General Linear Model) Procedure was used to fit the proportional hazards regression for the data. For ease of interpretation, sex was recorded as (1 = male, 0 = female) from the original coding of (1 = male, 2 = female). The results are given below:

**Proportional Hazards Model Fitted to the Smoking-Cessation Data**

| Risk factor | Regression coefficient ($\hat{\beta}_i$) | Standard error ($\widehat{SE}(\hat{\beta}_i)$) |
|---|---|---|
| $\log_{10}$ CO (adjusted)[a] | 0.833 | 0.350 |
| Sex (1 = M/0 = F) | −0.117 | 0.135 |

[a] This variable represents CO values adjusted for minutes elapsed since last cigarette smoke prior to quitting.

From Rosner, B. (1994). *Fundamentals of Biostatistics,* 4th ed., Duxbury Press. Belmont, CA, p. 623. With permission.

1. Carry out statistical tests of significance for each prognostic variable after controlling for the other variable and state results. Let $\alpha = 0.05$.
2. What do the statistical tests carried out in part (1) mean in this instance? State functional conclusions clearly and concisely.
3. Estimate the instantaneous relative risk of recidivism of two individuals of the same sex who differ by one unit on adjusted $\log_{10}$ CO concentration (i.e., who differ by tenfold in CO concentration), assuming that they have not started smoking up to time *t*.
4. Calculate 95% CI of the instantaneous relative risk using the estimate in part (3).

41. A proportional hazards regression was fitted to the smoking cessation data in the preceding exercise to assess the relationship of age, sex, number of cigarettes smoked, and $\log_{10}$ CO concentration, when considered simultaneously, to the ability to abstain from smoking. The results are given below:

**Proportional Hazards Regression Relating the Hazard of Recidivism to Age, Sex, Number of Cigarettes Smoked Prior to Quitting, and $\log_{10}$ CO Concentration**

| Risk factor | Regression coefficient ($\hat{\beta}_i$) | Standard error ($\widehat{SE}(\hat{\beta}_i)$) |
|---|---|---|
| Age | 0.0023 | 0.0058 |
| Sex (1 = M/0 = F) | –0.127 | 0.143 |
| No. of cigarettes smoked | –0.0038 | 0.0050 |
| $\log_{10}$ CO (adjusted)[a] | 0.912 | 0.366 |

[a] This variable represents CO values adjusted for minutes elapsed since last cigarette smoked prior to quitting.

From Rosner, B. (1994). *Fundamentals of Biostatistics,* 4th ed., Duxbury Press, Belmont, CA, p. 629. With permission.

1. Carry out statistical tests of significance for each prognostic variable after controlling for other variables and state results. Let $\alpha = 0.05$.
2. What do the statistical tests carried out in (1) mean in this instance? State functional conclusions clearly and concisely.
3. Estimate the effects of each variable in terms of relative risk on the instantaneous hazards or risk of recidivism (i.e., propensity to start smoking again).
4. Calculate 95% CIs of the instantaneous relative risks using the estimates in part (3).

## CHAPTER 9

42. Consider the data from a hypothetical study concerning the possible association between obesity and mortality from all causes among white women, aged 60 to 75 years, from a midwestern urban population, as described by Kleinbaum et al. (1982). The purpose of the study was to investigate the negative consequences of obesity among older women who, as a group, have not modified their weight-related behavior. The subjects for this hypothetical study entailed 450 Caucasian women between the ages 53 and 74, all of whom could contribute one or more years of observations to the age interval 60 to 75 years. The follow-up period was defined as the 8-year interval from 1960 through 1967, during which time 105 members of the cohort died. For each fatality, the year of death and obesity,

measured in 1960, by the Quetlet index, were recorded. The person-years data are summarized as follows:

| | Obesity | Nonobesity | Total |
|---|---|---|---|
| Deaths | 30 | 36 | 66 |
| Person-years | 699 | 1399 | 2098 |

Carry out the chi-square test of significance to evaluate the possible association between obesity and death from all causes among Caucasian women between 60 and 75 years of age. Calculate point estimates and 95% CIs of incidence rate difference (IRD) and incidence rate ratio (IRR) using the methods described in the text.

43. Consider the data on breast cancer cases and person-years of observations for women with tuberculosis frequently exposed to multiple X-ray fluoroscopies and women with tuberculosis not so exposed, as reported by Boice and Monson (1977) and by Rothman (1986). The data are summarized as follows:

| | Radiation exposure to multiple X-ray fluoroscopies | | |
|---|---|---|---|
| | Yes | No | Total |
| Breast cancer | 41 | 15 | 56 |
| Person-years | 28,010 | 19,017 | 47,027 |

Carry out the chi-square test of significance to evaluate the possible association between breast cancer and radiation exposure to X-ray fluoroscopies among women with tuberculosis. Calculate 95% CIs of IRD and IRR using the methods described in the text.

44. Consider a prospective study involving 117,156 U.S. women aged 30 to 55 years in 1970, who were free from CHD, as reported by Colditz et al. (1986). The purpose of the study was to investigate the impact of parental MI on the incidence of CHD. The results on parental history and other risk factors were obtained from questionnaires completed in 1976. The information on nonfatal CHD was taken from questionnaires administered in 1978 and 1980, and the fatal CHD cases were ascertained by searches of state vital records. All the women were followed until June 1, 1980. The incidence of CHD and the number of person-years of follow-up for the two endpoints for those women who reported no parental history of MI and a parental history of MI ≤60 years of age are shown below:

| | Parental history | | | | | |
|---|---|---|---|---|---|---|
| | Nonfatal MI | | | Fatal CHD | | |
| | None | ≤60(*e*) | Total | None | ≤60(*e*) | Total |
| Cases | 75 | 40 | 115 | 17 | 16 | 33 |
| Person-years | 304,203 | 59,386 | 363,584 | 330,997 | 64,275 | 395,272 |

Carry out the chi-square test of significance to determine whether there was an increased risk of both nonfatal MI and fatal CHD for women with a parental history of MI ≤60 years of age as compared to those with no family history. Calculate 95% CIs of IRD and IRR using the methods described in the text.

## CHAPTER 10

45. Consider the person-years data from the Framingham Heart Study, as presented in Kahn and Sempos (1989), comparing ages 55–62 to 45–49 and adjusted for blood pressure and sex. The basic data consist of eight 2 × 2 tables each comparing cases and person-year exposures for the two age groups and specific for systolic blood pressure (SBP) level, sex, and the two time intervals: 0-9 and 9-18. The results are summarized as follows:

| | | | Age 55–62 | | Age 45–49 | | Total |
|---|---|---|---|---|---|---|---|
| SBP | Sex | Observation period | Cases | Person-years | Cases | Person-years | person-years |
| <165 | M | 0–9 | 26 | 1408.5 | 12 | 1471.5 | 2880.0 |
| | | 9–18 | 23 | 877.5 | 24 | 1093.5 | 1971.0 |
| | F | 0–9 | 12 | 1368.0 | 1 | 1611.0 | 2979.0 |
| | | 9–18 | 13 | 954.0 | 12 | 1278.0 | 2332.0 |
| ≥165 | M | 0–9 | 17 | 265.5 | 3 | 202.5 | 468.0 |
| | | 9–18 | 4 | 94.5 | 6 | 103.5 | 198.0 |
| | F | 0–9 | 17 | 666.0 | 2 | 333.0 | 999.0 |
| | | 9–18 | 11 | 423.0 | 5 | 225.0 | 648.0 |
| Total | | | 123 | | 65 | | |

Carry out the chi-square test of significance to evaluate the possible association between the CHD and the age groups. Calculate overall point estimates and associated 95% CIs of IRD and IRR using the methods described in the text.

46. Consider the data on age-specific coronary disease deaths from cigarette smoking among British male doctors given in Example 10.3. Carry out the chi-square test of significance to evaluate the possible association between cigarette smoking and coronary deaths among doctors. Calculate overall point estimates and the associated 95% CIs of IRD and IRR using the methods described in the text.
47. Consider the data of incidence of thyroid neoplasms in females, by age and person-years exposed to <100 rad and those exposed to 300+ rad of radiation, as reported by Hempelman et al. (1975) and further discussed by Rothman (1986). The data are summarized as follows:

| | Age groups | | | | | |
|---|---|---|---|---|---|---|
| | 0–14 years | | 15–29 years | | 30+ Years | |
| **Exposure level** | **300+ rad** | **<100 rad** | **300+ rad** | **<100 rad** | **300+ rad** | **<100 rad** |
| Cases | 0 | 2 | 7 | 5 | 2 | 0 |
| Person-years | 1,054 | 9,942 | 2,665 | 15,410 | 2,217 | 1,530 |

Carry out the chi-square test of significance to evaluate the possible association between thyroid neoplasms in females and exposure to radiation. Calculate overall point estimates and associated 95% CIs of IRD and IRR using the methods described in the text.

## CHAPTER 11

48. Consider the data from a hypothetical study concerning the effect exposure on a disease state, as described in Kleinbaum et al. (1982). The results are summarized as follows:

| **Disease state** | **Exposed** | **Unexposed** | **Total** |
|---|---|---|---|
| Cases | 40 | 60 | 100 |
| Noncases | 80 | 320 | 400 |
| Total | 120 | 380 | 500 |

Calculate population attributable risk percent (PAR%) and the associated 95% CIs by first assuming that the data are taken from a retrospective case control study and then that they were taken from a prospective cohort study.

49. Consider the data from a large prospective study on smoking and lung mortality among U.S. war veterans, as reported by Kahn (1966) and further discussed by Kahn and Sempos (1989). The relevant data are summarized as follows:

| Smoking category | Lung cancer mortality Yes | No | Total |
|---|---|---|---|
| Current cigarette smokers | 1116 | 701 | 1817 |
| All others | 426 | 1016 | 1442 |
| Total | 1542 | 1717 | 3259 |

Calculate an estimated excess incidence rate (AR) and percent attributable risk (AR%) among those with the risk factor, including population attributable risk percent (PAR%) and the associated 95% CI.

50. Consider the Framingham data relating SBP to 18-year incidence of CHD, as described in Exercise 2. The data shown there used a single cut point, e.g., ≥165 compared to <165. The table below describes these data, with SBP divided in six classes as given in Kahn and Sempos (1989). Considering the persons with SBP <140 as the unexposed group, the relative risks for other SBP groups were calculated by comparing their risks to the risk for those with SBP <140. These results are shown in the last column of the table. Calculate the proportion of incidence rate 'due to' blood pressure (AR) for different SBP categories (SBP ≥180,...,SBP >140-149) relative to those with SBP <140.

| SBP (mmHg) | Coronary disease At risk | + | – | Risk | Relative risk |
|---|---|---|---|---|---|
| ≥180 | 158 | 54 | 104 | 0.342 | 2.65 |
| 170–179 | 98 | 31 | 67 | 0.316 | 2.45 |
| 160–169 | 127 | 29 | 98 | 0.228 | 1.77 |
| 150–159 | 181 | 39 | 142 | 0.215 | 1.67 |
| 140–149 | 231 | 42 | 189 | 0.182 | 1.41 |
| <140 | 568 | 73 | 495 | 0.129 | 1.00 |
| Total | 1363 | 268 | 1095 | 0.197 | — |

# References

**Armitage, P.** (1966). "The Chi-Square Test of Heterogeneity in Proportions After Adjustment for Stratification", *J. R. Stat. Soc.,* B, 26, 150–163.

**Armitage, P. and Berry, G.** (1994). *Statistical Methods in Medical Research,* 3rd ed. Blackwell Scientific, Oxford.

**Bain, C., Willett, W., Hennekens, C. H., Rosner, B., Belanger, C., and Speizer, F. E.** (1981). "Use of Post Menopausal Hormones and Risk of Myocardial Infarction", *Circulation,* 64, 42–46.

**Boice, J. D. and Monson, R. R.** (1977). "Breast Cancer in Women After Repeated Fluoroscopic Examinations of the Chest", *J. Nat. Cancer Inst.,* 59, 823–832.

**Cantor, K. P., Blair, A., Everett, G., Vanlier, S., Burmeister, L., Dick, F. R., Gibson, R. W., and Schuman, L.** (1988). "Hair Dye Use and Risk of Leukemia and Lymphoma", *Am. J. Publ. Health,* 78, 570–571.

**Colditz, G. A., Stampfer, M. J., Willett, W. C., Rosner, B., Speizer, F. E., and Hennekens, C. H.** (1986). "A Prospective Study of Parental History of Myocardial Infarction and Coronary Heart Disease in Women", *Am. J. Epidemiol.,* 123, 48–58.

**Cornfield, J.** (1956). "A Statistical Problem Arising from Retrospective Studies", In: *Proc. 3rd Berkeley Symp. Mathematical Statistics and Probability* (Ed. J. Neyman), pp. 135–148. University of California Press, Berkeley.

**Cot, T. R., Nelson, M. R., Anderson, S. P., and Martin, R. J.** (1990). "The Present and the Future of AIDS and Tuberculosis in Illinois", *Am. J. Publ. Health,* 80, 950–953.

**Cox, D. R.** (1966). "A Simple Example of a Comparison Involving Quantal Data", *Biometrika,* 53, 215–220.

**Dement, J. M., Harris, R. L., Symons, M. J., and Shy, C. M.** (1983). "Exposures and Mortality Among Chrysotile Asbestos Workers, II: Mortality", *Am. J. Ind. Med.,* 4, 421–433.

**Dorn, H. F.** (1954). "The Relationship of Cancer of the Lung and the Use of Tobacco", *Am. Stat.,* 8, 7–13.

**Fleiss, J. L.** (1984). "The Mantel-Haenszel Estimator in Case-Control Studies with Varying Numbers of Controls Matched to Each Case", *Am. J. Epidemiol.,* 120, 1–3.

**Gart, J. J.** (1962). "On the Combination of Relative Risks", *Biometrics,* 18, 601–610.

**Gart, J. J.** (1970). "Point and Interval Estimation of the Common Odds Ratio in the Combination of 2 × 2 Tables with Fixed Marginals", *Biometrika,* 57, 471–475.

**Gart, J. J.** (1979). "Statistical Analyses of the Relative Risk", *Environ. Health Perspect.,* 32, 157–167.

**Gaziano, J. M., Buring, J. E., Breslow, J. L., Goldhaber, S. Z., Rosner, B., VanDenburgh, M., Willett, W., and Hennekens, C. H.** (1993). "Moderate Alcohol Intake, Increased Levels of High-Density Lipoprotein and Its Subfractions, and Decreased Risk of Myocardial Infarction", *N. Engl. J. Med.,* 329, 1829–1834.

**Gordon, T. and Foss, B. M.** (1966). "The Role of Simulation in the Delay of Onset of Crying in the New-Born Infant", *Q. J. Exp. Psychol.,* 16, 79–81.

**Graham, S., Dayal, H., Rohrer, T., Swanson, M., Sultz, H., Shedd, D., and Fischman, S.** (1977). "Dentition, Diet, Tobacco, and Alcohol in the Epidemiology of Oral Cancer", *J. Nat. Cancer Inst.,* 59, 1611–1616.

**Haldane, J. B. S.** (1955). "The Estimation and Significance of the Logarithm of a Ratio of Frequencies", *Ann. Human Gen.,* 20, 309–311.

**Hayes, R. B., Raatgever, J. W., de Brkyn, A., and Gerin, M.** (1986). "Cancer of the Nasal Cavity and Paranasal Sinuses and Formaldehyde Exposure", *Int. J. Cancer,* 37, 487–492.

**Hempelman, L. H., Hall, W. J., Phillips, M., Cooper, R. A., and Ames, W. R.** (1975). "Neoplasms in Persons Treated with X-Rays in Infancy — Fourth Survey in 20 Years", *J. Nat. Cancer Inst.,* 55, 519–530.

**Henderson, B. E., Benton, B., Cosgrove, M., Baptista, J., Aldrich, J., Townsend, D., Hart, W., and Mack, T. M.** (1976). "Urogenital Tract Abnormalities in Sons of Women Treated with Diethylstibestrol", *Pediatrics,* 58, 505–507.

**Hiller, R. A. and Kahn, H. A.** (1976). "Senile Cataract Extraction and Diabetes", *Br. J. Ophthalmol.,* 60, 283–286.

**Hills, M.** (1974). *Statistics for Comparative Studies.* John Wiley & Sons, New York.

**Hoover, R. and Strasser, P. H.** (1979). "Progress Report to the FDA from NCI Concerning the National Cancer Study", National Cancer Institute, Bethesda, MD.

**Johnson, S. and Johnson, R.** (1972). "Tonsillectomy History in Hodgkin's Disease", *N. Engl. J. Med.,* 287, 1122–1125.

**Kahn, H. A.** (1966). NCI Monograph No. 19. National Cancer Institute, Bethesda, MD.

**Kahn, H. A. and Sempos, C. T.** (1989). *Statistical Methods in Epidemiology.* Oxford University Press, New York.

**Kleinbaum, D. G., Kupper, L. L., and Morgenstern, H.** (1982). *Epidemiologic Research: Principles and Quantitative Methods.* Lifetime Learning Publications, Belmont, CA.

**Lewak, N., van der Berg, B., and Beckwith, B.** (1979). "Sudden Infant Death Syndrome Risk Factors: Prospective Data Review", *Clin. Pediatr.,* 19, 404–411.

**Linn, S., Schoenbaum, S. C., Monson, R. R., Rosner, B., Stubblefield, P. C., and Ryan, K. J.** (1983). "The Association of Marijuana Use with Outcome of Pregnancy", *Am. J. Publ. Health,* 73, 1161–1164.

**Mintz, M.** (1980). "F. D. A. Panel is Given Reassuring Report on Bendectin-Safety", *The Washington Post,* Sept. 16, A 12 (Col. 1).

**Report of the Sixty Plus Reinfarction Study Research Group** (1980). "A Double-Blind Trial to Assess Long-Term Anticoagulant Therapy in Elderly Patients After Myocardial Infarction", *Lancet,* ii, 989–994.

**Rosner, B.** (1994). *Fundamentals of Biostatistics,* 4th ed. Duxbury Press, Belmont, CA.

**Ross, R. K., Pagamini-Hill, A., Gerkins, V. R., Mack, T. M., Pfeffer, R., Arthur, M., and Henderson, B. E.** (1980). "A Case-Control Study of Menopausal Estrogen Therapy and Breast Cancer", *J. Am. Med. Assoc.,* 243, 1635–1639.

**Rothman, K. J.** (1986). *Modern Epidemiology.* Little, Brown, Boston.

**Schatzkin, A., Cupples, L. A., Heeren, T., Morelock, S., and Kanmel, W. S.** (1984). "Sudden Death in the Framingham Heart Study: Differences in Incidence and Risk Factors by Sex and Coronary Disease Status", *Am. J. Epidemiol.,* 120, 888–899.

**Scott, J., Kopf, A. W., and Urbach, F.** (1974). "Non-Melanoma Skin Cancer Among Caucasians in Four Areas of the United States", *Cancer,* 34, 1333–1338.

**Selvin, S.** (1991). *Statistical Analysis of Epidemiologic Data.* Oxford University Press, New York.

**Shurtleff, D.** (1970). The Framingham Study: An Epidemiologic Investigation of Cardiovascular Disease, Section 26. U.S. Government Printing Office, Washington, D.C.

**Shurtleff, D.** (1974). The Framingham Study, NIH Publ. 74-599, Section 30, Department of Health Education and Welfare, Washington, D.C.

**Smith, A. H., Fisher, D. O., Pearce, N. E. et al.** (1982). "Do Agricultural Chemicals Cause Soft Tissue Sarcoma? Initial Findings of a Case-Control Study in New Zealand", *Commun. Health Stud.,* 6, 114–119.

**Smith, D. G., Prentice, R., Thompson, D. C., and Herrmann, W. L.** (1975). "Association of Exogenous Estrogen and Endometrial Carcinoma", *N. Engl. J. Med.,* 293, 1164–1167.

**Stewart, A., Webb, J., and Hewitt, D.** (1958). "A Survey of Childhood Malignancies", *Br. Med. J.,* 1, 1495–1508.

**Tarone, R. E.** (1981). "On Summary Estimators of Relative Risk", *J. Chronic Dis.,* 34, 463–468.

**Tyns, A. J., Pequignot, G., and Jenson, O. M.** (1977). "Le Cancer de l'oesphage en Ille-et-Vilaine en Fonction del Niveaux de Consommation d'Alcool et de Tabac", *Bull. du Cancer (Paris),* 64, 45–60.

**Vianna, N., Greenwald, P., and Davies, J.** (1971). "Tonsillectomy and Hodgkin's Disease: The Lymphoid Tissue Barrier", *Lancet,* 1, 431–432.

**Vollset, S. E. and Hirji, K. F.** (1991). "A Micro-Computer Program for Exact and Asymptotic Analysis of Several 2 × 2 Tables", *Epidemiology,* 2, 217–220.

**Woolf, B.** (1955). "On Estimating the Relation between Blood Group and Disease", *Ann. Human Gen.,* 19, 251–253.

# List of Symbols

| | |
|---|---|
| AR | Attributable risk |
| $\chi^2_v$ | Chi-square distributed random variable with $v$ degrees of freedom |
| $\chi^2_{\nu,\alpha}$ | 100($\alpha$)th upper percentile of the chi-square distributed random variable with $v$ degrees of freedom |
| ^ | When placed over a parameter, indicates an estimator of that parameter |
| $E(X)$ | Expected value of a random variable $X$ |
| $\chi^2_{\text{MH}}$ | Mantel-Haenszel chi-square |
| $F_{v_1,v_2}$ | $F$ distributed random variable with $v_1$ degrees of freedom in the numerators and $v_2$ in the denominator |
| $F_{\alpha,\nu_1,\nu_2}$ | 100($\alpha$)th upper percentile of the $F$ distributed random variable with $v_1$ and $v_2$ degrees of freedom |
| $h(t)$ | Hazard function |
| IRD | Incidence rate difference |
| IRR | Incidence rate ratio |
| ML | Maximum likelihood |
| OR | Odds ratio |
| PAR | Population attributable risk |
| POR | Prevalence odds ratio |
| PD | Prevalence difference |
| PR | Prevalence ratio |
| RD | Risk difference |
| RR | Risk ratio, relative risk |
| SE | Standard error |
| SRD | Standardized rate difference |
| SRR | Standardized rate ratio |
| SMR | Standardized mortality ratio |
| $\Sigma$ | Summation symbol |
| $S(t)$ | Survival function |
| Var$(X)$ | Variance of a random variable $X$ |
| $Z$ | Normally distributed random variable with mean zero and unit variance (standard normal distribution) |
| $Z_\alpha$ | 100($\alpha$)th upper percentile of the standard normal distribution |

# List of Symbols

# Subject Index

## A



## B



## C

## D



## E



## F



## H

## N



## O



## P

## U



## V



## W



## Z

# Author Index

## H



## I



## J

## K



## L



## M

## N



## O



## P



## Q



## R

## S



## T



## U



## V

## W



## Y



## Z

# Data Index